W9-BON-380

# HIKE LIST

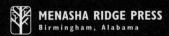

MENASHA RIDGE PRESS
Birmingham, Alabama

# 60 HIKES WITHIN 60 MILES

# PORTLAND

INCLUDES
THE COAST,
MOUNTS HOOD AND ST. HELENS,
AND THE
COLUMBIA RIVER GORGE

FOURTH EDITION

**PAUL GERALD**

Copyright © 2010 Paul Gerald
All rights reserved
Printed in the United States of America
Published by Menasha Ridge Press
Distributed by Publishers Group West
Fourth edition, first printing

Library of Congress Cataloging-in-Publication Data

Gerald, Paul, 1966–
    60 hikes within 60 miles, Portland : includes the coast, Mounts Hood and
    St. Helens, and the Columbia River Gorge / Paul Gerald. — 4th ed.
        p. cm.
    Includes index.
    ISBN-13: 978-0-89732-881-4
    ISBN-10: 0-89732-881-7
    1. Hiking—Oregon—Portland Region—Guidebooks. 2. Portland Region
    (Or.)—Guidebooks. I. Title.
    GV199.42.O72G47 2010
    796.5109795—dc22

                                        2010005804

Cover and text design by Steveco International
Cover photo by Paul Gerald
Author photo by Paul Gerald
All other photos by Paul Gerald
Maps by Steve Jones, Scott McGrew, and Paul Gerald

Menasha Ridge Press
P.O. Box 43673
Birmingham, AL 35243
www.menasharidge.com

DISCLAIMER
This book is meant only as a guide to select trails in the Portland area and does not guarantee hiker safety in any way—you hike at your own risk. Neither Menasha Ridge Press nor Paul Gerald is liable for property loss or damage, personal injury, or death that result in any way from accessing or hiking the trails described in the following pages. Please be aware that hikers have been injured in the Portland area. Be especially cautious when walking on or near boulders, steep inclines, and dropoffs, and do not attempt to explore terrain that may be beyond your abilities. To help ensure an uneventful hike, please read carefully the introduction to this book, and perhaps get further safety information and guidance from other sources. Familiarize yourself thoroughly with the area you intend to visit before venturing out. Ask questions, and prepare for the unforeseen. Familiarize yourself with current weather reports, maps of the area you plan to visit, and any relevant park regulations.

**WITH IMMENSE GRATITUDE AND RESPECT, I DEDICATE THIS BOOK TO THE PEOPLE WHO BUILD AND MAINTAIN THE TRAILS.**

**—PAUL GERALD**

# TABLE OF
# CONTENTS

# ACKNOWLEDGMENTS

**FOUR EDITIONS. UNBELIEVABLE.** When Menasha Ridge Press first asked me to write this book back in 2000, I said yes mainly so I could walk into Powell's one day, buy a latte, and see my book sitting on the shelf.

Frankly, I was setting my sights too low. I didn't realize all the wonderful things that would happen after I wrote it, primarily all the cool people I'd get to talk to, work with, and hike with.

For starters, of course, there are all the people at Menasha—none of whom I've ever even had the chance to meet! First and foremost is Molly Merkle, who for years has patiently answered all my tedious questions and put up with my somewhat adversarial relationship with deadlines. Then there are all the people who turn my Word files, photos, and GPS tracks into the book you're holding: Ritchey Halphen, Scott McGrew, and Alisha Gustin. And finally, many thanks to Mike Jones, who I'm lucky to have right here in Portland so he can act as my publishing guru—I can see him wince at that remark right now!

I processed a lot of information for this book, much of which came from the United States Forest Service, Oregon State Parks, PortlandHikers.org, the Columbia Gorge Visitors Center, the Mount Hood Visitors Center, the Mazamas, and the amazing book *Oregon Geographical Names* from the Oregon Historical Society Press. I own the sixth edition, revised and updated by Lewis L. McArthur, and I recommend it highly.

Once I put all of the information together, I needed somebody to make sure I wasn't completely out of touch with reality; enter a small army of patient employees of various federal, state, and private agencies who interrupted their busy schedules to review all the hiking text. My humble thanks to them all: Mark Marshall, Tom Robinson, Jacquelyn Oakes, Jane Dooley, Susan Freston, Gary Walker, Rick Swart, Breanne Jordan, Erik Plunkett, Pete Marvin, Gary McDaniel, Kevin Strandberg, Karen Houston,

Tom Atiyeh, Robin Jensen, Stephen Anderson, Heather Latham, Dean Robertson, Randy Peterson, Greg Hawley, Lynn Barlow, J. W. Cleveland, Bob Stillson, Brandon Haraughty, and Lorie Hutton.

Special thanks to Tom Kloster for all his help with the Old Vista Ridge Trail, and to Lee Davis and Peggie Schwarz at the Mazamas for letting me set up a small writing camp in their air-conditioned office during the hideous heat wave of 2009.

Of course, a hike is a lonely experience without good friends to share it with. Here—listed alphabetically to avoid controversy!—is a list of the folks who made "researching" this fourth edition such an enjoyable experience: Barbra Baker, Gene Blick, Jenny Boyce, Jim Chase, Tom Davidson, Tom Eggers, Rich Fuhs, Jane Garbisch, Sabrina Louise, Ben Maynard, Beth McNeil, Dean Meyerson, Maria Shindler, Alice Sufka, and Leslie Woods. I have done a horrendous job of keeping notes on who accompanied me along the way, and I probably left people out. Sorry.

And finally, a lifetime of love and thanks to my family back East: Marjorie and Barry Gerald; Lee, Lela, and Jack Gerald and Max Simpson; Lucy, Becky, David, Jeff, and Charlie Cook. Thanks also to my good friends and occasional housemates Joe and Vonne Williams. And a big hug to the Thursday Night Boys, for keeping me (reasonably) sane, one day at a time.

—Paul Gerald

# FOREWORD

Welcome to Menasha Ridge Press's *60 Hikes within 60 Miles*. Our strategy was simple: First, find a hiker who knows the area and loves to hike. Second, ask that person to spend a year researching the most popular and very best trails around. And third, have that person describe each trail in terms of difficulty, scenery, condition, elevation change, and all other categories of information that are important to hikers. "Pretend you've just completed a hike and met up with other hikers at the trailhead," we told each author. "Imagine their questions, and be clear in your answers."

An experienced hiker and writer, author Paul Gerald has selected 60 of the best hikes in and around his adopted home-town of Portland. From the civilized hikes of downtown Portland to the rugged trails of volatile Mount St. Helens, Gerald provides hikers (and walkers) with a great variety of trails—and all within 60 miles of the city.

You'll get more out of this book if you take a moment to read the introduction; though this is a "where-to" rather than a "how-to" guide, those of you who have hiked extensively will find it of particular value. The "Topographic Maps" section will help you understand how useful topos will be on a hike, and will also tell you where to get them.

As much for the opportunity to free the spirit as to free the body, let Paul Gerald's hikes elevate you above the urban hurry.

**All the best,**
**The Editors at Menasha Ridge Press**

# ABOUT THE AUTHOR

**PAUL GERALD**'s writing career began in the sports department of the much-missed *Dallas Times Herald*. He later worked for the *Memphis Commercial Appeal* and the *Memphis Flyer*. Since then, he has written some 300 travel articles for the *Flyer*, and along the way his work has also appeared in Northwest Airlines' *WorldTraveler*, and in Portland's *Willamette Week* and the *Oregonian*.

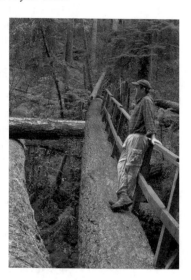

He's also worked in and around landscaping, public relations, social work, an amusement park, Alaskan fishing boats, the YMCA, and corporate marketing, and as a package handler for FedEx. Such is the life of a writer who wants to avoid having a regular job. He published *Breakfast in Bridgetown: The Definitive Guide to Portland's Favorite Meal* in 2008, under the name Bacon and Eggs Press.

Paul's hiking life started at age 12, when he went to a summer camp in the Absoraka Mountains of Wyoming. He became a trail and road hound at that point, and his hometown of Memphis never looked the same. He's hiked in the Rocky Mountains from New Mexico to Montana, and in Appalachia, Alaska, Nepal, and Argentina. In 1996 he moved to Portland to be close to the ocean, the mountains, the big trees, and the coffee shops.

This was his first book. He is also the author of *Day and Overnight Hikes: Oregon's Pacific Crest Trail* and revised *Best Tent Camping: Oregon* for Menasha Ridge in 2009.

Paul has greatly enjoyed meeting people using his books out on the trails; he's also grateful that none of them appeared to be lost or angry. He does hope, however, that any feedback will be directed to him, care of the publisher, or at **www.paulgerald. com**. And he hopes people will continue to enjoy and benefit from the fruits of his labor—if hiking and writing can truly be called labor.

# PREFACE

**HERE'S A FUNNY ADMISSION** from the author of a hiking book: There comes a time, almost every time I go hiking, when I kind of hate it.

Sometimes it's the weather, of course. I'm pretty much a fair-weather hiker. Sometimes it's the big uphills. Sometimes it's the big downhills. Sometimes it's the tedious drive back home (in particular the stretch of I-84 between Troutdale and I-205). Sometimes it's the early start, or the late return, or all the chatter on the trail.

Maybe I'm just getting old; my 43-year-old legs and back complain a little more than their 25-year-old versions did. Maybe it's the pounds I put on while writing a breakfast guidebook. And maybe I fell into the trap of letting my favorite pastime become part of my job; slogging up a viewless hill in the rain because I "have to do it for my book" hardly screams "glamorous life of a writer."

So why do it?

For the little moments in between.

Take Multnomah Falls, for example. You drive there, you see the falls, you fight the crowds, and maybe you drag yourself up the paved trail to the top of the falls for a look around. And yes, I am being a horribly jaded Oregonian, but there's an element of "been there, done that."

Ah, but if you keep going, there's a place just a little farther up, right past the old bridge over the creek, where the pavement ends, the crowds turn around, and it turns into a trail, a path leading into the woods, bound for miles away. And every time I go there, there's a little moment waiting for me, like a present I'm always getting for the first time. It's the moving on, the letting go, the opening up, the knowing that behind me is town, life, work, money, cars, computers . . . and ahead of me is only more trail and trees and creeks and birds and cliffs and mountains.

My brain knows that I can walk from that spot, using only forest trails, to Mount Hood, to countless other quiet, wild places—and that's a part of it. But it's my heart where the little moment happens, a kind of release and relaxation, a simple knowing that from here on, it's just me, or us, and the woods, and I can go wherever I feel, because I have everything I need right here with me.

Mountains have stirred my heart since I was a kid, and it's because they are filled with those little moments: walking over a ridge to see a great view, coming around a corner to surprise a deer on the path, catching a glimpse of an eagle or a big fish, or just sitting down for some peace next to a stream. Of course, it doesn't have to be in the mountains; much of Portland's magic lies in places like Macleay Park, where you leave "the city," in the metaphorical sense, and enter "the woods," where trout swim in the creek, massive trees are all around, and there's a bird sanctuary just up the hill. It's there in the wooded ravine around Marquam Trail, which was at one time to be filled with apartments but instead remains a quiet, shady way to reach the highest place in the city.

My original, superficial reason for writing this book, way back in 2000, was so that I could walk into Powell's, buy a latte, point at a book on the shelf, and say, "I wrote that." In other words, it was mostly ego. (Believe me, it wasn't the money!) There was something deeper, though. I have always wanted to visit interesting places, meet interesting people, and do interesting things, then tell people about them. Part of that is still ego, sure, but a bigger part is that I just think life is cool, and I want to share that coolness with people. I think hiking is particularly cool, even when I hate it—because, after all, don't you feel a little more satisfaction walking to the top of, say, Larch Mountain than driving up there? Especially if you start by the banks of the Columbia and walk to the top of a Cascades peak? The work, if you can do it, enhances the payoff. You get a connection with the whole mountain.

Over the years, the deeper reason for writing this book has really come to the surface. Thousands of people have bought it, which amazes and humbles me, and more than a few have told me they like and enjoy it. Ego again, sure, but also something else: they (you) are having those little moments, too! To think that I drove all the ridiculous way to Whetstone Mountain to that somewhat boring hike—ah, but to get that mind-boggling view—and then somebody else read about it, made the same drive, and got the same view . . . well, it makes me feel warm and fuzzy. People often thank me for writing the book, and all I can think to say is, "Thanks for enjoying it."

And that's when they ask me the Question: "What's your favorite hike?" (Everybody asks it, and if you do, too, it's not a problem.) And I, being a wordy writer (have you noticed?) always say, "Well, that depends." Depends, in my case, almost entirely on what month it is. I often think of Catherine Creek, Coyote Wall, and the Labyrinth, hikes that in April and May are awash in flowery, sunny, breezy, bird-songy little moments . . . and which in July or August would probably kill you with heat and boredom. My "favorite" also depends on what mood I'm in. Sometimes I want a big adventure like Trapper Creek Wilderness, maybe even an overnight, and sometimes I just want to stroll along the Salmon River for a couple of miles, to gaze at the big trees and look for salmon.

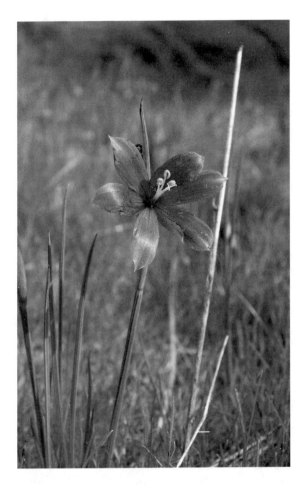

Grass widow

I have written this book, four times now, with one intention: to help my fellow humans get out to some cool spots so they can experience those little moments. (It still isn't about the money. Well, not much.) I wrote it as if you're going to actually carry the book along with you, so I can point stuff out along the way and give you some things to think about while you're doing the dull stuff. I'll tell you why Ramona Falls is called that (it's a sweet story), where the Throne of the Forest King sits, and why there are cables around stumps high above the Clackamas River. I assume you want to know these things.

What I also assume is that, like most people I talk to, you may want to know what my favorite hike is. Like I said, that depends! So here, by way of introduction to the book, is my Personal Hiking Calendar. I don't stick to this, or anything else in life, very strictly, but I bet that if you follow it you'll have a fine year of hiking, and there's a decent chance we'll bump into each other.

I get through winter the way most outdoorsy Portlanders do: I'll go up the Macleay or Marquam Trail to stretch my legs, and maybe out to Angels Rest for a sunset, but otherwise it's snowshoes, coffee, and planning for better weather. For this edition, I've even included a list of good snowshoeing hikes, and if you want a list of breakfast places, I've got that in another book.

What I really look for, usually on **PortlandHikers.org**, is the first picture of a grass widow. What's a grass widow? Well, objectively speaking, it's a small, unassuming, mostly purple flower, barely six inches tall. But to the hiker's heart, it's the Beginning of It All, the first spring wildflower that blooms where such flowers bloom. Most often, the grass widow is first seen in March at Catherine Creek, and its appearance means that we can now leave rainy old Portland, drive an hour east, and listen to the meadowlarks while we look for the rest of the hundreds of types of flowers that will soon drape the slopes at Coyote Wall and McCall Nature Preserve.

That show goes until May, and in the meantime, the few dry days offer a chance to go to Silver Falls State Park, where you can walk 7 miles, see ten full-tilt waterfalls, and get a latte before and/or after you go. It's also time to start getting into shape, and for that there is Hamilton Mountain, itself a flowery scene by April, when flowers on the Oregon side of the gorge have yet to bloom but the Washington side is catching rays. I also use, as a conditioner and a reminder of why I live here, the loop from Wahkeena Falls over to Multnomah Falls. You might like it as well, if you're into stuff like creeks and waterfalls and springs and views and soft ice cream.

Other April favorites? The plunging waters of Herman Creek, Eagle Creek, or Falls Creek; the high water and birds at Oaks Bottom; or the irises out at the end of Cape Falcon.

By May, in theory, I'm getting in pretty good shape, and the sun is starting to win its annual battle against the clouds. Barely. But May means one big thing in my hiking life: Dog Mountain. It's physically big, but psychologically bigger. The flower show up there from mid-May to mid-June wipes me out every year, and whenever I tell people the balsamroot is a "sea of yellow," it's an understatement. Really, if you do one hike this year, go up Dog Mountain in late May or so. Well, first do some other hikes to prepare.

By June the bloom is spreading, and the clouds clearing. June can be maddening, though; you want to get up high, but most years the snow still blankets those trails. June is about transition and mid-elevation: too late for spring flowers, too early for Mount Hood . . . just right for being around 2,000 to 3,000 feet for the first blast of summer. My June favorites are Silver Star Mountain for the flowers, Salmon Butte for the rhododendrons, and Kings Mountain or Saddle Mountain for both the flowers . . . and breakfast at Camp 18.

In July I play two little games called "Beat the Heat" and "Follow the Mosquitoes." See, for the first month after the snow melts, the mosquitoes will make you hate life. And July tends to be pretty warm. So I wait for word that the little varmints are gone from various shady forests, then I move in to hike. This leads me to lower-elevation places like Breitenbush, Opal Creek, and Lewis River, or the ever-cool coast, where July means the big bloom at Cascade Head, and July 16 the opening of the upper trailhead there.

August is what it's all about around here. The snow and mosquitoes are gone everywhere, and my hiker's life is all about getting as high as possible. For me, this means it's Mount Hood Time: Vista Ridge barely edges out McNeil Point, Paradise Park, and Lookout Mountain as a favorite, but anything in the "Around Mount Hood" section will be a day well spent.

For a lot of hikers, September is the best month. The weather is cooling, the crowds are gone, and there will just start to be some fall colors somewhere. I like Cooper Spur this time of year, because at about 8,000 feet, you can just barely sense winter coming over the ridge. It's also your last shot at the high stuff, so it's a good time to hit Bull of the Woods for that big view, as well.

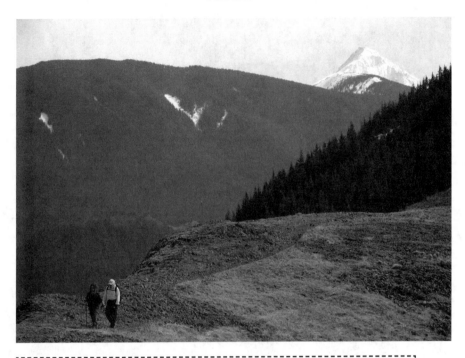

**Walking north off the "back side" of Hamilton Mountain.**

For this hiker, October is the big show. You're in shape, you've got your hiking crowd of friends, you can still do any hike in the book, and there's a sweet sadness, plus a sense of rush to get it all in, before the snow blows. For highlights, it's all about two things: salmon and fall colors. October is when the ocean-run fish make it into the Salmon River and the Wilson River, and when the vine maples at Trapper Creek or Ape Canyon will blow your mind.

After a year like that, frankly, I'm more interested in watching college football for November and December than I am in hiking. And I know that I just listed at least a third of the book as a "favorite," but what can I say? The whole book is favorites! I have done close to 100 different hikes around here, and these are the 60 I believe anyone will enjoy.

So please do enjoy them. And take care of them. And remember, if you have one of those moments where you hate hiking, just keep truckin', and you'll soon get to one of those other little, but glorious, moments in between.

I hope to see you out there on the trail.

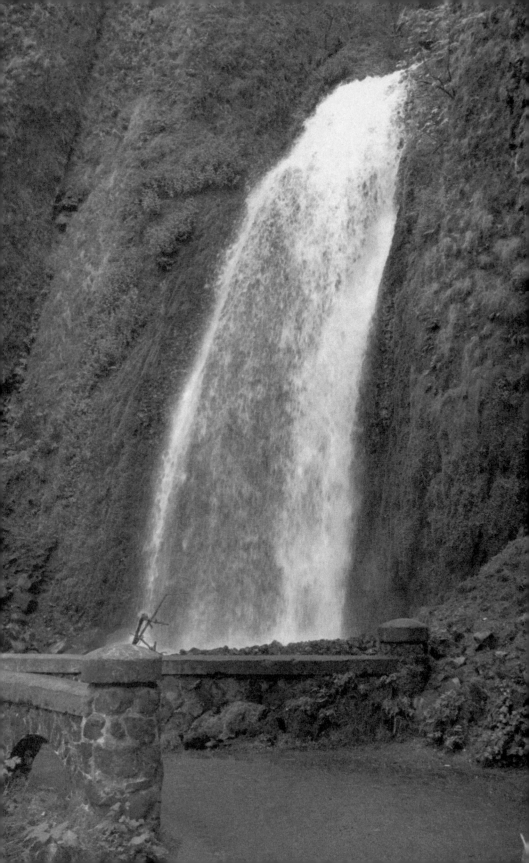

# HIKING RECOMMENDATIONS

## HIKES GOOD FOR CHILDREN

## FLAT HIKES

## STEEP HIKES

Wahkeena Falls

## STEEP HIKES (*continued*)

## URBAN HIKES

## BEST FOR BACKPACKING

## SECLUDED HIKES

## HIKES GOOD FOR WATCHING WILDLIFE

## HIKES WITH BIG-TIME VIEWS

## TRAILS GOOD FOR RUNNERS

## MULTIUSE TRAILS

## HISTORIC TRAILS

## TRAILS FEATURING WATERFALLS

## BEST FOR WHEELCHAIRS

## BEST FOR SNOWSHOES

*In the following categories, parentheses indicate a shorter option within a longer hike.*

## HIKES LESS THAN 1 MILE

12. Triple Falls (to Upper Horsetail Falls) (page 59)
17. Lava Canyon (upper loop) (page 80)
18. Lewis River (to Lower Falls) (page 84)
28. Breitenbush Hot Springs Area (several options) (page 129)
33. Elk Meadows (to Newton Creek) (page 154)
42. Timberline Lodge (to White River Canyon overlook) (page 190)
46. Wildwood Recreation Area (two loops) (page 208)
58. Silver Falls State Park (South Falls Loop) (page 261)
59. Tryon Creek State Park (several options) (page 265)
60. Washington Park–Hoyt Arboretum (several options) (page 268)

## HIKES 1 TO 3 MILES

2. Beacon Rock–Hamilton Mountain (Beacon Rock or Rodney Falls) (page 16)
7. Eagle Creek (to Punchbowl Falls) (page 38)
10. McCall Nature Preserve (page 52)
18. Lewis River (to Middle Falls) (page 84)
22. Bagby Hot Springs (page 102)
23. Bull of the Woods (to Pansy Lake) (page 106)
25. Roaring River Wilderness (to Shellrock Lake) (page 114)
34. Lookout Mountain (from High Prairie) (page 159)
37. Mirror Lake (to lake) (page 172)
42. Timberline Lodge (to Silcox Hut) (page 190)
43. Trillium Lake (page 195)
48. Cascade Head (upper trailhead) (page 218)
54. Macleay Trail (to Audubon Society) (page 246)
56. Oaks Bottom Wildlife Refuge/Willamette River (Oaks Bottom) (page 254)
57. Sauvie Island (to Oak Island) (page 257)
58. Silver Falls State Park (several options) (page 261)
59. Tryon Creek State Park (page 265)

## HIKES 3 TO 6 MILES

1. Angels Rest–Devils Rest (to Angels Rest) (page 12)
3. Catherine Creek (page 20)
4. Chinidere Mountain (page 25)
5. Coyote Wall–The Labyrinth (page 30)
8. Herman Creek (to creek crossing or PCT Falls) (page 42)
12. Triple Falls (page 59)

## HIKES 3 TO 6 MILES (CONTINUED)

## HIKES MORE THAN 6 MILES

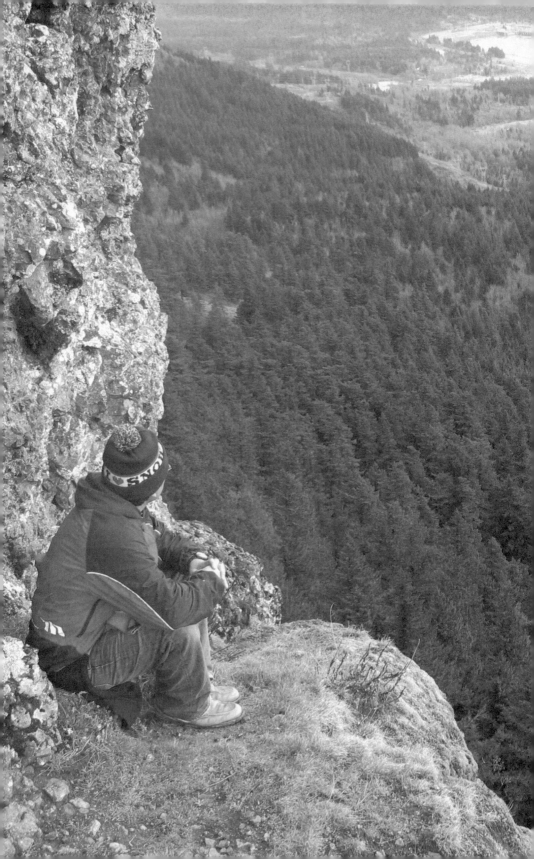

# 60 HIKES
## WITHIN 60 MILES

### PORTLAND

INCLUDES

**THE COAST,
MOUNTS HOOD AND ST. HELENS,
AND THE COLUMBIA RIVER GORGE**

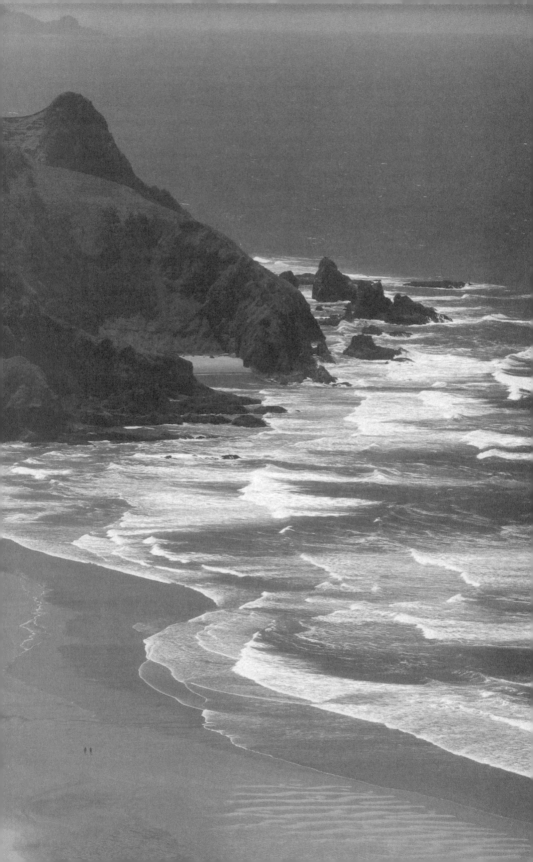

# INTRODUCTION

Welcome to *60 Hikes within 60 Miles: Portland!* If you're new to hiking, or even if you're a seasoned trailsmith, take a few minutes to read the following introduction. We'll explain how this book is organized and how to get the best use of it.

## HOW TO USE THIS GUIDEBOOK
### THE OVERVIEW MAP AND OVERVIEW MAP KEY

Use the overview map on the inside front cover to find the exact location of each hike's primary trailhead. Each hike's number appears on the overview map, on the map key facing the overview map, and in the table of contents. As you flip through the book, you'll see that a hike's full profile is easy to locate by watching for the hike number at the top of each page. The book is organized by region as indicated in the table of contents. A map legend that details the symbols found on trail maps appears on the inside back cover.

### REGIONAL MAPS

The book is divided into regions, and prefacing each regional section is an overview map of that region. The regional map provides more detail than the overview map does, bringing you closer to the hike.

### TRAIL MAPS

Each hike contains a detailed map that shows the trailhead, route, significant features, facilities, and topographic landmarks such as creeks, overlooks, and peaks. The author gathered map data by carrying Garmin eTrex or Garmin 60CS GPS units while hiking. This data was downloaded into the digital mapping program Topo USA and processed by expert cartographers to produce the highly accurate maps found in this book. Each trailhead's GPS coordinates are included with each profile (see page 2).

Beach view from Cascade Head

## ELEVATION PROFILES

Corresponding directly to the trail map, there is a detailed elevation profile for each hike. The elevation profile provides a quick look at the trail from the side, enabling you to visualize how it rises and falls. Key points along the way are labeled. Note the number of feet between each tick mark on the vertical axis (the height scale). To avoid making flat hikes look steep and steep hikes appear flat, height scales are used throughout the book to provide an accurate image of the hike's climbing difficulty.

## GPS TRAILHEAD COORDINATES

In addition to highly specific trail outlines, this book also includes the GPS coordinates for each trailhead in two formats: latitude/longitude and UTM. Latitude/longitude coordinates tell you where you are by locating a point west (latitude) of the 0° meridian line that passes through Greenwich, England, and north or south of the 0° (longitude) line that belts the Earth, also known as the equator.

Topographic maps show latitude/longitude as well as UTM grid lines. Known as UTM coordinates, the numbers index a specific point using a grid method. The survey datum used to arrive at the coordinates in this book is WGS84 (versus NAD27 or WGS83). For readers who own a GPS unit, whether handheld or onboard a vehicle, the latitude/longitude or UTM coordinates provided on the first page of each hike may be entered into the GPS unit. Just make sure your GPS unit is set to navigate using WGS84 datum. Now you can navigate directly to the trailhead.

Most trailheads, which begin in parking areas, can be reached by car, but some hikes still require a short walk to reach the trailhead from a parking area. In those cases a handheld unit is necessary to continue the GPS navigation process. That said, readers can easily access all trailheads in this book by using the directions given, the overview map, and the trail map, which shows at least one major road leading into the area. But for those who enjoy using the latest GPS technology to navigate, the necessary data has been provided. A brief explanation of the UTM coordinates from Angels Rest–Devils Rest (page 12) follows.

UTM Zone (WGS84)   10T<br>
Easting   564632<br>
Northing   5045586

The UTM zone number **10** refers to one of the 60 vertical zones of the Universal Transverse Mercator (UTM) projection. Each zone is 6 degrees wide. The UTM zone letter **T** refers to one of the 20 horizontal zones that span from 80 degrees south to 84 degrees north. The easting number **564632** indicates in meters how far east or west a point is from the central meridian of the zone. Increasing easting coordinates on a topo map or on your GPS screen indicate that you are moving east; decreasing easting coordinates indicate that you are moving west. The northing number **5045586** references in meters how far you are from the equator. Above and below the equator, increasing northing coordinates indicate that you are traveling north; decreasing northing coordinates indicate that you are traveling south. To learn more about how to enhance your outdoor experiences with GPS technology, refer to *GPS Outdoors: A Practical Guide for Outdoor Enthusiasts* (Menasha Ridge Press).

# HIKE DESCRIPTIONS

Each hike contains six key items: an **In Brief** description of the trail, a **Key-at-a-Glance Information** box, **directions** to the trail, a **locator map**, a **trail map**, and a **hike description**. Combined, the maps and information provide a clear method to assess each trail from the comfort of your favorite chair.

## IN BRIEF

Here you'll get a "taste of the trail." Think of this section as a snapshot of the historical landmarks, beautiful vistas, and other interesting sights you might encounter on the trail.

## KEY-AT-A-GLANCE INFORMATION

The Key at-a-Glance Information boxes give you a quick idea of the specifics of each hike, covering 18 basic elements.

**LENGTH** The length of the trail from start to finish. There may be options to shorten or extend the hikes, but the mileage corresponds to the hike described. Consult the hike description to help decide how to customize the hike for your ability or time available.

**CONFIGURATION** A description of what the trail might look like from overhead. Trails can be loops, out-and-backs (taking you in and out via the same route), figure eights, or balloons.

**DIFFICULTY** The degree of effort an "average" hiker should expect on a given hike. For simplicity, difficulty is described as "easy," "moderate," or "strenuous."

**SCENERY** Rates the overall environs of the hike and what to expect in terms of plant life, wildlife, streams, and historic buildings.

**EXPOSURE** A quick check of how much sun you can expect on your shoulders during the hike. Descriptors used are self-explanatory and include terms such as shady, exposed, and sunny.

**TRAFFIC** Indicates how busy the trail might be on an average day, and if you might be able to find solitude out there. Trail traffic, of course, varies from day to day and season to season.

**TRAIL SURFACE** Indicates whether the trail is paved, rocky, smooth, or composed of a mixture of elements.

**HIKING TIME** How long it took the author to hike the trail. Paul Gerald is a self-described dawdler who often fritters away time eating or admiring wildflowers. On average, he covers 2 miles an hour (faster downhill, slower on steady ascents, particularly during hot weather). If you're an experienced hiker in great shape, you'll finish the hikes with time to spare, but if you're a beginner or like to stop to take in the views, allow a little extra time.

**DRIVING DISTANCE**   and time are both measured from Pioneer Square in downtown Portland. Not that you'd start there, necessarily, but it should help you compare travel times to the trailheads from where you live.

**SEASON**  Time of year when a particular hike is accessible. In most cases, the determining factor is snow.

**BEST TIME**  If you want to save this hike for when it's at its best, this is the time to shoot for.

**BACKPACKING OPTIONS**  Feel like spending the night out? Here's a quick glance; more details are in the text.

**ACCESS**  Notes fees or permits needed to hike the trail.

**WHEELCHAIR ACCESS**  Many trails have a small paved section.

**MAPS**  Which map is the best or easiest (in the author's opinion) for this hike.

**FACILITIES**  What to expect at the trailhead or nearby in terms of restrooms, phones, water, and other niceties.

**INFO**  What's the number to call for up-to-date conditions?

**SPECIAL COMMENTS**  Provides you with those little extra details that don't fit into any of the above categories. Here you'll find assorted nuggets of information, including whether or not your dog is allowed on the trails.

## DIRECTIONS

The directions will help you locate each trailhead. When pertinent, numbered exits are included in the driving directions for each hike.

## DESCRIPTIONS

In the trail description, the author summarizes the trail's features and highlights any special sights or activities along the hike. Ultimately, the hike description will help you choose which hikes are best for you.

## NEARBY ACTIVITIES

Not every hike will have recommended nearby attractions. For those that do, look here for information on places of interest near, or on the way to or from, the trail. In Paul's case, many of these have to do with food.

# WEATHER

For most folks, hiking season around Portland starts in March or April, when flowers bloom and temperatures start to rise. Unfortunately, that's the least stable of seasons, where the weather is concerned. Weather forecasts are notoriously off the mark during spring, so if they aren't absolutely, positively sure it will be clear, plan for 50-something degrees and drizzling into June.

Snow is a different matter; the higher hikes in this book won't be completely clear most years until July. Also beware that in the Columbia River Gorge, wind is a constant reality, so even on a sunny June day a hike such as the one to Dog Mountain can have you reaching for a hat and gloves. By mid- to late June, and all the way into October, you'll see mostly sunny skies, mild temperatures, and happy hikers. Then winter comes and, for all intents and purposes, it rains until spring. We try to think of it as "waterfall loading."

## AVERAGE DAILY (HIGH) TEMPERATURE BY MONTH

| | JAN | FEB | MAR | APR | MAY | JUN |
|------|------|------|------|------|------|------|
| HIGH | 46° F | 51° F | 56° F | 60° F | 68° F | 74° F |
| | JUL | AUG | SEP | OCT | NOV | DEC |
| HIGH | 80° F | 81° F | 75° F | 64° F | 53° F | 46° F |

## TOPOGRAPHIC MAPS

The maps in this book have been produced with great care and, used with the hiking directions, will help you stay on course. But as any experienced hiker knows, things can get tricky off the beaten path.

The maps in this book, when used with the route directions in each hike profile, are sufficient to direct you to the trail and guide you on it. However, you will find superior detail and valuable information on the United States Geological Survey's 7.5-minute series topographic maps. Topo maps are widely available online. The single easiest-to-use Web resource is **terraserver.microsoft.com**. You can view and print topos of the entire United States there, and view aerial photographs of the whole country, as well. The downside to topos is that most of them are outdated, having been created 20 to 30 years ago. But they still provide excellent topographic detail.

If you're new to hiking, you might be wondering, "What's a topographic map?" In short, a topo indicates not only distance but elevation, using contour lines. Contour lines spread across the map like dozens of intricate spider webs. Each line represents a particular elevation, and at the base of each topo a contour's interval designation is given. If the contour interval is 200 feet, then the distance between each contour line is 200 feet. Follow five contour lines up on a map and the elevation has increased by 1,000 feet.

In addition to outdoors shops and bike shops, you'll find topos at major universities and some public libraries, where you might try photocopying the ones you need to avoid the cost of buying them. But if you want your own and can't find them locally, contact map retailers (see Appendix B).

# WATER

"How much is enough? One bottle? Two? Three? But think of all that extra weight!" Well, one simple physiological fact should convince you to err on the side of excess when it comes to deciding how much water to pack—a hiker working hard in 90-degree heat needs approximately ten quarts of fluid every day. That's two-and-a-half gallons—12 large water bottles or 16 small ones. In other words, pack along one or two bottles even for short hikes.

Serious backpackers hit the trail prepared to purify water found along the route. This method, while less dangerous than drinking it untreated, comes with risks. Purifiers with ceramic filters are the safest, but also the most expensive. Many hikers pack along the slightly distasteful tetraglycine hydroperiodide tablets (sold under the names Potable Aqua, Coughlan's, and others).

Probably the most common waterborne "bug" that hikers face is giardia, which may not hit until one to four weeks after ingestion. It will have you passing noxious rotten-egg gas, vomiting, shivering with chills, and living in the bathroom. But there are other parasites to worry about, including *E. coli* and *cryptosporidium* (both of which are harder to kill than giardia).

For most people, the pleasures of hiking make carrying water a relatively small price to pay to remain healthy. If you're tempted to drink "found" water, do so only if you understand the risks. Better yet, hydrate prior to your hike, carry (and drink) six ounces of water for every mile you plan to hike, and hydrate after the hike.

# FIRST-AID KIT

A typical kit might contain more items than you think necessary. But these are just the basics:

- **Ace bandages or Spenco joint wraps**
- **Antibiotic ointment (Neosporin or the generic equivalent)**
- **Aspirin or acetaminophen**
- **Band-Aids**
- **Benadryl or the generic equivalent, diphenhydramine (an antihistamine, in case of allergic reactions)**
- **Butterfly-closure bandages**
- **Gauze (one roll)**
- **Gauze compress pads (a half-dozen 4-by-4–inch pads)**
- **Hydrogen peroxide or iodine**
- **Matches or pocket lighter**
- **Moleskin/Spenco "Second Skin"**
- **A prefilled syringe of epinephrine (for those known to have severe allergic reactions to such things as bee stings)**
- **Snakebite kit**
- **Sunscreen**
- **Water purification tablets or water filter (see section, Water, above)**
- **Whistle (more effective in signaling rescuers than your voice)**

Pack the items in a resealable waterproof bag. You will also want to include a snack for hikes longer than a couple of miles. A bag full of GORP ("good ol' raisins and peanuts") will kick up your energy level fast.

# SNAKES

The most common snakes you'll encounter in and west of the Cascades are non-poisonous garter snakes. The only venomous snakes in Oregon are rattlesnakes, but sightings of these pit vipers are generally infrequent, occurring most commonly in dry, rocky, or exposed zones east of the mountains. The standard rules for hiking in rattlesnake territory are:

- **Do not put your hands (or feet) where you can't see them—for example, on top of a rock outcrop or in a log pile.**
- **Be extra cautious in hot weather, as snakes are more active then.**
- **Scan the trail continuously as you hike.**
- **Keep children from running ahead on trails. Bites to children are more severe than to adults.**
- **Avoid tall grass where you can't see your feet (or a potential snake).**

Should you encounter a rattler, its body language will reveal its mood. A coiled rattler is primed for a strike, while a stretched rattler is more sanguine (although snakes have been reported to "lunge"). If the snake is within striking distance, stand motionless and wait for it to calm down and move. Taking small, slow steps backward is also an option. If you're out of immediate range, you can either skirt the snake or wait for it to move. Some people believe that tapping the ground with a stick (from a safe distance, rather than in the snake's face) will encourage the snake to move on.

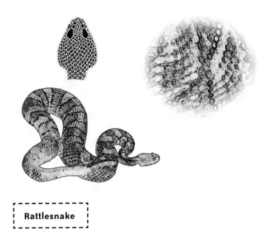

Rattlesnake

# TICKS

Ticks like to hang out in the brush that grows along trails. I've noticed ticks mostly in the eastern gorge, but you should be tick-aware during all months of the spring, summer, and fall. Ticks—actually arthropods and not insects—are ectoparasites, which need a host for the majority of their life cycle in order to reproduce. The ticks that light onto hikers will be very small, sometimes so tiny that you won't be able to spot them. Primarily of two varieties, deer ticks and dog ticks, both need a few hours of attachment before they can transmit any disease they may harbor. I've found ticks in my socks and on my legs several hours after a hike that have not yet anchored. The best strategy is to visually check every half hour or so while hiking, do a thorough check before you get in the car, and then, when you take a post-hike shower, do an even more thorough check of your entire body. Ticks that haven't latched on are easily removed, though not easily killed. If I pick off a tick in the woods, I just toss it aside. If I find one on my person at home, I make sure to dispatch it down the toilet. For ticks that have embedded themselves, it's best to remove them with tweezers.

## POISON OAK

Poison oak is a deciduous plant that grows as sparse ground cover, vine, or shrub; regardless of its form, poison oak always has three leaflets. It is easiest to spot in summer and early autumn, when the leaves flush bright red. Beware of unknown bare-branched shrubs and vines in winter—the entire plant can cause a rash no matter what the season.

The rashes are caused by urushiol, the oil in the sap of poison oak. Reactions may start almost immediately, or may not appear until a week after exposure: raised lines and/or blisters are accompanied by a terrible itch. Refrain from scratching because bacteria under fingernails may cause infection. Wash and dry the rash thoroughly, and apply a calamine lotion to help dry out the rash. If itching or blistering is severe, seek medical attention.

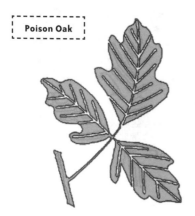

Poison Oak

Recognizing and avoiding poison oak is the most effective way to prevent painful, itchy rashes. Most people come into contact with the plant while they're bushwhacking or traveling off trail, so you can minimize your encounters with poison oak by staying on established trails. If you do knowingly contact poison oak, you must remove the oil within 15 to 20 minutes to avoid a reaction. Showering on the trail with cool water (hot water spreads the oil) is impractical, but some commercial products, such as Tecnu, clean the oil off skin.

If you come into contact with poison oak, remember that oil-contaminated clothes, pets, or hiking gear can easily inflict an irritating rash on you or someone else, so wash not only any exposed parts of your body but also clothes, gear, and pets, if applicable.

## HIKING WITH CHILDREN

No one is too young for a hike in the woods or through a city park. Be careful, though. Flat, short trails are probably best with an infant. Toddlers who have not quite mastered walking can still tag along, riding on an adult's back in a child carrier. Use common sense to judge a child's capacity to hike a particular trail, and be prepared for the possibility that the child will tire quickly and need to be carried.

When packing for the hike, remember the needs of the child as well as your own. Make sure children are adequately clothed for the weather, have proper shoes, and are protected from the sun with sunscreen. Kids dehydrate quickly, so make sure you have plenty of fluid for everyone.

To help you determine which trails are suitable for children, there's a list of hike recommendations on page xvii.

Finally, when hiking with children, remember that the trip will be a compromise. A child's energy and enthusiasm alternate between bursts of speed and long stops to examine snails, sticks, dirt, and other attractions.

## THE BUSINESS HIKER

Whether you're visiting or a resident in the Portland area, these hikes are the ideal opportunity for a quick getaway from everyday demands. Many of the hikes are classified as urban and are easily accessible from downtown areas.

Instead of grabbing a burger down the street, pack a lunch and head out to one of the area's many urban trails for a relaxing break from the office or that tiresome convention. Or plan ahead and take a small group of your business comrades on a nearby hike in one of the area forests. A well-planned half-day getaway is the perfect complement to a business stay in Portland.

## TRAIL ETIQUETTE

Whether you're on a city, county, state, or national park trail, always remember that great care and resources have gone into creating these trails. Treat the trail, wildlife, and fellow hikers with respect.

Here are a few general ideas to keep in mind while on the trail.

- **Hike on open trails only. Respect trail and road closures (ask if you're not sure), avoid trespassing on private land, and obtain all permits and authorization as required. Also, leave gates as you found them or as marked.**

- **Leave no trace of your visit other than footprints. Be sensitive to the ground beneath you. This also means staying on the trail and not creating any new ones. Be sure to pack out what you pack in. No one likes to see the trash someone else has left behind.**

- **Never spook animals. An unannounced approach, a sudden movement, or a loud noise startles most animals. A surprised snake or skunk can be dangerous to you, to others, and to themselves. Give animals extra room and time to adjust to your presence.**

- **Plan ahead. Know your equipment, your ability, and the area in which you are hiking —and prepare accordingly. Be self-sufficient at all times; carry necessary supplies for changes in weather or other conditions. A well-executed trip is a satisfaction to you and to others.**

- **Be courteous to other hikers, or bikers, you meet on the trails.**

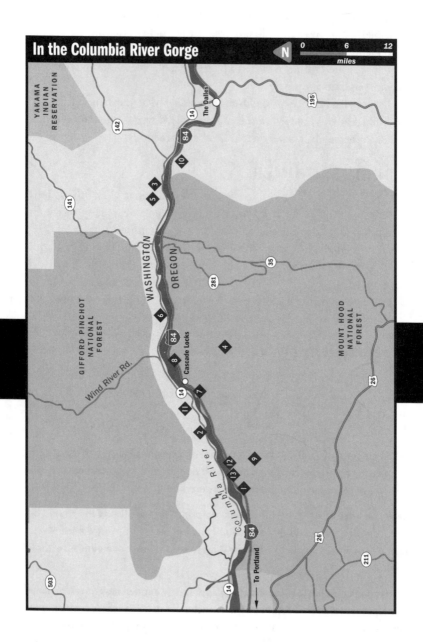

# In the Columbia River Gorge

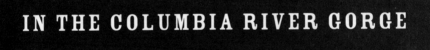

IN THE COLUMBIA RIVER GORGE

# 01 ANGELS REST-DEVILS REST

## IN BRIEF

There's a reason for all the parking at this trailhead: it's one of the finer hikes around, with a gentle grade to a spectacular lookout point above the Columbia River. It also connects with Wahkeena Trail, making longer loops or one-way hikes with shuttles possible.

## DESCRIPTION

As you drive out I-84, you can actually see Angels Rest, a flat-topped rock outcropping sticking out over the road at the end of a ridge. What looks like a building on top is in fact a clump of trees. And if it looks like it's way up there, just remember that if you take your time on the way up you'll have plenty of breath left to be taken away by the view up top.

The trail starts with a climb that is steep only for a moment and leads through the woods to an early reward: a rare view from above a waterfall, in this case the 100-foot Coopey Falls, named for a Portland tailor who owned land here. A short way past this, the trail crosses a wooden bridge over Coopey Creek and then starts climbing just a little more steeply.

After about a mile, you'll start switchbacking through an area that burned in 1991; note the blackened trunks of some of the

---

## GPS Trailhead Coordinates

UTM Zone (WGS84) 10T

Easting 564632

Northing 5045586

Latitude N 45.56081°

Longitude W 122.17184°

## *Directions* ———————➤

**Take I-84 from Portland, driving 21 miles east of I-205 to Exit 28/Bridal Veil. Drive less than a mile and park in the parking area at the intersection with the Historic Columbia River Highway; there's a second parking lot down the road to the right. The signed trailhead is on the old highway between the two parking lots.**

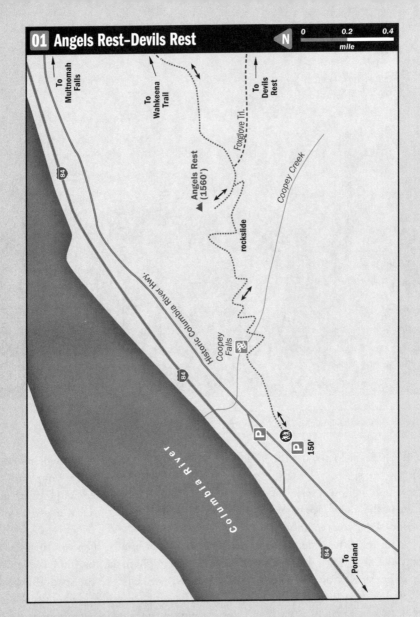

N

0        0.2        0.4

mile

To
Multnomah
Falls

To
Wahkeena
Trail

To
Devils
Rest

Foxglove Trl.

Coopey Creek

▲ Angels Rest
(1560')

rockslide

Historic Columbia River Hwy.

Coopey
Falls

84

84

P

P    150'

Columbia River

84

To
Portland

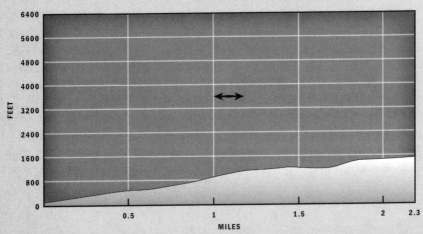

FEET

6400
5600
4800
4000
3200
2400
1600
800
0

0.5        1        1.5        2    2.3

MILES

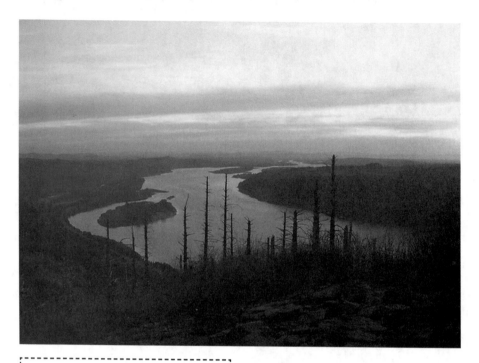

Looking down the Columbia from Angels Rest

bigger trees. Mostly just the underbrush and smaller trees burned, which opened up the forest floor to the sun and let wildflowers come in to take your mind off the climb. Follow a series of small switchbacks into more-open country, getting a view of the rocky face of Angels Rest as you go. When the trail traverses 100 yards of rockslide, you're almost done.

Just past the slide, the trail reenters the woods briefly, then you turn left out onto the final ridge. This last stretch of the trail might make you think twice about bringing small children: it gets a little narrow, with cliffs to the east falling away a few hundred feet, and in one spot you'll have to scramble up about ten feet of rock. When a trail goes back and to the right on the ridgetop, continue straight.

The reward for your effort is a view to rival any other in the gorge. To the east you can see Beacon Rock and the high walls on either side of the river. To the west you can see Vista House (built in 1916 as a pioneer memorial and rest stop for travelers, now an interpretive center, museum, and gift shop) and the hills falling away toward Portland and the Willamette Valley. The Columbia River, right below you, seems close enough that if you got a running start you could jump into it. You might see some windsurfers out there; on one trip, I watched a floatplane practicing touch-and-go landings on this stretch of the river. You can also see two other hikes from this book: right next to Beacon Rock is the step-shaped Hamilton Mountain, and the big flat-topped mountain looming behind that is Table Mountain. There's even a nice bench to sit on out there. Around to the left of the summit there is a notch in some rocks that offers shelter from frequently high winds. All in all, it's hard to imagine a better place to have lunch.

If you're up for more hiking, you can turn this into a longer out-and-back or do a one-way hike with another car parked farther east. To do either, as you walk back down the ridge, veer left (east) instead of continuing straight, which is where you came from. After a few minutes you'll come to a junction; go left for Wahkeena Trail or continue straight 1 mile up Foxglove Trail to reach Devils Rest.

If you turn left, you'll soon pass a nice campsite and then come to Wahkeena Spring in 2.6 miles; 0.1 mile later you'll intersect Wahkeena Trail (420). Here, you can turn left (downhill) and follow Wahkeena Creek 1.6 miles to the picnic area at Wahkeena Falls, or you can go straight and, in 1.2 miles, intersect Larch Mountain Trail. Go down that one 1.8 miles, and you'll be at Multnomah Falls. There's a more detailed description of this trail section in the Wahkeena Falls to Multnomah Falls profile (hike 13, page 62).

## NEARBY ACTIVITIES

Vista House, and the road that leads to it, are both worth a visit. To get there, simply drive back toward Portland on the Historic Highway, rather than on I-84. Follow the pre-1920 road past a few other waterfalls and then up the hill to Crown Point, where you can step into Vista House and take in a postcard view and historic displays about the building of the road. Keep going west on that road, pass Vista House, and in a couple of miles you'll see a sign down a steep hill back to I-84.

# 02 BEACON ROCK– HAMILTON MOUNTAIN

## KEY AT-A-GLANCE INFORMATION

**LENGTH:** 1.8 miles round-trip to top of Beacon Rock; 8 miles to Hamilton Mountain

**CONFIGURATION:** Out-and-back, loop

**DIFFICULTY:** Beacon Rock easy–moderate; Hamilton Mountain strenuous

**SCENERY:** Overlooks of river, waterfall, spring wildflowers

**EXPOSURE:** Hamilton is mostly shady, with one rocky section near cliff tops; Beacon Rock is on the side of a cliff, but there are handrails.

**TRAFFIC:** Heavy on weekends, moderate otherwise

**TRAIL SURFACE:** Packed dirt with rocks, some pavement

**HIKING TIME:** 1 hour for Beacon Rock, 3.5 hours for Hamilton Mountain

**DRIVING DISTANCE:** 51 miles (1 hour 10 minutes) from Pioneer Square

**SEASON:** Year-round; call for trail conditions in winter

**BEST TIME:** April–May

**ACCESS:** No fees or permits needed

**WHEELCHAIR ACCESS:** On Hadley Trail, and a 1-mile loop at the Doetsch Day-Use area

**MAPS:** Green Trails #428 (Bridal Veil); state park map at Park Headquarters

**FACILITIES:** Water and restrooms at the trailhead

**INFO:** Beacon Rock State Park, (509) 427-8265

---

## GPS Trailhead Coordinates

UTM Zone (WGS84) 10T

Easting 576229

Northing 5053231

Latitude N 45.62844°

Longitude W 122.02206°

## IN BRIEF

One of the most recognized symbols of the Columbia River Gorge, Beacon Rock is also an amazing, if short, hiking experience—and it's not even all this state park has to offer. There's also a rigorous climb to the scenic Hamilton Mountain, with an amazing waterfall along the way.

## DESCRIPTION

Beacon Rock got its name—well, its white man's name—on Halloween 1805, when William Clark described it in his journal. For the Corps of Discovery and the people who then lived along the Columbia River, Beacon Rock meant two important things: the last of the rapids on the Columbia and the beginning of tidal influence on the river. Today, it means a unique hiking experience to its summit, and the state park around it means a chance to take in more nice views of the Columbia River.

To climb Beacon Rock, which ascends nearly 600 feet in less than a mile, start at a sign on the south side of WA 14, and get

---

## Directions ⟶

Take I-84 from Portland, driving 37 miles east of I-205 to Exit 44/Cascade Locks. As soon as you enter the town, take your first right to get on Bridge of the Gods, following a sign for Stevenson, Washington. Pay a $1 toll on the bridge, and at the far end turn left (west) on WA 14. Proceed 6.9 miles to Beacon Rock State Park. To hike up Beacon Rock, park on the left; to go toward Hamilton Mountain, turn right on the access road to the campground and drive 0.4 miles to the trailhead. The gate to the upper trailhead is closed in winter, but the trail is open; you'll just have to park on the south side of WA 14 and walk up the access road.

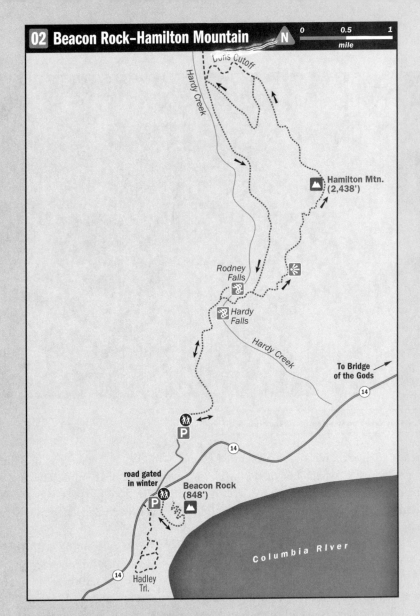

N

0        0.5        1

mile

Doris Cutoff

Hardy Creek

Hamilton Mtn.
(2,438')

Rodney
Falls

Hardy
Falls

Hardy Creek

To Bridge
of the Gods

14

14

road gated
in winter

Beacon Rock
(848')

14

Hadley
Trl.

Columbia River

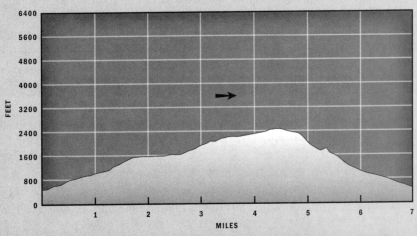

FEET

6400
5600
4800
4000
3200
2400
1600
800
0

1        2        3        4        5        6        7

MILES

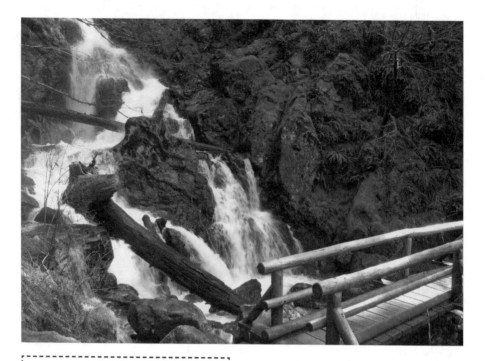

Hardy Creek on the Hamilton Mountain Trail

ready to give thanks to a man named Henry J. Biddle. It was he who bought the rock (which is what's left of the inside of an ancient volcano) in 1914 to save it from being blasted to pieces for jetty material. He said his purpose was simply to build the trail you're about to hike, and he never charged hikers a penny. Eventually, the land was donated by his family to the state.

The trail is something of an engineering wonder, beginning with the fact that the builders couldn't scout the route; they had to just build a section, then figure out where to take it next. The finished product is 4,500 feet long and 4 feet wide, and includes 52 switchbacks, 100 concrete slabs, and, originally, 22 wooden bridges. Some of the original work remains, such as wrought-iron handrails at some switchbacks and steel eyebolts in the rock wall.

To get to the top, just persevere and, if heights bother you, don't look down. It's virtually all rails and bridges and platforms until you're just below the summit, where you'll have a view east to Bonneville Dam, north to Hamilton Mountain, and straight down the other side to the boat docks of the state park. Keep an eye out for rock climbers, and don't throw anything from the top.

For a more challenging and more rewarding hike, drive (or walk, if the gate is closed) up the road across WA 14 to the campground and the Hamilton Mountain trailhead. From here, you'll climb gently through forest until you reach a bench to take a break; the power lines you're under here aren't all that scenic, but you do get a view ahead to the summit of Hamilton. At 0.5 miles, continue straight at a trail leading left to the campground and a rock formation called Little Beacon Rock; 0.4 miles later you'll come to a trail leading down and to the right 100 yards to two viewpoints overlooking Hardy Falls. A minute past that on the main trail, you'll see a sign that says "Hamilton Mountain"; oddly enough, it points downhill.

For a sight to remember, and a soak to cool you down (if you'd like), walk a couple hundred yards to the left and check out Rodney Falls (also known as the Pool of Winds), which almost explodes out of a bowl in the rock face. You can get right in its spray, if you don't mind essentially wading the last part of the trail.

If you don't feel like climbing anymore, turn back here—it gets tougher quickly. For Hamilton Mountain, follow the signed trail as it descends to, then crosses, Hardy Creek and then heads up the hill. After 0.2 miles of climbing, you'll come to a trail junction with two wonderful options: "Difficult" and "More Difficult." To the left is the return portion of a possible loop hike, but keep right (taking the more difficult way), and after 0.3 miles of sturdy climbing you'll reach a spectacular rock lookout. There's nothing wrong with turning back here, but do be careful as you walk around on these rocks—in some spots it's more than 200 feet straight down.

If you want the real views, keep climbing. In just a few minutes you'll see side trails on the right leading to the top of the ridge. (You can take one of the side trails to get a view of the river. Along the main trail, a little farther up, you reach the views mentioned of the rock face of Hamilton.) You'll pass two fantastic viewpoints of the mountain's rocky face while gaining 700 feet in just over a mile, bringing you to a mountaintop junction. The view south is somewhat blocked by brush, but you can see up to Table Mountain (hike 11, page 55) to the northeast, Mount Adams just east of that, and Mount St. Helens to the northwest. You should also be able to make out Dog and Wind mountains up the river, Eagle Creek and the Benson Plateau across it, and the town of Cascade Locks.

The scenery is better on the route you just climbed, but if you want to make it a loop, continue 0.9 miles north along the ridge, turn left onto an old road, and go 100 yards to Dons Cutoff Trail. Take this scenic but uneventful side trip, named for Don Cannard—cofounder of the Chinook Trails Association, trail builder, and visionary, down to Hardy Creek Trail, which at this point looks like a road. Turn left, follow the trail downhill past a picnic table, and after another mile you'll be back at the junction mentioned above, just east of Rodney Falls. Turn right and you'll reach the trailhead in 1.6 miles.

## NEARBY ACTIVITIES

The Columbia Gorge Interpretive Center, 10 miles east on WA 14 in Stevenson, features historical displays ranging from the geological (descriptions of the formation of the gorge) to the mechanical (examples of steam engines used on railroads a bit more recently).

# 03   CATHERINE CREEK

## KEY AT-A-GLANCE INFORMATION

**LENGTH:** Up to 4.1 miles

**CONFIGURATION:** Loop

**DIFFICULTY:** Easy–moderate

**SCENERY:** Wide-open vistas, a geological curiosity, and (in spring) flowers, flowers everywhere!

**EXPOSURE:** Out in the open most of the way, optional trip to a cliff top

**TRAFFIC:** Heavy on weekends in late spring and early summer, light otherwise

**TRAIL SURFACE:** Dirt and some rock, also a small paved section

**HIKING TIME:** 30 minutes–4 hours

**DRIVING DISTANCE:** 72 miles (1 hour 30 minutes) from Pioneer Square

**SEASON:** Year-round

**BEST TIME:** Late March–early June

**ACCESS:** No fees or permits

**WHEELCHAIR ACCESS:** A series of loops below the parking area offers access to flowers, birds, views of the Columbia River, and a waterfall on Catherine Creek.

**MAPS:** None

**FACILITIES:** Portable restroom at the trailhead, but no drinkable water around

**INFO:** Columbia River Gorge National Scenic Area, (541) 308-1700

## IN BRIEF

For about ten months of the year, there's really no reason to go to Catherine Creek, but in April and May, there's no better place to be, for Catherine Creek at that time is wildflower heaven, with close to 100 species in bloom.

## AUTHOR'S NOTE

In 2010, as this book went to press, the trails around Catherine Creek were subject to a large-scale planning process that may have resulted in significant changes. I am writing this chapter based on what was being planned at the time. Call ahead or check the National Scenic Area Web site to get the latest info.

## DESCRIPTION

In a typical hiking year, there are usually some hikes that I do before Catherine Creek, but my personal hiking season really starts when the grass widow blooms at Catherine Creek in late March. It gets serious when the camas blooms in early April; my personal Easter Sunday tradition is to pack a lunch, hike up the hill to a certain spot, spread out my food, take in the view, and listen to the meadowlarks. Then I go back to (usually) rainy old Portland.

There's really not much to this hike,

## GPS Trailhead Coordinates

UTM Zone (WGS84) 10T

Easting 627516

Northing 5063180

Latitude N 45.71043°

Longitude W 121.36172°

## *Directions*

Take I-84 from Portland, driving 57 miles east of I-205 to Exit 64, the third exit for Hood River, Oregon. Turn left at the end of the ramp, following signs for White Salmon, Washington. Pay a 75-cent toll to cross the Columbia River, then turn right on WA 14. Travel 5.9 miles and turn left onto Old Highway 8. The parking area is 1.5 miles ahead, on the left.

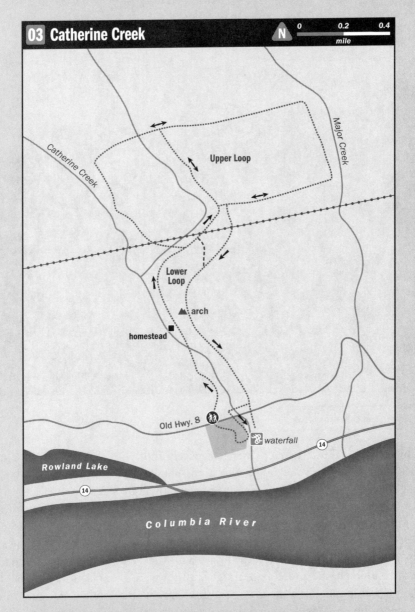

N

0       0.2       0.4

*mile*

Catherine Creek

Major Creek

Upper Loop

Lower Loop

▲ arch

■ homestead

Old Hwy. 8

waterfall

14

Rowland Lake

14

*C o l u m b i a   R i v e r*

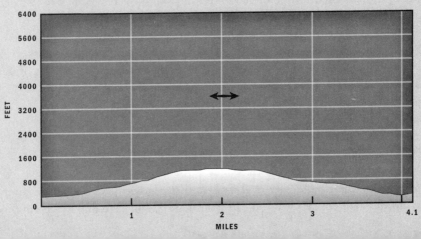

FEET

6400
5600
4800
4000
3200
2400
1600
800
0

1          2          3          4.1

MILES

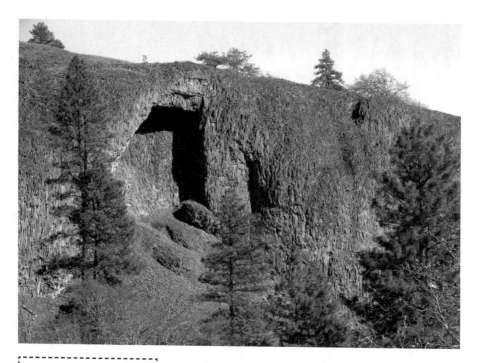

The arch at Catherine Creek

physically speaking. In fact, there's a paved and wheelchair-accessible section below the road that you could knock out in about 15 minutes. It's really all about the flowers and the wide-open vistas uncommon elsewhere in our hiking world.

From the road, walk through a gate and choose a path that tends to the right toward a small canyon just up the hill. If you're like me, you'll stop within a few feet and start admiring flowers. One enthusiast has counted as many as 82 species in bloom here on an April day, with such fantastic names as chocolate lily, common bastard toad flax, rough wallflower, Columbia Gorge lupine, least hop clover, poet's shooting star, rigid fiddleneck, great hound's tongue, slender popcorn flower, small-flowered blue-eyed Mary, and chickweed monkey flower. (I didn't make up any of those names!)

Follow a gravel road into the canyon and up the creek. Watch out for poison oak; it's everywhere—there's an "old-growth" stand of it on the right as you near the creek. After 0.25 miles, cross the creek on a cool, bouncy plank bridge and, 100 yards later, you'll arrive at an old homestead. Above you now is a geological curiosity, a natural arch we'll visit later.

Past the homestead, staying to the right, go up a slight rise and into a meadow. In May, under some of the bushes, you'll find dense thickets of irises—technically not wildflowers, but lovely nonetheless. When you reach the power lines, a total of 0.8 miles from the car, you'll have your first decision to make. You can go left here and take a trail that parallels Catherine Creek before climbing into the high country, or you can continue straight here and make another

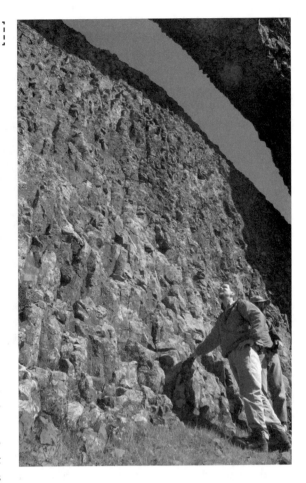

Looking up through the arch

decision in a minute, which is what I recommend.

At the second junction, moments later, you have two options: a lower loop and an upper loop. For the lower loop, follow a trail to the right and then along the top of a little ridge, and your hike will be less than a mile. I'll describe that section later, because you really should at least do part of the upper loop.

For that, follow a trail east and across the meadows to eventually reach an overlook of Major Creek. From a junction there, go down to the old highway and back toward the car, or take a trail that goes up to the tree line, where it turns to the west, crosses another line of trees, and enters yet another huge meadow. Here, if you look up and to the right, you'll see a clump of trees that shelters a tiny spring. Just below that is a berm that gathers the spring water into a surprising pond. And on that berm a guy could have himself quite a fine Easter picnic, with the Columbia River laid out at his feet, flowers all around, and Mount Hood across the way.

From that point, the trail continues west, reaches an overlook of Catherine Creek, and then drops back to the place where you made your first decision on this hike, down below the power lines.

OK, now for the "lower loop." From the second decision point you reached, just follow a trail that eventually hugs the top of the ridge above Catherine Creek. Following this, you'll get a view into the canyon where the homestead is, and then you'll be at the top of the arch. You can get out on top of it (it's wider than it looks, but be careful), and you can also walk down through it to get back to the homestead. But why should you? There's more to see up here.

Keep descending the hill, following the trail near the cliff's edge. You'll cross a little draw filled with purple camas (in April), with creek access on your right, and a few minutes later you'll be at the road—and probably as close to power lines

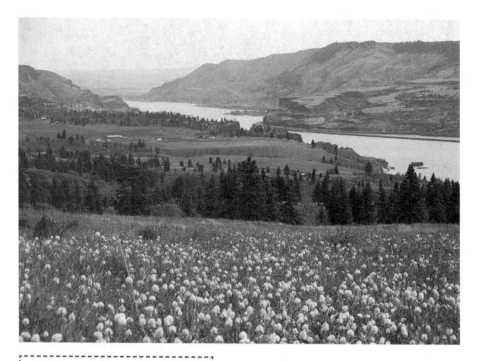

Camas on the Catherine Creek upper loop

as you'll ever be in your life. Turn right; a little rock scramble will put you on the road's shoulder. Cross the creek again and see the parking lot, just up the hill.

And yet there's more! Catherine Creek has a neighbor hike to the west called Coyote Wall (hike 5, page 30), with a neat area called the Labyrinth in between, and the two hikes share a kind of secret door to one another. I shall now give the secret away. From the Catherine Creek trailhead, go left on another old road, which climbs gently through marshy areas and over small hills. After 0.25 miles, it arrives at an uphill turn back to the right, near the top of a cliff. For many years, a big dead tree has lain here, and if you go behind that tree, you'll see a small trail heading down to the west, along the face of the cliff. Didn't see *that,* did you?

This little trail hugs a steep, rocky hillside for a short time, then drops down into a grassy bowl, where it intersects yet another old road heading steeply uphill. Follow this road as it climbs then swings to the left and becomes a trail. You'll pass a series of rock pits that Native Americans used as vision quest sites— don't disturb them!—as the trail keeps winding west, up through the oaks. I call it a "faith trail," because it seems to be going nowhere. Trust me, it isn't.

It eventually leads through several meadows some 700 feet above Rowland Lake, then past a freaky tree known as the Coyote Tree (complete with bones hanging in it), and finally down into a mess of trails, all of which lead into an area called the Labyrinth. For a description of that area, see the Coyote Wall–The Labyrinth trip (hike 5, page 30). Combining these two hikes as an out-and-back or with an easy car shuttle is one of my absolute favorites and an April tradition.

# CHINIDERE MOUNTAIN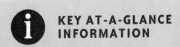

## IN BRIEF

Unless you're spending the night, you might spend more time in the car than on the trail for this one. But the view from the top of Chinidere is more than worth it, and Wahtum Lake is a fine destination as well. Still, consider making this part of a longer trip to Lost Lake or the Hood River Valley.

## DESCRIPTION

If you're using a view-for-effort scale to measure your hikes, Chinidere Mountain ranks 11 out of 10—once you get there. It's a two-hour drive from Portland, but the roads are all paved, and you'll be rewarded with a fairly easy hike, a beautiful mountain lake with camping and fishing, and a view that stretches hundreds of miles.

If you're wondering, *Chinidere* is pronounced "SHIN-uh-deer," and it's named for the last reigning chief of the local Wasco tribe. And *Wahtum* is a local Native American word meaning "pond" or "body of water." So you're looking through the trees here at "Lake Lake."

From the trailhead, walk through the campground (not down the road near the

### KEY AT-A-GLANCE INFORMATION

**LENGTH:** 4 miles
**CONFIGURATION:** Loop
**DIFFICULTY:** Easy, then moderate right at the end
**SCENERY:** Old-growth forest, a deep mountain lake, and a panoramic view
**EXPOSURE:** Mostly shady, nothing exposed except on top
**TRAFFIC:** Light
**TRAIL SURFACE:** Packed dirt, roots, rocks
**HIKING TIME:** 2.5 hours
**DRIVING DISTANCE:** 87 miles (2 hours) from Pioneer Square
**SEASON:** July–mid-October
**BEST TIME:** August–September
**BACKPACKING OPTIONS:** Two good areas on the lake
**ACCESS:** Northwest Forest Pass required
**WHEELCHAIR ACCESS:** None
**MAPS:** Green Trails #429 (Bonneville Dam)
**FACILITIES:** Outhouse at trailhead
**INFO:** Hood River Ranger District, (541) 352-6002
**SPECIAL COMMENTS:** Wahtum Lake is at the very top of Eagle Creek Trail, so consider doing a fantastic, one-way, downhill 14-miler with a car shuttle.

## *Directions* ⟶

From I-84, take Exit 62, then turn right on Country Club Road. After 3 miles, turn left at a stop sign, onto Barrett Drive. After 1.3 miles, turn right on Tucker Road, which turns into Dee Highway. Go 8.5 miles to Dee and turn right on Lost Lake Road. After 4.8 miles, turn right on FS 13. Drive 4.4 miles farther, then make a right on FS 1310. Stay on the pavement, driving 6 miles to find parking (on the right). If the pavement ends, you've passed the parking area.

### GPS Trailhead Coordinates

UTM Zone (WGS84) 10T
Easting 594190
Northing 5047826
Latitude N 45.57760°
Longitude W 121.79273°

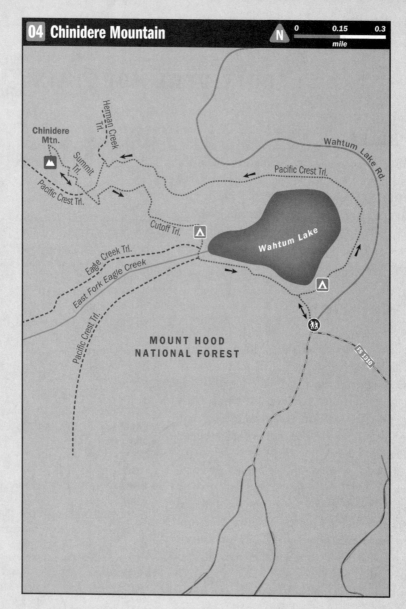

N

0          0.15          0.3

*mile*

Chinidere
Mtn.

Herman Creek Trl.

Summit
Trl.

Pacific Crest Trl.

Pacific Crest Trl.

Wahtum Lake Rd.

Cutoff Trl.

Eagle Creek Trl.

East Fork Eagle Creek

Pacific Crest Trl.

Wahtum Lake

MOUNT HOOD
NATIONAL FOREST

FS 1310

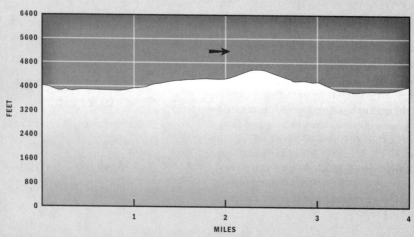

FEET

6400
5600
4800
4000
3200
2400
1600
800
0

1          2          3          4

MILES

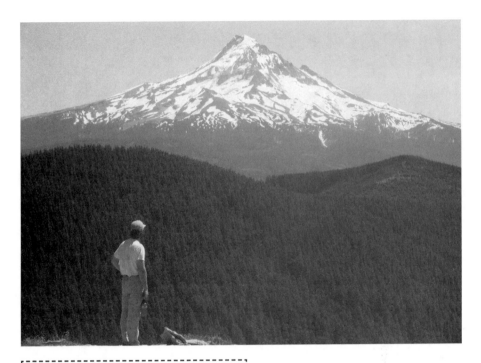

Looking at Mount Hood from Chinidere Mountain

outhouse) and follow a trail called the Wahtum Express, which includes 250 wooden stairs. (You can skip this by following a parallel horse trail to the right, if you wish.) At the bottom of the Express, turn left and walk 100 feet down to a big tree with two Pacific Crest Trail (PCT) signs on it. You'll be right by the lake, with a picnic area in front of you—and also in the middle of several nice lakeshore campsites. Turn right here, heading north on the PCT.

The trail meanders along at first, near the lake, weaving through a lovely forest of hemlocks interspersed with bunchberry, thimbleberry, vanilla leaf, columbine, huckleberry, and salmonberry. Look along the near shore for a small island with about four trees on it. There's also, around half a mile up, some impressive trail construction to let water pass. Tiny springs and other mossy, flower-covered babbling brooks will keep you entertained and charmed.

After about 1 flat mile, you'll come into more-open forest, with beargrass that blooms in July, and you'll start climbing gradually on some classic Oregon PCT: wide trails over soft ground covered in pine needles and traversing thick forest. At a total of 1.75 miles, you'll cross a creek that dries up by midsummer, and at 1.9 miles (now having climbed only 400 feet) you'll intersect Herman Creek Trail (hike 8, page 42), which leads all the way down to the outskirts of Cascade Locks.

A tenth of a mile later, you'll see Chinidere Cutoff Trail (406M) plunging down to the left; we'll take that one back. For now, go another 100 feet and

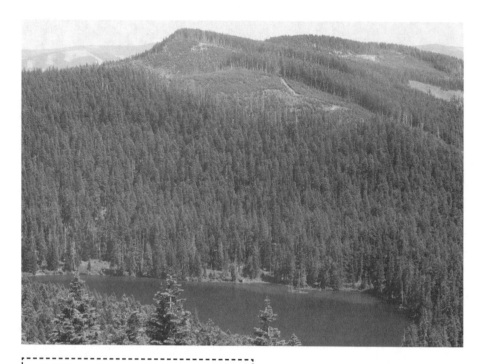

A view of Wahtum Lake from Chinidere Mountain

leave the PCT, taking Chinidere Mountain Trail. Starting here, you'll put in the climbing you've been warming up for, picking up 400 feet in a third of a mile to eventually reach the rocky summit. You might want to watch for a side trail from one of the first switchbacks, heading out into the open; this path leads to a rocky scramble up the west side of the mountain, where you'll find some interesting rock benches made by industrious hikers.

After you've caught your breath, stop to enjoy the view. Mount Hood rises to the south. To the right of that is Mount Jefferson, and just to the left of "Jeff" is Olallie Butte.

To the east, beyond "Lake Lake," you can see the upper parts of Hood River Valley, and to the left of that is Dalles Mountain and the desert of Central Oregon. The big peak with all the radio towers is Mount Defiance, the highest spot in the Gorge, and Mount Adams is to the left of that. The bald ridge directly between you and Adams is Tomlike Mountain (named for Chief Chinidere's son), and to the left of that is the Herman Creek drainage. Off in the distance are Mounts Rainier and St. Helens, and right in line with the latter is the broad, flat Benson Plateau. Immediately below you, to the west, is the Eagle Creek Canyon (the East Fork drains Wahtum Lake straight away from your feet), and in the distance beyond that is Tanner Butte. On a really clear day on Chinidere, I once saw Saddle Mountain, which is about 10 miles this side of the coast!

While we're up here, how about a little introduction to the PCT, a 2,600-mile trail from Mexico to Canada? The northbound PCT, which stretches some

460 miles across Oregon, comes up the right (west) side of Jefferson, then past the right side of Hood, mostly in the trees. In its approach to Wahtum Lake, the PCT rounds an open ridge between you and Hood called Indian Mountain, and from Chinidere it heads north across the Benson Plateau and down, heinously, into Cascade Locks. But most thru-hikers take Eagle Creek Trail, since it's well-graded and has about a dozen waterfalls; then they walk the few miles along the road into Cascade Locks. After crossing Bridge of the Gods, the trail passes the west side of Table Mountain (which looks like a big gash from Chinidere), then heads around the north side of it before making a swing east toward Adams, the Goat Rocks, and Rainier. So, from Mount Jefferson to Mount Rainier, you're effectively looking at about 280 miles of PCT—slightly more than 10 percent of it!

And by the way, the rusty cables atop Chinidere are from an old Forest Service fire lookout, and the pits are tent sites, not Indian vision quest sites. Sorry it's nothing more romantic than that.

Head back down to the PCT, turn left, and take Chinidere Cutoff Trail, which will seem more like Chinidere Dropoff Trail for its steep descent to the lake. You'll cross a creek or two along the way, depending on the season, and you'll even see a pipe along the trail that used to carry water down to some campsites on the north shore of the lake. When you reach these campsites, stay on the main trail to where it crosses the East Fork of Eagle Creek on an impressive (and fun) logjam.

Cross the creek, and in 200 yards you'll hit the top of Eagle Creek National Recreation Trail, which was built before 1920 and connects Wahtum Lake with the Columbia River Highway, 14 miles below. (A 12-mile roundtrip hike is described on page 38.) Turn left onto this trail and follow it a couple hundred yards back to the PCT, which leads 0.25 miles past campsites, swimming holes, and even the occasional beach, back to the bottom of the Wahtum Express—whose 250 steps will seem much less appealing to you now, no doubt.

# 05 COYOTE WALL-THE LABYRINTH

## KEY AT-A-GLANCE INFORMATION

**LENGTH: 4.6 miles just to the top of the wall, 5.2 miles to include the Labyrinth**

**CONFIGURATION: Out-and-back with optional side loop**

**DIFFICULTY: Moderate**

**SCENERY: Cliff-top vistas, wide-open country, spring wildflowers**

**EXPOSURE: Along a cliff at times, and out in the open almost the whole way**

**TRAFFIC: Heavy on spring weekends, light otherwise**

**TRAIL SURFACE: Dirt; can be slick when wet**

**HIKING TIME: 3 hours**

**DRIVING DISTANCE: 69 miles (1 hour 15 minutes) from Pioneer Square**

**SEASON: Year-round**

**BEST TIME: March–May**

**ACCESS: No fee**

**WHEELCHAIR ACCESS: First half mile on an old paved road**

**MAPS: USGS White Salmon**

**FACILITIES: None at the trailhead**

**INFO: Columbia River Gorge National Scenic Area, (541) 308-1700**

## IN BRIEF

Let's say it's springtime, at least according to the calendar, but Portland is socked-in and wet. Go east, young hiker!—to the high and dry lands of the Columbia River Gorge, where flowers bloom, birds croon, and Coyote Wall looms.

*Note:* In 2010, as this book went to press, the trails around Coyote Wall and the Labyrinth were subject to a large-scale planning process that may have resulted in significant changes. Call ahead or check online to get the latest information.

## DESCRIPTION

Standing at the trailhead, looking up at Coyote Wall, one might feel a bit intimidated. Fear not, for the way is gradual and the work much rewarding. Just walk around the gate and follow the old road along Locke Lake, and eventually around the base of the wall itself. Turn left at the first cairn leading uphill, and immediately you're faced with numerous trailheads. Mountain bikers zip through here in every direction, but our path is always the one to the left and uphill.

Soon, the trail you're on (actually an old jeep road) is the only one around; you'll

---

## GPS Trailhead Coordinates

UTM Zone (WGS84) 10T

Easting 624310

Northing 5059990

Latitude   N 45.68231°

Longitude  W 121.40371°

## *Directions* ⟶

**Take I-84 from Portland, driving 57 miles east of I-205 to Exit 64, the third exit for Hood River, Oregon. Turn left at the end of the ramp, following signs for White Salmon, Washington. Pay a 75-cent toll to cross the Columbia River, then turn right on WA 14. Go 4.6 miles, turn left onto Courtney Road, and look for parking 100 yards ahead on the left.**

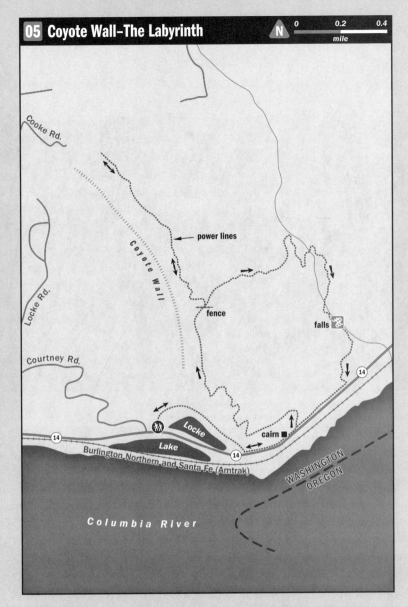

N

0    0.2    0.4
mile

Cooke Rd.

Locke Rd.

Courtney Rd.

Coyote Wall

power lines

fence

falls

14

14

14

cairn

Locke
Lake

Burlington Northern and Santa Fe (Amtrak)

WASHINGTON
OREGON

Columbia River

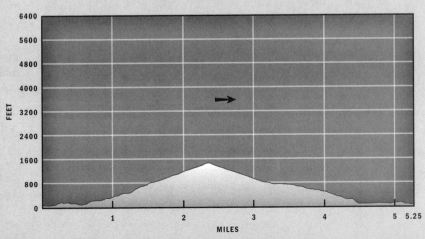

6400
5600
4800
4000
3200
2400
1600
800
0

FEET

1    2    3    4    5  5.25

MILES

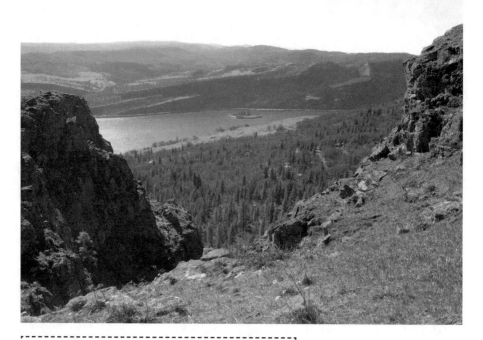

The Columbia River, as seen through a notch in Coyote Wall

follow it up the edge of the wall—though rarely too close to the edge to be of concern. Just less than a mile up, you reach a fence, where you have to make a choice. You can keep going up the wall or cut over to the Labyrinth—or, of course, go up the wall and then come back here and add the loop. This final loop is what the elevation profile for this hike shows.

If you're going up, stay to the left and follow a switchbacking trail that's more scenic (and less destructive) than the super-steep jeep road. After 1.2 miles of steep and steady climbing, generally through a sea of flowers with views behind you to the Columbia and Mount Hood, you'll reach a junction with several old roads at the head of the wall, close to an area with plenty of big logs to rest on. In the olden days (well, in earlier editions of this book), I encouraged hikers to explore various roads and trails in this area before connecting to the Catherine Creek trip (hike 3, page 20). But concerns about erosion and private-land rights caused the Forest Service to reevaluate the whole thing, and so, to avoid conflict, and to avoid the hassle of describing an unsigned network of social trails and private land, I'll just say, "Enjoy the view and then head back down the trail you came up." However, if they have added official trails by the time you get there, explore on your own; it's a great area.

Back at the fence, follow a trail leading east into the Labyrinth. I will, again, not try to describe an unsigned (in 2009, anyway) network of trails, and instead I'll just say, "Go wandering around in the Labyrinth; it's really cool." True to its

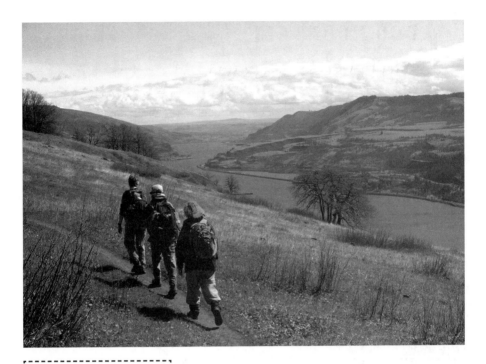

Headed toward the Labyrinth

name, this area can get confusing, with trails weaving between basalt pillars and through pocket meadows. The bottom line, though, is that if you keep heading downhill and to the right, you will emerge on the abandoned highway very near where you first left it to head up Coyote Wall.

The Labyrinth is filled with hidden wonders: waterfalls, a small cave, small buttes to climb, and hidden meadows filled with flowers. So take your time, have faith, and enjoy yourself. And if, since this book was published, the Forest Service has built and signed trails in the area, you'll have an easier time finding your way around. But I also think you (we) will perhaps have lost some opportunity for adventure.

## NEARBY ACTIVITIES

Bingen is worth a stop on the way home, especially for its slightly bizarre combination coffee–antiques shop, called Antiques and Oddities.

# 06  DOG MOUNTAIN

*Don't really want to do it again*

## KEY AT-A-GLANCE INFORMATION

**LENGTH:** 6.9 miles
**CONFIGURATION:** Loop
**DIFFICULTY:** Strenuous — *big time*
**SCENERY:** Second-growth forest, wildflowers, and a panoramic view of the Columbia River Gorge
**EXPOSURE:** Alternates between shady and open
**TRAFFIC:** Very heavy on weekends, especially in early summer; moderate otherwise
**TRAIL SURFACE:** Packed dirt with rocks, some gravel
**HIKING TIME:** 4 hours
**DRIVING DISTANCE:** 56 miles (1 hour 30 minutes) from Pioneer Square
**SEASON:** Year-round, but occasional snowfall on top
**BEST TIME:** Mid-May–early June
**ACCESS:** Northwest Forest Pass required
**WHEELCHAIR ACCESS:** None
**MAPS:** Trails of the Columbia Gorge; Green Trails #430 (Hood River)
**FACILITIES:** Toilets at the trailhead, but no water
**INFO:** Columbia River Gorge National Scenic Area, (541) 308-1700
**SPECIAL COMMENTS:** Start early in the day on this one, if only to make sure you get a parking spot.

## IN BRIEF

This is probably the most popular of the real hiking trails in the Columbia River Gorge—"real" meaning it requires some real effort. But with an easy-access trailhead, great views of the river, and sunshine and wildflowers at a time when it's still raining in Portland, it's no wonder everybody on Earth comes here.

## DESCRIPTION

It seems that every hiker around Portland has been up Dog Mountain, or heard about it. Climbers use it as an early-season conditioner. Wildflower enthusiasts flock to it in early summer. In spring, when it's still raining in Portland, it is often sunny here. But most people take the main Dog Mountain Trail, which is therefore crowded, and which was also designed, it seems, to punish the legs and lungs of those who would hike it. This thing is steep! You can come down this way, if you want, but it's no bargain then, either.

From the parking lot, you have a choice to make, and it boils down to this: When hiking a loop of a steep trail and a *really* steep trail, which one would you rather go up, and which down? Do you prefer the more gradual up, or the more gradual down?

I prefer the gradual up (take my time) and the steep down (get it over with), so I'll

## GPS Trailhead Coordinates

UTM Zone (WGS84) 10T
Easting 600519
Northing 5061450
Latitude   N 45.69931°
Longitude  W 121.70882°

## *Directions* ⟶

**Take I-84 from Portland, driving 37 miles east of I-205 to Exit 44/Cascade Locks. As soon as you enter the town, take your first right to get on Bridge of the Gods, following a sign for Stevenson, Washington. Pay a $1 toll on the bridge, and at the far end turn right, onto WA 14. Proceed 12 miles to the trailhead, on the left.**

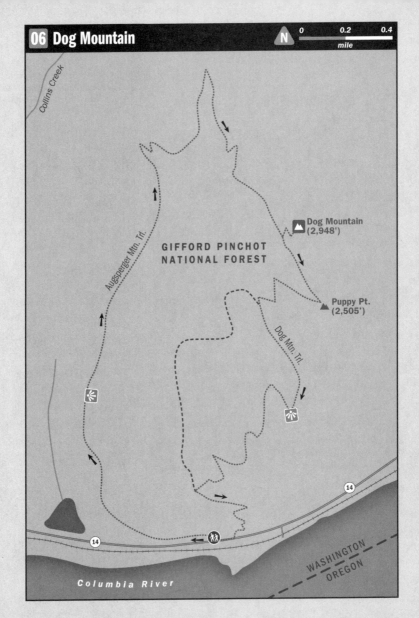

N

0          0.2          0.4
*mile*

Collins Creek

Augsperger Mtn. Trl.

**GIFFORD PINCHOT NATIONAL FOREST**

Dog Mountain
(2,948')

Puppy Pt.
(2,505')

Dog Mtn. Trl.

14

14

WASHINGTON
OREGON

*Columbia River*

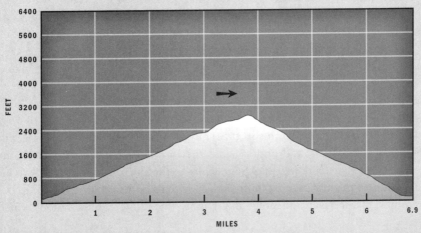

FEET

6400
5600
4800
4000
3200
2400
1600
800
0

1          2          3          4          5          6     6.9

MILES

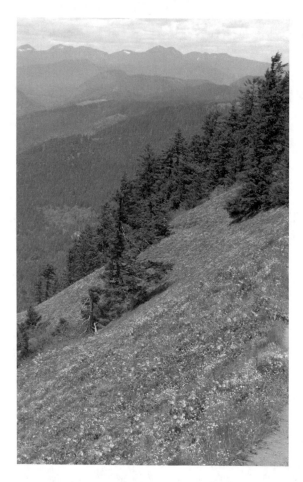

describe that here. To do the opposite, walk up to the bathroom and follow the main (crowded) trail, turning right at all junctions until you're out in the open at "Puppy Point," just below the summit. Then aim for the top. To come down the other way, make two rights below the summit and stick with Augsperger Trail back to the trailhead.

For the other way, from the trailhead, take the trail on the left, Augsperger Mountain Trail. It's 0.6 miles longer, but whoever designed it had a much better grasp of the concept of "grade." That's not to say it's easy—it's 3.7 uphill miles, gaining 2,700 feet. But it's steady, whereas parts of the other trail are insane, and on this trail you'll spend more time in the meadows up top. So take this one as it contours left, with ever-improving views of the river and Wind Mountain. When you turn right and away from the river, you will have gone 0.9 miles and gained 600 feet. Not so bad, right? In the next 1.3 miles you'll gain 1,000 feet. That's when the switchbacks start—and remember, this is the *easier* way. The next half mile gains some 500 feet. Then you'll turn right at a junction toward Dog Mountain.

I'd like to take this moment to explain why Dog Mountain is called Dog Mountain. It's neither because of all the dogs on the trail, nor because the hike is a real "bitch." It's because some pioneers in the area were forced to eat dog meat to avoid starvation. The town of Hood River, Oregon, was in fact first called Dog River, but the name was changed because nobody liked it. Imagine that.

Try to forget you know this so that you can enjoy a few minutes of flat trail before you climb again and pop out into the sun. Now it's time to claim your reward for all that climbing. In May and June, the open slopes of Dog Mountain are awash in flowers, especially big yellow balsamroot; but year-round, the views here of the river and other mountains—including Mount Hood, which

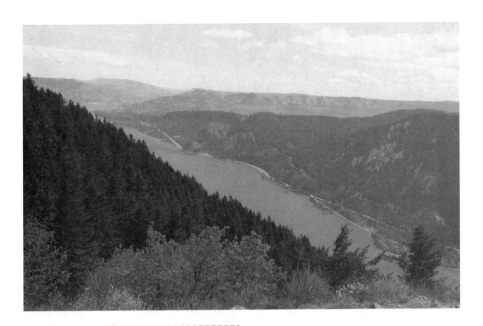

Looking 3,000 feet down at the Columbia River

peeks its head over the far side—are sublime. Stroll through this area and know that virtually all your climbing is done. You'll intersect Dog Mountain Trail after 0.9 miles; turn left and, just 0.1 mile up, you'll be at the top of a sloped meadow with everybody else and their dogs.

The view here stretches from the high desert of central Oregon to Beacon Rock in the west—look how small it is! Way to the right is Mount St. Helens. Directly opposite is the 4,960-foot Mount Defiance, the one with radio towers on top—look how big it is! The highest point in the gorge, it seems to taunt, "Yeah right, you've climbed barely half of me."

To descend Dog Mountain, either follow the crowds down through the meadows to your left, or take an alternate loop. From the summit, head left on a trail that soon ducks into the trees, some of which are surprisingly large. Keep an eye out for Mount Adams to the north. This trail rejoins the other branch of Dog Mountain Trail at a lookout that's actually called Puppy Point (2,505 feet). Then the bottom drops out, and you lose 600 feet in the next half mile before a junction. You'll save 0.2 miles by going right, but it's worth it to head left for one last view of the river 0.6 miles down. Stay left at a junction 1 mile ahead, and after a final 0.5 miles you can finally rest your throbbing feet.

## NEARBY ACTIVITIES

When you get back across to Cascade Locks, take a ride on the sternwheeler *Columbia Gorge,* which makes several scenic trips per day from mid-June through September. For more information, see **www.portlandspirit.com.**

# 07 EAGLE CREEK

## KEY AT-A-GLANCE INFORMATION

**LENGTH:** 4 miles round-trip to Punchbowl Falls; 12.5 miles round-trip to Tunnel Falls

**CONFIGURATION:** Out-and-back

**DIFFICULTY:** Easy–moderate, depending on how far you go

**SCENERY:** Waterfalls, old-growth forest, spawning salmon in the fall

**EXPOSURE:** Several sections of trail along the tops of ledges and cliffs, only sometimes with cables to hold onto; not the trail to hike if you're afraid of heights

**TRAFFIC:** Heavy all summer, moderate in spring and fall

**TRAIL SURFACE:** Packed dirt and rocks

**HIKING TIME:** 2 hours to Punchbowl Falls, 5.5 hours to Tunnel Falls

**DRIVING DISTANCE:** 41 miles (45 minutes) from Pioneer Square

**SEASON:** Year-round, but muddy in winter and spring and could get snow

**BEST TIME:** Spring for big water flows, fall for colors and fish

**BACKPACKING OPTIONS:** Several sites starting a few miles up, access to more

**ACCESS:** Northwest Forest Pass required

**WHEELCHAIR ACCESS:** A road along and bridge over Eagle Creek near trailhead

**MAPS:** Trails of the Columbia Gorge

**FACILITIES:** Toilets at trailhead; no water

**INFO:** Columbia River Gorge National Scenic Area, (541) 308-1700

- - - - - - - - - - - - - - - - - - - - - - -

## GPS Trailhead Coordinates

UTM Zone (WGS84) 10T

Easting 584214

Northing 5054233

Latitude N 45.63653°

Longitude W 121.91947°

## IN BRIEF

One of the classic and most popular hikes in Oregon, seemingly everybody has done part of Eagle Creek. That's because this hike's easy to get to, easy to hike, and beautiful in several ways. With that in mind, start early, or go on a weekday, so you won't have to share the trail with everyone in Oregon.

## DESCRIPTION

The magic of this hike, at certain times of the year, begins before you even hit the trail itself. Eagle Creek has a small run of fall chinook salmon—fish that spend their adult lives in the ocean, come more than 70 miles up the Columbia, swim the fish ladder at Bonneville Dam, and then arrive here to spawn. A small dam blocks their further progress up Eagle Creek, but in October and November they spawn in little round pools cleared by volunteers to simulate conditions of a wild mountain stream.

The trail was built before 1920 to coincide with the opening of the Columbia River Highway. Although that historic roadway has mostly been gobbled up by I-84, the section from Bonneville Dam to Cascade Locks (which passes right by Eagle Creek) has been converted into a hiking and biking trail, as have a few other sections.

Eagle Creek Trail is a heroic feat resulting from a lot of hard work. The trail builders chipped the path into cliff faces, built High

- - - - - - - - - - - - - - - - - - - - - - - - - - - - - -

## *Directions* ———————————➤

**Take I-84 from Portland, driving 34 miles east of I-205 to Exit 41/Eagle Creek. Go 0.2 miles, turn right, and drive 0.6 miles to the end of the road. If it's crowded, you might have to park closer to the highway and hike that much farther.**

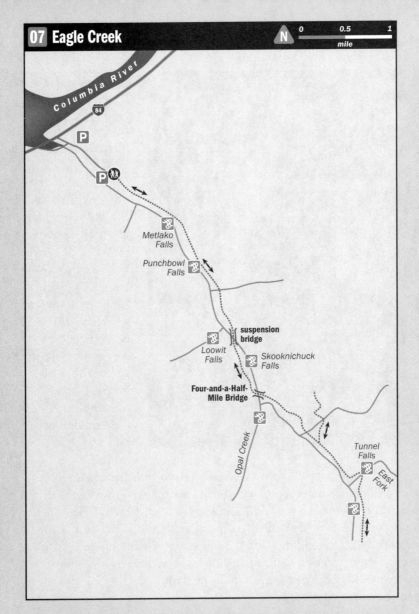

Columbia River

84

P

P

Metlako
Falls

Punchbowl
Falls

suspension
bridge

Loowit
Falls

Skooknichuck
Falls

Four-and-a-Half-
Mile Bridge

Opal Creek

Tunnel
Falls

East
Fork

N

0        0.5        1
mile

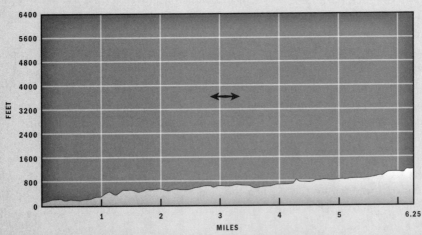

FEET

6400
5600
4800
4000
3200
2400
1600
800
0

1        2        3        4        5        6.25

MILES

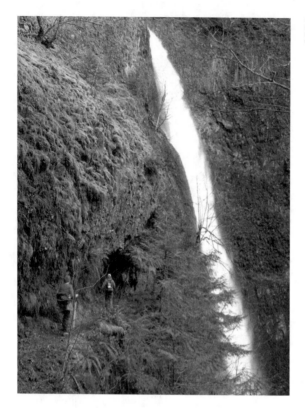

Bridge over the gorge, and blasted a tunnel behind a falls 6 miles up. It's work like this that inspired me to write this book.

At just under 1 mile, you'll come to the first of several places where you walk a ledge—in this case, but not all, with a cable to hang on to. If it's a summer weekend, things can get interesting here while you are competing for cable space with dozens of other hikers. But the importance of being careful cannot be overstated: people have fallen to their deaths from this trail.

At 1.5 miles, you'll have a view of Metlako Falls (named for a Native American goddess of salmon), the first of many such sights. Just past the viewpoint is a bench, if you need a rest. At 1.8 miles is another bench; from here a side trail leads down to Punchbowl Falls, a must-see sight and the end of the line for a lot of people. Descend this trail 0.2 miles to reach an unnamed falls; just above that is a large clearing that's often filled with swimmers and sunbathers. At the upstream end of the clearing is a lovely (and often photographed) view of Punchbowl Falls (see opposite page).

If you turn back here, you will have hiked 4 miles, but it's not much more work to go at least as far as High Bridge, another 1.2 miles up. If you continue, you'll get a bird's-eye view of Punchbowl Falls just 0.3 miles ahead; then the gorge narrows considerably. You'll see Loowit Falls on the right just before High Bridge; if you turn around at the bridge, you'll have a 7-mile day. But before you turn back, put in another 0.3 miles to reach a great picnic spot on the left and, 100 yards farther, enjoy this rare chance for creek access, at the top of Skooknichuck Falls. Just past that are some very impressive Douglas firs right on the trail.

Continuing up the trail, you'll soon cross what is officially known as Four-and-a-Half-Mile Bridge. Now, even the map acknowledges that this is exactly 4 miles from the trailhead, so what's with the name? Well, the fish hatchery back at the trailhead wasn't there when the trail was built (there was no need for it, because Bonneville Dam didn't exist yet), so the trailhead used to be half a mile

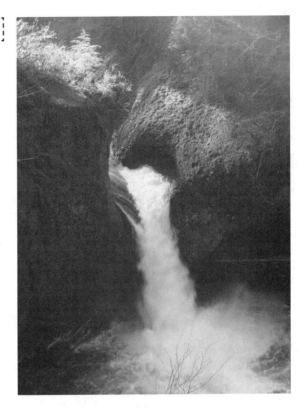

Punchbowl Falls

farther north, at the edge of the Columbia River Highway.

Just past the bridge, look on the right for a double waterfall; that's Opal Creek, but it shouldn't be confused with the world-famous Opal Creek described elsewhere in this book (hike 29, page 134). About half a mile above that waterfall, a sign explains that the area you're now entering was burned in a 1902 fire; there are still some charred stumps around. So all the trees you'll see in this area are less than 100 years old.

Hiking another 1.5 miles brings your total to 6 miles hiked, and you'll come into a deep gorge, where Tunnel Falls plunges 130 feet and the trail continues behind it through a 35-foot tunnel. Tunnel Falls is actually on East Fork Eagle Creek, which flows from Wahtum Lake. You could get to Wahtum Lake by hiking another 8 miles (and several thousand feet) up this trail or by following the directions in our Chinidere Mountain profile on pages 25 to 29.

To return to Eagle Creek and see one final, dramatic falls, hike on about 0.2 miles. This falls doesn't have an official name, but it does have an interesting crisscross feature in its upper section, leading many people to call it Crisscross Falls or Crossover Falls.

If you're backpacking, you'll find good camping at 7.5 Mile Camp (7 miles up) and at Wahtum Lake. Otherwise, if you head back at this point, you'll wind up having put in 12 miles—which should be enough for a day. Besides, you'll get to see everything again on your way back.

## NEARBY ACTIVITIES

Stop at the fish hatchery at Bonneville Dam on the way home. They have a fish ladder where, at certain times of year, you can see salmon and steelhead swimming up past the dam to spawn, and year-round ponds where you can view big trout and sturgeon. It's 1 mile west on I-84, and admission is free.

# 08 HERMAN CREEK

## KEY AT-A-GLANCE INFORMATION

**LENGTH:** Anything from 6–20 miles
**CONFIGURATION:** Out-and-back or loops
**DIFFICULTY:** Easy–strenuous
**SCENERY:** Old-growth forest, a clear stream, waterfalls, views of mountains and the gorge
**EXPOSURE:** Almost all shaded, with one optional bit of very exposed rock
**TRAFFIC:** Moderate on weekends, light otherwise
**TRAIL SURFACE:** Dirt, rocks
**HIKING TIME:** 2 hours–2 days
**DRIVING DISTANCE:** 46 miles (50 minutes) from Pioneer Square
**SEASON:** Year-round for the lower hikes, but snow possible; Nick Eaton Ridge likely snow-free April–November
**BEST TIME:** April–May, or October
**BACKPACKING OPTIONS:** Everywhere!
**ACCESS:** Northwest Forest Pass required at summer trailhead only
**WHEELCHAIR ACCESS:** None
**MAPS:** USFS Trails of the Columbia Gorge
**FACILITIES:** Restroom and water at summer trailhead
**INFO:** Columbia River Gorge National Scenic Area, (541) 308-1700
**SPECIAL COMMENTS:** May–September, when Herman Creek Campground is open, park at the official trailhead. Otherwise, park along Forest Lane and walk 0.5 miles up the access road, staying to the right for the trailhead.

## IN BRIEF

More of a hub than a hike, Herman Creek offers something for everyone, be it a midwinter riverside stroll, a spring get-in-shape workout, or a long summer backpack hike. The prize of the area, though, is Indian Point. That's the hike shown on the elevation profile; none of the others described here are nearly as steep as this one.

## DESCRIPTION

Each spring, we Portland hikers get our annual itch. But with snows still blanketing the high hills, the question is where to go. We're tired of the crowds at Eagle Creek. Dog Mountain isn't in flower yet. The eastern gorge isn't challenging enough to get us in shape. The coast is still miserable.

Every spring, at some point, most of us trail hounds will wind up at the Herman Creek trailhead—probably more than once. There are just so many options here, and so few people compared with other gorge locations, that whatever you're looking for, you can find it on these forested slopes. Stroll a few easy miles to a creek and waterfall, test out your backpacking gear at one of countless campsites, or—this is my favorite—see how your conditioning survived the winter by pushing yourself up

## GPS Trailhead Coordinates

UTM Zone (WGS84) 10T

Easting 590173

Northing 5059403

Latitude N 45.68231°

Longitude W 121.84207°

## *Directions*

**Take I-84 from Portland, driving 37 miles east of I-205 to take Exit 44/Cascade Locks. Go 1.3 miles to the other side of town and turn left onto Forest Lane. It's another 1.3 miles to the access road.**

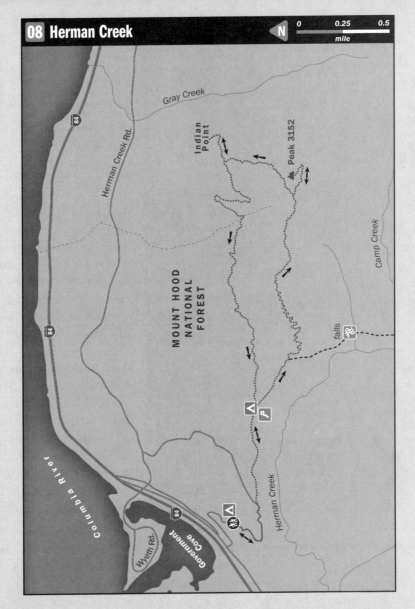

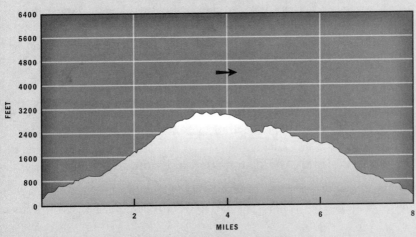

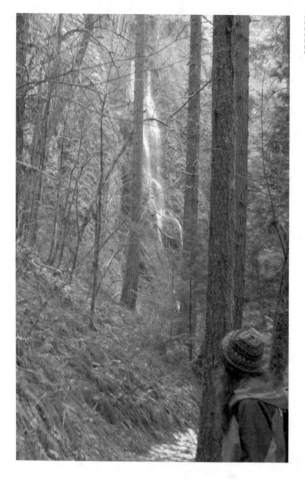

Nick Eaton Ridge to Indian Point.

So, rather than one hike, here are a few options, from easiest to hardest, with enough variations that you may not know which to choose—and *that's* why so many of us return to Herman Creek time and time again.

All the hikes start at the same place, the Herman Creek trailhead, which until May 1 will mean a half-mile walk from Forest Lane. From the trail sign, hike a short, steep section to some power lines and follow the trail past them, for a total of 0.6 miles, to a junction. The options start here, as do the mileage counts.

**PACIFIC CREST FALLS AND THE PINNACLES (4.1 MILES; EASY):** From this junction, turn right and descend 0.4 miles to cross Herman Creek on a large metal bridge. This creek does get runs of anadromous fish (which live in the ocean and spawn in the rivers). Steelhead enter from June through October, and salmon are in from August to November. Perhaps you can spot one of these, or the large trout that inhabit the deeper pools.

Beyond the bridge, climb again for 0.8 miles to reach an intersection with the PCT. Turn right here, pass through a rockslide, and in 0.5 miles arrive at the two-tiered Pacific Crest Falls, which is much more impressive in winter and spring than in summer or fall.

Continue 0.2 miles and you'll catch a glimpse of the Herman Creek Pinnacles, basalt cones that can be tough to spot through summer brush.

Hike another 1.5 miles along the PCT to Dry Creek, which isn't dry; a side trail leads 0.2 miles to the equally wet Dry Creek Falls.

**HERMAN CREEK TRAIL (UP TO 20.8 MILES ROUND-TRIP):** Think of Herman Creek Trail as a highway of sorts—not because it's boring or crowded, but because it leads to

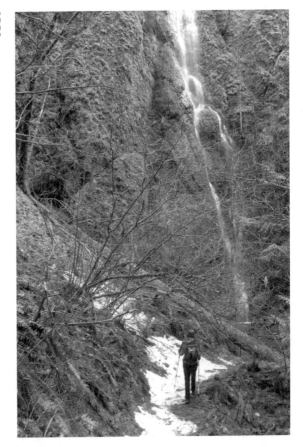

Herman Creek Trail in winter

several side trips, many nice places, and one spectacular destination. Best of all, the average elevation gain here is a paltry 350 feet per mile. So you can do as little or as much as you want—and there's a *lot* to do.

From the same junction referenced above, continue uphill and to the left, and you'll climb (briefly on a road) 0.7 miles, to reach Herman Camp and a big trail intersection. From left to right, the trails are Gorge Trail, Gorton Creek Trail, and Herman Creek Trail. (If you're looking for a campsite, you can do a lot better than Herman Camp.)

Keep climbing Herman Creek Trail, which still looks like a road, and in 0.3 miles you'll pass the Nick Eaton Way junction (more on that later). After this, your trail is more, well, trail-like, and begins a lazy climb in and out of small side canyons, though never near Herman Creek. Over the course of 2.4 miles, you'll pass a series of creeks and waterfalls until, at 4 miles total (3.4 since the first junction), you'll hit Casey Creek Camp and two trails.

For your first real view of Herman Creek on this hike, head down and to the right for a steep 0.3 miles to the confluence of Herman Creek's east and west forks. It's a fine place to have lunch and turn around for an 8-mile round-trip stroll.

If you keep going, you'll pass more creeks and falls over the next 3.5 miles (notice a pattern?) and arrive at Cedar Swamp Camp, the first of three sites, in half a mile. Things start to open up a bit here, and 3 more miles (a total of 11 since the car) puts you at the PCT just below Chinidere Mountain and just above Wahtum Lake, where campsites and deep, blue water beckon. For details on that scenic, trail-filled area, see page 25.

**NICK EATON WAY TO INDIAN POINT (8 MILES; STRENUOUS):** This is the big dog of the area, at least for day-hikers. It's also the hike shown on the elevation profile for this chapter. Nick Eaton Way (it and the ridge are named for a pioneer-era farmer) is among the steeper paths around. I often use it to see what kind of shape I'm in by April; usually the answer is "not good."

From its start at Herman Creek Trail just above Herman Camp, Nick Eaton Way ascends as abruptly as an airplane taking off. If you want numbers, it climbs 1,960 feet in 2 miles, making it steeper than Dog Mountain. But hey, it's only 2 miles, and along the way you'll traverse hanging meadows with flowers and great views. The meadow at 1 mile has a view down the Columbia to Bonneville Dam and Bridge of the Gods, and another, 0.2 miles on, has a rare view south—in this case, up Herman Creek's drainage.

After 2 miles of this, you'll enter Hatfield Wilderness, named for a Republican U.S. senator (how times have changed!), and hit Ridge Cutoff Trail. Your path here is on the left, but if it's clear, it's worth staying on Nick Eaton Way 0.25 miles to a saddle; there, look for a trail heading up to what's known as simply Peak 3152 (its elevation). The view is better than the name.

To continue the loop, take Ridge Cutoff Trail 0.6 miles to Gorton Creek Trail, where you have more choices. One option is to turn right and hike 6.5 miles, passing various camps and trails in a swing around to Wahtum Lake. The first campsite you encounter is Deadwood Camp, 0.8 miles along, which has a year-round stream.

If you're feeling slightly adventurous, your second option is to go about 50 yards right, then look for a seriously steep trail descending to the left. This path goes out toward Indian Point, a dramatic rock outcrop hundreds of feet above the Columbia. It's about 0.25 miles down to a flat spot with a view of the point and the river; going any farther is enthusiastically discouraged if you have even the slightest fear of heights or lack balance.

Back on Gorton Creek Trail, hike 2.6 mellow, lusciously green miles to Herman Camp, then turn right, on Herman Creek Trail, to return to the official trailhead after hiking another 1.3 uneventful miles.

# LARCH MOUNTAIN 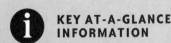 09

## IN BRIEF

Sure, you can drive almost to the top of Larch Mountain, but the trail between there and Multnomah Falls is one of the classic walks in Oregon—from the shores of the Columbia River to a high lookout in the Cascades, with old-growth forest on the way up and a view from the top that takes in everything from Portland to several volcanoes. There's even a shorter loop hike that encompasses the upper parts of the mountain only.

## DESCRIPTION

Pick a clear day to get the best view; or think about timing your arrival at the top to coincide with sunset—you'll get to see Mount Hood bathed in pink light, and the lights of Portland are spectacular from the summit. Consider doing this one in late August, when the upper parts of the hill are awash in huckleberries.

You can actually see Larch Mountain as you drive out I-84; it's just to the left of Mount Hood and has a notch in the top. The top of that notch is where you're headed.

------------------------------------

### *Directions* ──────────────➤

**To start at Multnomah Falls, take I-84, driving 24 miles east of I-205 to Exit 31/Multnomah Falls, the exit for the parking lot. Park and walk under the expressway to the historic lodge. For the upper trailheads, take I-84, driving 15 miles east of I-205, and take Exit 22/Corbett. At the intersection with Historic Columbia River Highway, turn left. Drive 2 miles, then veer right on Larch Mountain Road. The uppermost trailhead is in the parking lot at the end of the road, 14 miles up. The middle trailhead is 11.5 miles ahead, on the left, where Larch Mountain Road heads right and a gravel road takes off to the left.**

### (i) KEY AT-A-GLANCE INFORMATION

**LENGTH: 6.8 miles one-way with a car shuttle, 13.6 miles out-and-back, 6-mile optional upper loop**

**CONFIGURATION: Out-and-back or one-way**

**DIFFICULTY: Moderate–strenuous**

**SCENERY: Waterfalls, creeks in wooded canyons, colossal trees, view from top**

**EXPOSURE: Mostly shady (until summit)**

**TRAFFIC: Always heavy on lower stretches**

**TRAIL SURFACE: Pavement, packed dirt, some gravel**

**HIKING TIME: 5 hours one-way, 8 hours round-trip, 4 hours for upper loop**

**DRIVING DISTANCE: 31 miles (40 minutes) to lower trailhead or 36 miles (1 hour) to upper trailheads from Pioneer Square**

**SEASON: June–October**

**BEST TIME: Late August (for amazing huckleberries)**

**ACCESS: No fees or permits**

**WHEELCHAIR ACCESS: Only first 0.2 miles to Benson Bridge**

**MAPS: Trails of the Columbia Gorge; USGS Multnomah Falls**

**FACILITIES: Full services at Multnomah Falls trailhead; restrooms atop Larch Mountain**

**INFO: Columbia River Gorge National Scenic Area, (541) 308-1700**

------------------------------------

### GPS Trailhead Coordinates

UTM Zone (WGS84) 10T

Easting 571215

Northing 5042155

Latitude  N 45.52929°

Longitude W 122.08800°

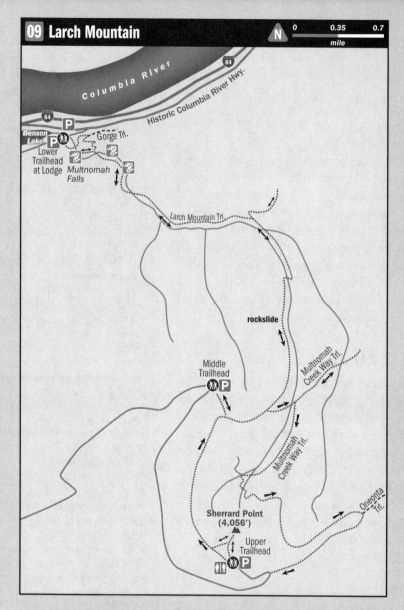

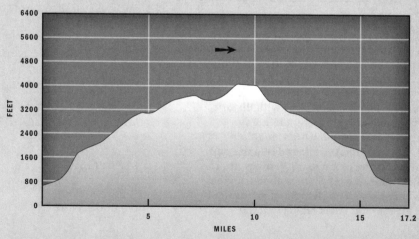

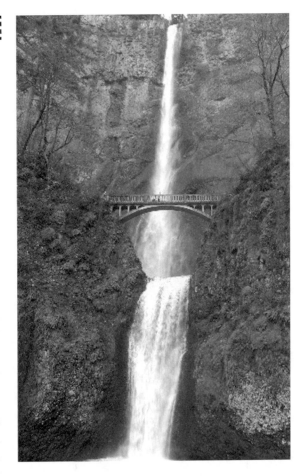

Benson Bridge and Multnomah Falls

As for the hike, I confess a bias in favor of walking up hills as opposed to walking down them. It seems easier to recover from losing your breath while climbing than to recuperate from pounding your knees and feet while you descend. Still, you've got three options here, all quite worthwhile. You can start at the top or at the bottom and put in 6.8 miles (assuming you have a second car for a shuttle), or you can start in the middle and do a loop that takes in the view but with less work. Or you can combine these.

For our purposes, let's assume you put a second car at the top parking lot, and we'll start at the bottom, then include the upper loop on the way. From Multnomah Falls Lodge, walk with the masses up the paved trail that leads over Benson Bridge and covers 1 mile (climbing 600 feet) to reach a junction with a side trail leading to the viewing platform at the top of the falls. Continuing past this point, you'll leave 90 percent of your comrades behind so that, for the next several miles, you may well have Larch Mountain Trail (441) to yourself. You will also enter one of the few areas of old-growth forest in the Columbia River Gorge.

The trail was built in the early 1900s to coincide with the opening of the Columbia River Highway. One thing we should get straight is that there are no larch trees on Larch Mountain. The name stuck after old-time loggers confused the noble fir with the larch, which grows only east of the Cascade Range (although they have a few in the Washington Park–Hoyt Arboretum; see hike 60, page 268).

Staying on this trail, you'll cross Multnomah Creek and pass two lovely waterfalls. At 1.6 miles, ignore Wahkeena Trail (420), on the right. At 2 miles you'll cross Multnomah Creek again, then at 3 miles traverse the East Fork of

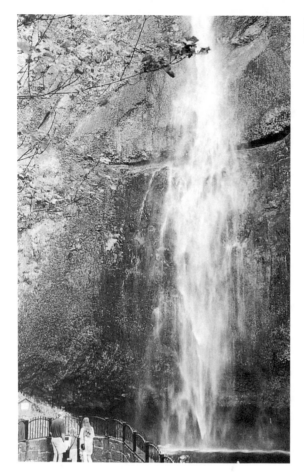

Multnomah Creek. Just 0.6 miles later you'll cross a one-log footbridge, which, by pure coincidence, my friend Christie and I were the first people to cross in 2000. (The workers had just set the log in place, and they allowed us to cross before they started on the handrails.)

At 3.9 miles you'll cross a rockslide and then start climbing through an old-growth forest of western hemlock and Douglas fir trees that get as thick as five and six feet in diameter and as old as 400 years. In late summer, this area abounds with huckleberries, and in autumn the red, yellow, and orange vine maple is astounding.

At 4.8 miles you'll come to a junction with Multnomah Creek Way Trail (444), and you'll have the option to simply stay on Larch Mountain Trail (441) (to reach the top in 2 miles) or to take Trail 444, to the left, a more scenic route to the top but one that is 0.7 miles longer. If the latter sounds OK, follow the trail 0.2 miles, cross Multnomah Creek, then turn right and go 2.8 miles, through a marsh and up the ridge of Larch Mountain. When you come to Oneonta Trail (424) at the top of the ridge, turn right and follow it 0.9 miles to the parking area atop Larch Mountain. You'll follow the road for the last little bit. Then take a signed, paved trail to Sherrard Point for the big view. It's 0.7 miles from where you enter the road to Sherrard Point—a total of 7.5 miles from the trailhead at Multnomah Falls.

Now, as for your other hiking options on Larch Mountain, you can either start at the top and descend to Multnomah Falls (following Larch Mountain Trail all the way down or taking the loop described, which uses Multnomah Creek Way Trail), or you can park at the middle trailhead described above. The middle trailhead accesses the upper part of Larch Mountain, saving you from climbing 3,000 feet from the Columbia. From that trailhead, either walk 1.5 miles up Larch Mountain Trail to reach the top, or descend it half a mile and take Multnomah Creek Way Trail (444) and the loop described above.

Any way you go, make sure that when you hit the top you go out the paved trail to Sherrard Point and have a look around. You'll see (if it's clear) Portland, Mount Hood, Mount Jefferson, Mount Adams, Mount St. Helens, and Mount Rainier. You'll also notice that you're at the top of a cliff on a semicircular ridge. That's because Larch Mountain is what remains of an ancient volcano, and what you're looking down into is a crater of that volcano.

Millions of years ago lava flows from volcanoes like this one used to periodically dam the Columbia River, forming lakes that stretched back into Montana and occasionally caused catastrophic floods. At such times there would have been some 400 feet of water where Portland is now—just a little something to think about as you walk back to your car.

## NEARBY ACTIVITIES

If you did the one-way car shuttle, stop on the way to or from Multnomah Falls at the Portland Women's Forum Viewpoint on Historic Columbia River Highway. Because it's a little farther west than the more famous Vista House, it's a less-visited spot for viewing the Columbia River Gorge.

# 10 MCCALL NATURE PRESERVE

## KEY AT-A-GLANCE INFORMATION

**LENGTH:** McCall Point Trail 3 miles long, Plateau Loop 2 miles

**CONFIGURATION:** Out-and-back to McCall Point, balloon to Plateau

**DIFFICULTY:** McCall Point is moderate (due to the climb); Plateau is easy.

**SCENERY:** Wildflowers, the Columbia River below, 2 volcanoes, old oak trees

**EXPOSURE:** Wide open most of the time

**TRAFFIC:** Moderate when flowers are out, light otherwise

**TRAIL SURFACE:** Packed dirt

**HIKING TIME:** 1.5 hours to McCall Point, 1 hour for Plateau Loop

**DRIVING DISTANCE:** 76 miles (1 hour 30 minutes) from Pioneer Square

**SEASON:** McCall Point open May–November, Plateau Loop year-round

**BEST TIME:** April–May

**ACCESS:** No fees or permits

**WHEELCHAIR ACCESS:** None

**MAPS:** USGS Lyle; map at the trailhead

**FACILITIES:** None

**INFO:** Columbia River Gorge National Scenic Area office, (541) 308-1700; or The Nature Conservancy, (503) 802-8100

**SPECIAL COMMENTS:** Consider wearing long pants; there are ticks, poison oak, and rattlesnakes in the area. Dogs are not allowed on either trail.

## IN BRIEF

McCall Nature Preserve is in a different world from most of the hikes in this book. It's a glimpse into central Oregon, a land of wide-open vistas, grass blowing in the nearly constant wind, and semiarid forests of oaks and ponderosa pine. It also has panoramic vistas of the Columbia and Mounts Adams and Hood, and more than 300 species of plants, some of them unique to the Columbia River Gorge.

## DESCRIPTION

OK, so this one is more than 60 miles from Portland, even as the crow flies. But it's truly worth the extra bit of easy driving, especially in the spring and early summer. At those times of the year, there is a kind of rain shroud somewhere between Cascade Locks and Hood River; while it's still pouring in Portland, places like the McCall Preserve are bathed in sunlight and carpeted in a few dozen kinds of wildflowers all blooming at once.

Start with McCall Point Trail and get your exercise out of the way. The trail, which climbs about 1,000 feet in 1.5 miles, starts out nearly flat and on an old jeep road, winding through the kind of open space that is so rare in the western part of the state. The trees you eventually encounter are oaks, most of

## GPS Trailhead Coordinates

UTM Zone (WGS84) 10T

Easting 632144

Northing 5058635

Latitude N 45.66867°

Longitude W 121.30352°

## Directions

Take I-84 from Portland, driving 62 miles east of I-205 to Exit 69/Mosier. Turn right and follow Historic Columbia River Highway (US 30) 6.5 miles through Mosier to Rowena Crest Viewpoint. McCall Point Trail begins at a sign at the end of the stone wall. Plateau Loop begins across the highway, where a set of steps leads over a fence.

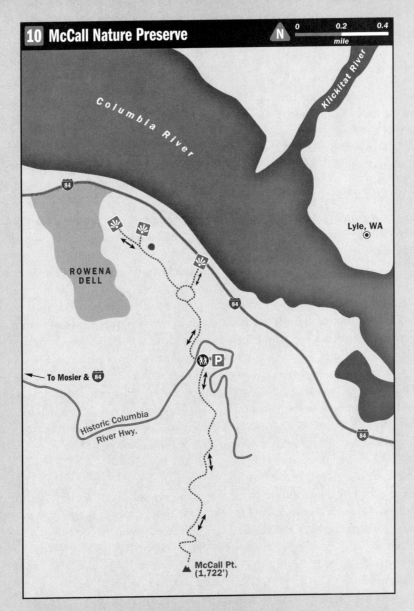

N

0     0.2     0.4
mile

Columbia River

Klickitat River

84

Lyle, WA

ROWENA DELL

84

To Mosier & 84

Historic Columbia River Hwy.

P

84

McCall Pt. (1,722')

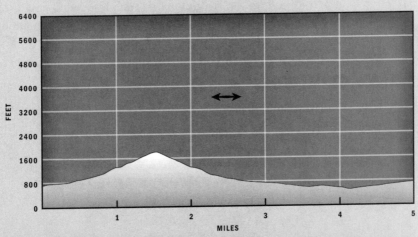

them Oregon white oak, and some as much as 800 years old. The trail ascends slightly when it gains the edge of the ridge, with ever-more-impressive views out to the east. Keep an eye out for Mount Adams as its summit comes into view across the river.

The second half of the trail is a little steeper, and after a rain it might be slick and muddy, so add solid boots to your clothing list. But soon enough you'll come to McCall Point, an open hilltop with a sprawling view from Mount Hood to Mount Adams; you're actually about halfway between the two peaks, each of which is roughly 35 miles away. Looking west, you can see into the Columbia River Gorge; just to the left of it, the high peak with the towers on top is Mount Defiance, the highest point in the gorge.

Now, you summit hounds out there might stand at McCall Point and notice there's some more trail going south, through a notch, and then climbing again. I walked about a mile down (and then up) that trail, through some very peaceful oak stands, but technically speaking it didn't go anywhere special before it got pinched between a fence and the edge of a cliff. My advice is to have yourself a picnic at McCall Point and don't worry about that other trail.

Back at the highway, use the steps over the fence to begin Plateau Loop. This wide, easy path (which actually drops 100 feet in elevation) traverses flower and grass country to loop around a pond. Early in the year, there will be numerous other little ponds and wet areas, each supporting their own microhabitats. The small canyon below you on your left is called Rowena Dell.

When a sign reading "Trail" indicates a right turn, you'll notice a trail that continues straight out into the grasslands. There is another pond out there among the trees, in addition to other viewpoints out over the river. But the most dramatic view is on the official trail to your right. After that trail has passed the pond, it turns right again. A small trail to the left leads to the top of a cliff that is not for the acrophobes among us—it's a sheer drop of 500 feet from where you stand (without a railing, so keep an eye on the kids) down to the railroad tracks and the river. The town across the river is Lyle, Washington, which lies on a gravel bar formed by catastrophic floods more than 10,000 years ago.

To return to the trailhead, follow the trail back around the pond, and turn left (uphill) at the sign. Or wander farther to your right toward the viewpoint of Lyle to keep exploring.

## NEARBY ACTIVITIES

As long as you're this far east, keep going to the Dalles to visit the Columbia Gorge Discovery Center, where displays range from a working model of the Columbia before and after the Dalles Dam to a Living History Center with presentations on the life of the Oregon Trail pioneers.

# TABLE MOUNTAIN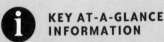

## IN BRIEF

This leg-buster of a climb has a great reward on top: one of the best panoramas in the whole Columbia River Gorge, including a bird's-eye view of Bonneville Dam, from a lunch spot atop 800-foot cliffs. And there are hot springs at the trailhead!

## DESCRIPTION

You have two options for where to start this hike. Using the "official" trailhead on WA 14 at North Bonneville makes it about a 14-mile tromp, though it does visit a lake and an additional viewpoint along the way. If that's what you're after, take the trail 0.6 miles from WA 14 up to the PCT and turn left, following the PCT 1.9 miles to Gillette Lake, then 1.3 miles to Greenleaf Overlook, then 1.7 miles to the top of the road, where the other route comes in.

As for that other route, which is the highly recommended one, it's almost 6 round-trip miles shorter and starts at a hot-springs resort. The only concern is that the resort has

### KEY AT-A-GLANCE INFORMATION

**LENGTH:** 8.5 miles

**CONFIGURATION:** Out-and-back

**DIFFICULTY:** Strenuous

**SCENERY:** A tumbling stream, 5 volcanoes, some of the steepest trail around, and a bird's-eye view of the Columbia River Gorge

**EXPOSURE:** Mostly shady but with rocky slopes to climb and descend, open rock at the top; extreme cliff-top exposure in places

**TRAFFIC:** Moderate on summer weekends, light otherwise

**TRAIL SURFACE:** Grass, packed dirt with rocks, then just (sometimes loose) rocks

**HIKING TIME:** 7 hours

**DRIVING DISTANCE:** 45 miles (50 minutes) from Pioneer Square

**SEASON:** April–November

**BEST TIME:** May

**BACKPACKING OPTIONS:** One poor site

**ACCESS:** No fee

**WHEELCHAIR ACCESS:** None

**MAPS:** Green Trails #429 (Bonneville Dam), though only the PCT appears on it

**FACILITIES:** Trailhead for longer hike has toilets; the other one has no facilities other than those at the resort

**INFO:** Columbia River Gorge National Scenic Area, (541) 308-1700

### Directions

Take I-84 from Portland to Exit 44/Cascade Locks. As soon as you enter the town, take the first right to get on Bridge of the Gods, following a sign for Stevenson, Washington. Pay a $1 toll to cross the bridge, and at the far end, turn left onto WA 14. North Bonneville Trailhead is 1.5 miles ahead on the right—this is the starting point for the longer hike and also has the only public toilet in the area. For the shorter hike, continue another 1.2 miles on WA 14 and turn right, crossing under the railroad tracks. Just beyond the tracks, turn right on Hot Springs Way. The entrance to the resort is 0.9 miles ahead.

### GPS Trailhead Coordinates

UTM Zone (WGS84) 10T

Easting 581121

Northing 5056367

Latitude  N 45.65611°

Longitude W 121.95879°

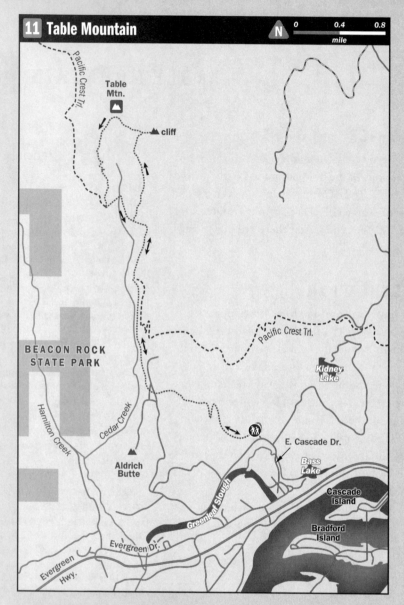

N

0        0.4        0.8

*mile*

Pacific Crest Trl.

Table
Mtn.

▲ cliff

BEACON ROCK
STATE PARK

Hamilton Creek

Cedar Creek

Pacific Crest Trl.

*Kidney
Lake*

▲
Aldrich
Butte

E. Cascade Dr.

*Bass
Lake*

Greenleaf Slough

Evergreen Dr.

Evergreen
Hwy.

*Cascade
Island*

*Bradford
Island*

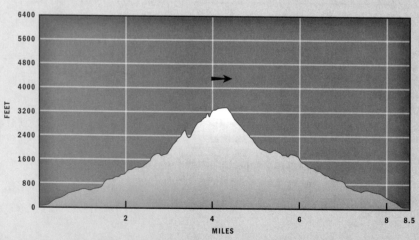

6400

5600

4800

4000

3200

2400

1600

800

0

FEET

2        4        6        8   8.5

MILES

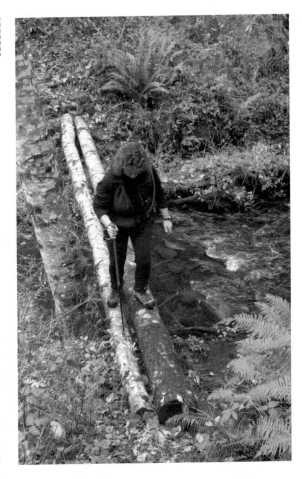

Stream crossing on the way to Table Mountain

become weary of hikers stomping around with their muddy boots. So call them ahead of time to see if their lot is available, and please treat the place with respect so they'll let us keep parking there.

To begin the hike, from the parking lot, head for the far west end of the pavement, beyond the rock wall surrounding the bath area, and look for an old road ascending the hill. Climb it 100 yards to a T-intersection, then take a little trail bound for a tree with a sign that says "PCT" and "Table Mountain."

Follow that trail as it winds up, steeply at times, through a young forest choked with vine maple, and pass a tiny lake on the right after 0.5 miles. Just under 1 mile, top out over a ridge, and 0.2 miles later cross a tiny creek on the logs placed there.

A few steps later, take a moment to look up toward Table Mountain and Sacajawea Rocks beyond the meadow. Yes, that's where we're headed. See if you can also spot a "rabbit ears" rock formation up there. Just past this area, turn right at a road junction, go 100 yards, turn left onto another road, and then, after taking a swooping switchback to the right, continue straight, through yet another junction. If all that gets confusing, remember this: your goal here is to climb on an old jeep road with the meadow below you and on your right.

Climb up from that meadow, in which lies the tough-to-spot Carpenters Lake, and just less than half a mile up (about 1.5 miles since the trailhead), cross the ridge to climb along Cedar Creek, which is lined almost exclusively with alder and Douglas fir. Go figure.

When you've gone a total of 2.3 miles—that is, about a mile past the meadow—you'll arrive in what looks like a campground area at an intersection with the PCT. (This is the spot that's 5.5 miles from the North Bonneville trailhead.) Turn left on the PCT, which goes left from the road and climbs a moderate grade through a more interesting forest. There are a few Douglas firs of decent size, but this whole area has been logged, much of it more than once. After you've gone 0.3 miles, you'll see a side trail leading left to a poor campsite; stay right, on the PCT. About 0.4 miles later, our summit trail enters from the right.

This is the old "Heartbreak Ridge" Trail, reopened in 2007 to give hikers a way to get to the top without traversing fragile meadows. You'll soon see how the trail got its name. If I had to rank the steepest sections of trail in this whole book, this stretch would easily make the top three. If you want stats, it's a 1,600-foot climb over the 1.3 miles from here to the summit, but there's actually a smidgen of *downhill* in there! So take your time and have faith; it's worth it.

After 0.6 miles (and 800 feet of gain!), you'll reach a tiny saddle with a big-time view of Table's rocky face, then you'll descend briefly and head to the base of a talus slope. Climb straight up that (lovely!), staying generally left and watching for the occasional sign. At the top, find the trail in the woods, turn right, and climb a bit more to reach the top.

When you get up there and catch your breath, you'll find that trails actually crisscross the broad summit. Head left for views of Mounts St. Helens, Rainier, and Adams. Go right (toward the Columbia River) for a spectacular view that ranges from Dog Mountain and Mount Defiance to Mount Hood, looking right up the Eagle Creek drainage. Beware that the final portions of this trail literally take you a foot away from a drop of hundreds of feet, and there's no protection.

Those cliffs are part of Table Mountain's fascinating geological history. As you look out toward the Columbia, you might realize that the southern half of Table Mountain actually slid into the river, leaving behind the cliffs and narrowing the Columbia to just a hundred yards at the most (at the point where Bridge of the Gods crosses). This slide, spanning more than 10 square miles, occurred about 550 years ago—basically yesterday, in geologic time. It first created a natural dam that blocked the river, and then the Cascades of the Columbia, which were submerged when Bonneville Dam went in.

Now look up at Mount Hood. On the left skyline you can see a ridge leading up to a bump just below the snow line. That's Cooper Spur (hike 32, page 150). For a real adventure, hike up that one and look for Table Mountain.

To finish the loop, head west. All trails lead to the way down—and the way down is scary, especially when wet. This steep, rocky scramble along the spine of the ridge eventually drops you back, exhausted, onto the PCT. Turn left to retrace your steps to your car.

## NEARBY ACTIVITIES

Now, about that hot-springs resort. It's a giant, lush place with a restaurant, rooms ($139 and up per night), and a day spa with hot tubs, massage, skin treatments, and so on. Your basic soak starts at $15 for 25 minutes. For more information, call (509) 427-7767 or visit **www.bonnevilleresort.com.**

# TRIPLE FALLS  12

## IN BRIEF

A unique waterfall lies at the end of this moderate hike, but you don't have to go that far to see some fine Columbia River Gorge scenery. You can, in fact, just drive by the trailhead and admire Horsetail Falls.

## DESCRIPTION

If all you do is slow down while driving by Horsetail Falls, you'll be pleased. But at least cross the parking area to pick some blackberries over by the railroad tracks; they're ripe in late summer. The great thing about this trail is that the farther you go, the better it gets, and you never have to work very hard at all.

From Horsetail Falls, follow the gravel trail behind the sign describing some of the animals that live in the area. At 0.2 miles, stay right at a trail junction. A few hundred yards later you'll come around a bend and see Upper Horsetail Falls. A popular turnaround spot because it's so near the car, these falls are also a hit with kids, who, with supervision, can get under them and catch some spray. The falls seem to shoot out of a basalt cliff face, and the area behind them is a grotto through which the trail passes. If you get under them, some smaller streams will trickle down onto your head (and your dog's). Just don't get directly under the main stream of water; even this relatively small waterfall is extremely powerful.

-------------------------------------------

*Directions* ———————————➤

**Take I-84 from Portland, driving 21 miles east of I-205 to Exit 28/Bridal Veil. Turn left onto Historic Columbia River Highway and continue 5.2 miles to the signed parking area at Horsetail Falls.**

---

### ⓘ KEY AT-A-GLANCE INFORMATION

**LENGTH: 4.5 miles**

**CONFIGURATION: Out-and-back or loop**

**DIFFICULTY: Moderate**

**SCENERY: Four waterfalls, a spectacular gorge, a view of the Columbia River**

**EXPOSURE: In the forest all the way, with some cliff-top walking**

**TRAFFIC: Moderate on summer weekends, light otherwise**

**TRAIL SURFACE: Gravel and packed dirt; roots, rocks**

**HIKING TIME: 2.5 hours**

**DRIVING DISTANCE: 33 miles (40 minutes) from Pioneer Square**

**SEASON: Year-round, though it gets muddy in winter and spring**

**BEST TIME: April for water flow and flowers, October for colors**

**ACCESS: No fees or permits**

**WHEELCHAIR ACCESS: None**

**MAPS: Trails of the Columbia Gorge; Green Trails #428 (Bridal Veil)**

**FACILITIES: None at the trailhead; water and restrooms 0.5 miles east, at Ainsworth State Park**

**INFO: Columbia River Gorge Visitors Association, (800) 984-6743**

- - - - - - - - - - - - - - - - - - - - - - -

### GPS Trailhead Coordinates

UTM Zone (WGS84) 10T

Easting 569447

Northing 5047289

Latitude  N 45.57567°

Longitude  W 122.10991°

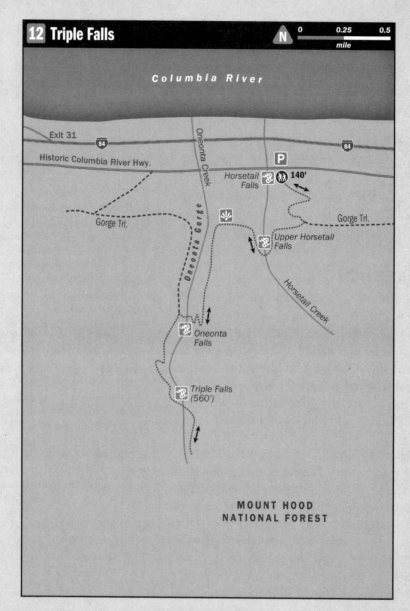

0    0.25    0.5

*mile*

N

**Columbia River**

Exit 31

84

Historic Columbia River Hwy.

Oneonta Creek

P

Horsetail Falls

140'

Gorge Trl.

Oneonta Gorge

Gorge Trl.

Upper Horsetail Falls

Horsetail Creek

Oneonta Falls

Triple Falls (560')

**MOUNT HOOD NATIONAL FOREST**

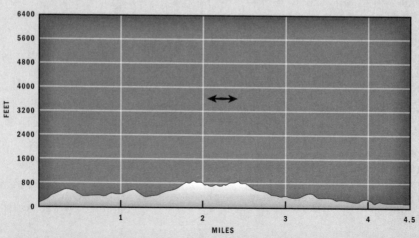

FEET

6400
5600
4800
4000
3200
2400
1600
800
0

1    2    3    4    4.5

**MILES**

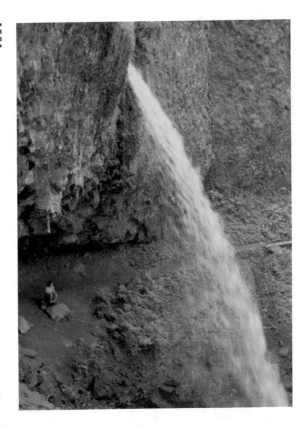

Hanging out behind Ponytail Falls

To keep going, simply follow the trail as it contours around the gorge wall. It soon comes to a brushy area on the right, through which several trails lead out to cliff-top viewpoints over the Columbia River. You can make a side loop out there and work your way back to the main trail as it turns away from the river. There's a network of trails in this tiny area, but they all lead to the same place, so you won't get lost.

A mile past Upper Horsetail Falls, after you pass under a mossy "weeping" rock face, you'll descend to a bridge spanning the spectacular Oneonta Gorge. A geological and biological wonder, Oneonta alone is worth a visit; from here, you're looking down into it, with waterfalls above and below you. Just across the bridge (and after a little climbing) is another junction; you can loop back to the highway by going right (you'll have to walk nearly half a mile along the road, however, to get back to your car), or you can turn left and head up toward Triple Falls. The trail is rocky in places, and there's a little more elevation gain, but nice views of the narrow gorge will help keep you moving.

About a mile up you'll see Triple Falls. It's actually just one creek (Oneonta), but it divides into three just before it goes over the edge. So take your pictures from here, and then walk another minute or two to a wooden bridge across the wide stream just above the falls. Across the bridge are some nice rocks for picnicking, and just upstream are some pools the kids can jump in, if you've managed to get them this far.

## NEARBY ACTIVITIES

You can get about a quarter of a mile into Oneonta Gorge, but not without getting wet. Even in late summer, adults will find themselves wading in waist-high water or climbing rocks to avoid it. (So put on your swimsuit, along with some shoes you don't mind soaking, and explore this official U.S. Forest Service Botanical Area.

# 13 WAHKEENA FALLS TO MULTNOMAH FALLS

### KEY AT-A-GLANCE INFORMATION

**LENGTH:** 5.2 miles

**CONFIGURATION:** Loop

**DIFFICULTY:** Moderate

**SCENERY:** Waterfalls, canyons, river views, flowers, a spring, big trees

**EXPOSURE:** In the forest all the way, nothing dangerous

**TRAFFIC:** Heavy, especially on weekends and around Multnomah Falls; moderate on weekdays

**TRAIL SURFACE:** Pavement, gravel, packed dirt with some rocky sections

**HIKING TIME:** 3 hours

**DRIVING DISTANCE:** 31 miles (35 minutes) from Pioneer Square

**SEASON:** Year-round (muddy and possibly icy in spots in winter and spring)

**BEST TIME:** Whenever you can get out there!

**BACKPACKING OPTIONS:** A couple of sites along the trail toward Angels Rest

**ACCESS:** No fees or permits

**WHEELCHAIR ACCESS:** The first section of trail heading up from either falls is paved.

**MAPS:** Trails of the Columbia Gorge, Green Trails #428 (Bridal Veil)

**FACILITIES:** Full service at Multnomah Falls

**INFO:** Columbia River Gorge National Scenic Area, (541) 308-1700

## IN BRIEF

Just off I-84 and bookmarked by two beautiful waterfalls, this is the ideal introduction to all that the Columbia River Gorge has to offer, including great scenery, big crowds, and nice steep climbs.

## DESCRIPTION

When hiking friends come to visit Oregon, this is where I take them first. They get to see the scenic spectacle that is the Columbia River Gorge, they get to view the highest waterfall in Oregon, they get to see old-growth Douglas firs, and they get their hearts pumping—from excitement and, at times, from effort.

You can hike either way on this trail and park at either falls; my preference is to park at Multnomah Falls and start the hike at Wahkeena Falls. I'll tell you why later.

To do this, walk 100 yards down the historic highway to the west of Multnomah Falls Lodge and take Return Trail (442), which parallels the road 0.6 miles to Wahkeena Falls. Along the way you'll pass under a rock and be cooled by a mossy, "weeping" rock wall.

Actually several falls in one, Wahkeena Falls encompasses everything from sheer drops to cascades to misty sprays. This creek, by the way, comes primarily from a spring up

## GPS Trailhead Coordinates

UTM Zone (WGS84) 10T

Easting 568035

Northing 5047230

Latitude N 45.57528°

Longitude W 122.12801°

## Directions ⟶

Take I-84 east 21 miles to Exit 28/Bridal Veil. Turn left onto Historic Columbia River Highway and proceed 2 miles to the signed parking area at Wahkeena Falls or continue another 0.7 miles to Multnomah Falls.

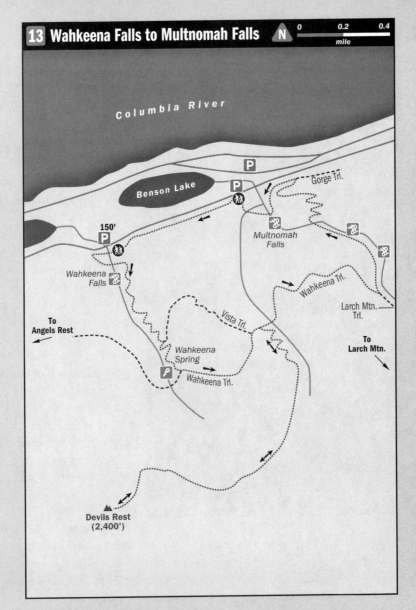

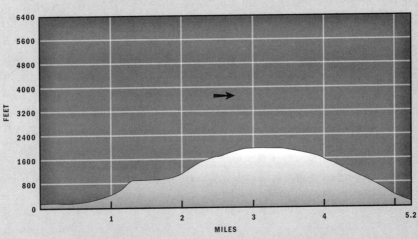

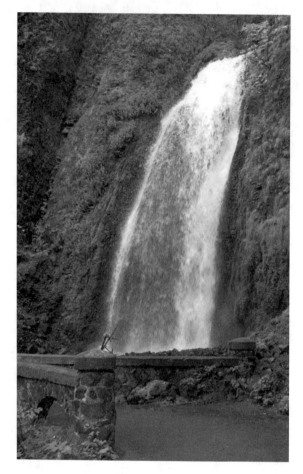

Halfway up Wahkeena Falls

on the ridge that you'll see later. To start the loop, follow the paved trail across the creek and then 0.2 miles up to a footbridge at the base of the upper falls. Take a nice deep breath of that cool, moist air; your workout is about to begin.

In the next 0.4 miles of paved switchbacks, you'll gain about 400 feet; such quick climbs are the trademark of gorge hikes. When you get to a lookout point on the right with a great view of the Columbia, the worst is over. You can rest later for a few minutes on a bench at the lovely Fairy Falls, sort of a miniature version of Ramona Falls (hike 38, page 175).

There's still some climbing to do; it's just that now it's more gradual and you have the creek and some lovely old forest to take your mind off it. Fairly recent fires took out smaller growth, blackened the trunks of bigger trees, and opened the forest floor for berries and wildflowers to move in. Just above Fairy Falls, you'll encounter Vista Point Trail; turn right here, staying on Wahkeena Trail (420). After another 0.4 miles you'll come to an intersection with Angels Rest Trail (415). The sign here was helpfully edited: because it lacked the word "Trail" after Vista Point, Devils Rest, and Larch Mountain (the distances listed are to those trails, not to the destinations), somebody came by and scratched "Trail" after each name. At any rate, you should at least take a 100-yard detour here on Angels Rest Trail to see Wahkeena Spring. There are also some campsites a bit farther down this trail.

At the intersection of the Wahkeena and Angels Rest trails, back near the spring, take Wahkeena Trail up the hill 0.4 miles to a four-way intersection. Ascending the hill from your left is Vista Point Trail; ignore it. Ascending the hill to your right is Devils Rest Trail, which climbs briefly and then heads over to what, frankly, is a disappointing viewpoint. So unless you just want some more exercise, continue straight on Wahkeena Trail.

This eastbound stretch on Wahkeena Trail soon descends and, in 0.9 miles, intersects Larch Mountain Trail (441), which connects Multnomah Falls with Larch Mountain (hike 9, page 47). For our purposes, turn left and head down the rock-filled Multnomah Creek. In the next mile, you'll pass several waterfalls in a gorge filled with ferns and large, old-growth Douglas firs.

A well-marked (and well-traveled) paved trail to the left leads 0.1 mile to the top of Multnomah Falls, where a wooden platform offers an ego-building view of the camera-toting throngs below. "Yeah," you can say later at the bottom, "I've been up there." This brings me to why I like to do the hike this way. From this point on, especially on a weekend, you'll be among hundreds of people. From my perspective, it's better (faster) going downhill than uphill through such a mob. Multnomah Falls and Benson Bridge is just 1 mile on.

The highest falls in Oregon, at 542 feet, upper Multnomah Falls is quite a sight. Be sure to stop at the information office at the lodge to see pictures of the various floods and a massive rockfall that have occurred there. Now, for the final reason I like to start this hike at Wahkeena Falls but park at Multnomah Falls: When you're all done, you can get yourself an ice cream cone or an espresso, or cruise the gift shop, if you're into that, and your car is right there waiting for you.

## NEARBY ACTIVITIES

The 1925 Multnomah Falls Lodge is well worth checking out, with its skylights and fireplace in the restaurant and its old-style stone-and-wood construction. The food is not as good as the setting, but the Sunday brunch is massive.

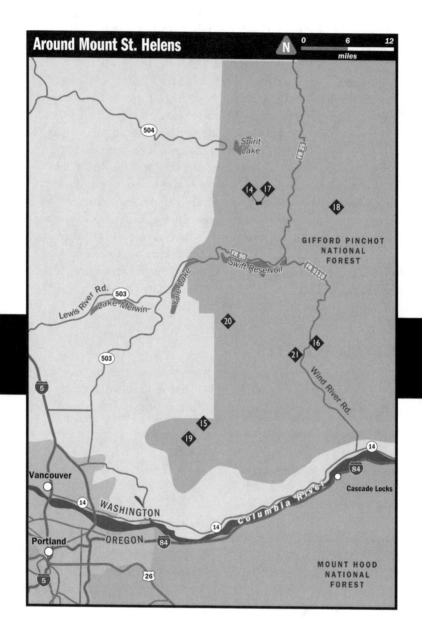

0    6    12
miles
N

504

Spirit
Lake

FR 25

14  17

18

GIFFORD PINCHOT
NATIONAL
FOREST

FR 90

Swift Reservoir

FR 5110

Lewis River Rd.
503
Lake Merwin

Yale Lake

20

16

503

21

Wind River Rd.

5

15

19

14

84

Vancouver

Cascade Locks

14

WASHINGTON

Columbia River

14

OREGON   84

Portland

MOUNT HOOD
NATIONAL
FOREST

5

26

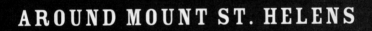

AROUND MOUNT ST. HELENS

# 14 APE CANYON

### KEY AT-A-GLANCE INFORMATION

**LENGTH:** 11.6 miles

**CONFIGURATION:** Out-and-back

**DIFFICULTY:** Moderate

**SCENERY:** Old-growth forest, a volcanic mudflow, a narrow canyon

**EXPOSURE:** Shady and open areas on the way up, then wide open at the top

**TRAFFIC:** Moderate on summer weekends, light otherwise

**TRAIL SURFACE:** Packed dirt with roots and rocks, rock at the top

**HIKING TIME:** 5.5 hours

**DRIVING DISTANCE:** 66 miles (1 hour 35 minutes) from Pioneer Square

**SEASON:** Late June–October

**BEST TIME:** September–October

**BACKPACKING OPTIONS:** Poor

**ACCESS:** Northwest Forest Pass required

**WHEELCHAIR ACCESS:** None, but some of the nearby Lava Canyon Trail is accessible

**MAPS:** USFS Mount St. Helens National Volcanic Monument

**FACILITIES:** None at trailhead; toilets at Lava Canyon trailhead; no water at trailhead or on trail

**INFO:** Mount St. Helens National Volcanic Monument, (360) 449-7800

**SPECIAL COMMENTS:** In June, call the monument to make sure FS 83 is open and snow-free. This trail gets a lot of mountain-bike traffic.

## IN BRIEF

This trail visits two worlds not ordinarily seen: the upper reaches of a volcano and the edge of what they call the "blast zone." Without too much climbing, you can stand in a wonderful old-growth forest and be about 20 feet from an area that was completely obliterated in 1980. At the top, you'll have a sweeping view highlighted by an amazing geological oddity.

## DESCRIPTION

You'll get your first glimpse of the contrasts ahead when you have walked only 500 feet on this trail. At that point you'll be at the top of a little bluff, looking out over a wide area of rocks. Those rocks used to be on the upper slopes of Mount St. Helens, but on May 18, 1980, they tumbled down the hill at about 45 miles per hour, part of a landslide triggered when most of Shoestring Glacier melted a moment after the volcano erupted. But the mudslide stayed generally within the boundaries of the Muddy River, so the forest you're standing in—even though it was within feet of the slide—was spared. You'll spend the next 5 miles climbing this ridge, but don't worry: you'll gain only a little more than 1,300 feet along the way.

Before you leave this viewpoint, look down. You're standing on several layers of

## GPS Trailhead Coordinates

UTM Zone (WGS84) 10T

Easting 570090

Northing 5112807

Latitude  N 46.16523°

Longitude  W 122.09212°

## *Directions*

**Take I-5 from Portland, driving 21 miles north of the Columbia River to Exit 21/Woodland. Turn right onto WA 503 (Lewis River Road), which after 31 miles (2 miles past Cougar) turns into FS 90. Continue 3.3 miles, then turn left onto FS 83. The trailhead is 11.2 miles ahead on the left, just before the Lava Canyon trailhead.**

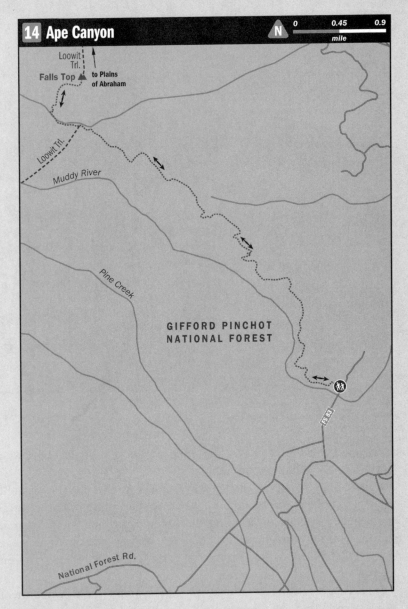

N   0   0.45   0.9
mile

Loowit
Trl.
Falls Top ▲   to Plains
of Abraham

Loowit Trl.

Muddy River

Pine Creek

**GIFFORD PINCHOT
NATIONAL FOREST**

FS 83

National Forest Rd.

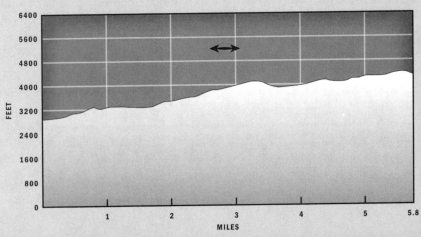

6400
5600
4800
4000
3200
2400
1600
800
0

FEET

1       2       3       4       5    5.8

MILES

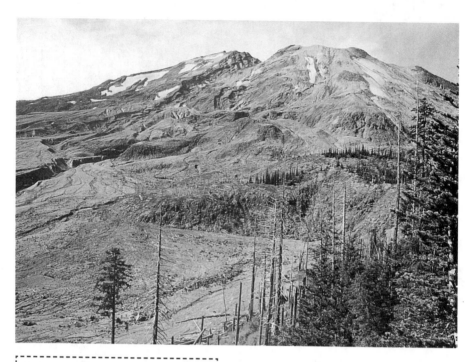

Mount St. Helens from the Ape Canyon Trail

rock, the result of a 1980 mudflow that exposed the rock, giving scientists clues to the volcano's history of eruptions.

If you're on this trail in September or October, you'll be in the world of the vine maple; its red and orange explosion contrasts beautifully with the evergreen canopy. Keep an eye out for deer and elk. At a quarter mile, look for an island of trees on the edge of the mudflow, and after a half mile, enjoy your first view south to Mount Hood. Ahead, on the slopes of Mount St. Helens, you can see the canyon left behind by Shoestring Glacier.

At 1.2 miles, you'll reach a little ridge, then soon after make a switchback to the right and climb a bit more; you'll also notice some social trails heading out to brushy viewpoints facing east to Mount Adams. At around 2 miles starts a series of switchbacks, now well within the old-growth forest of towering hemlocks and thick vine maple. Just past 3 miles, you'll actually lose some elevation before a viewpoint that takes in two-humped Mount Rainier off to your right. From here, you can also make out a large waterfall (probably dry by late summer) on an eastern ridge of St. Helens; we'll be at the top of that soon!

At 4.4 miles you'll be out in the open at the head of Ape Canyon proper—and in the "blast zone" itself. There you'll see trees that were killed by the super-heated gases produced when the mountain blew in 1980, and to the north (ahead of you) you will see the utter desolation the eruption created. (The volcano exploded in that direction.)

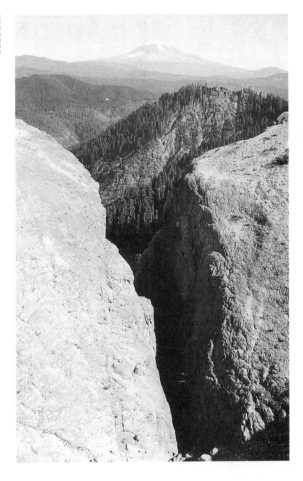

Ape Canyon, with Mount Adams in the distance

When you come to a lookout point on the right, you can scramble down a bit (be very careful) and look into the 300-foot slot at the head of Ape Canyon, which now stretches away to your right. If you work it right, it makes a heck of a foreground for a picture of Mount Adams. It's also visible from a little farther up the trail.

Just 0.2 miles farther up is an intersection with Loowit Trail, which goes all the way around Mount St. Helens. Stay to the right here, wind through another lahar, and half a mile later you'll climb out of it to the east, where a series of rock cairns marks the trail's path across the moonlike Plains of Abraham. When the trail dips to the cliff edge, you'll be at the top of that waterfall, with a sweeping view south.

If you're wondering about the name of this hike, it recalls a 1920s incident in which an apelike "Bigfoot" (decades later found to be a kid playing a prank) threw rocks at some miners in the area. The only connection between Ape Canyon and Ape Cave is in the name. The Mount St. Helens Apes, a local Boy Scout troop that took its name from the Ape Canyon legend, discovered Ape Cave.

## NEARBY ACTIVITIES

On the way back down FS 83, you'll pass a sign for Ape Cave, which is actually a long lava tube divided by an access ladder. Exploring the lower cave involves a 1.6-mile round-trip walk through a large cavern. Taking in the upper, 2.3-mile cave is trickier, requiring some rock scrambling here and there. Take two flashlights if you go.

# 15 BLUFF MOUNTAIN TRAIL

### KEY AT-A-GLANCE INFORMATION

**LENGTH:** 13.2 miles
**CONFIGURATION:** Out-and-back
**DIFFICULTY:** Strenuous
**SCENERY:** Wide-open, flower-covered ridges; exposed mountainsides; waterfalls; a panoramic vista
**EXPOSURE:** Open almost the whole way, occasionally on knife-edge ridges
**TRAFFIC:** Light
**TRAIL SURFACE:** Rocky
**HIKING TIME:** 7.5 hours
**DRIVING DISTANCE:** 55 miles (1 hour 45 minutes) from Pioneer Square
**SEASON:** Late June–October
**BEST TIME:** July for flowers, October for fall colors
**BACKPACKING OPTIONS:** Poor
**ACCESS:** No fee
**WHEELCHAIR ACCESS:** None
**MAPS:** Green Trails #396 (Lookout Mountain, WA) and #428 (Bridal Veil, OR)
**FACILITIES:** None at the trailhead; restrooms and water in Sunset Falls Campground on the way
**INFO:** Mount Adams Ranger District, (509) 395-3400
**SPECIAL COMMENTS:** FS 41, while passable to all vehicles, is rife with potholes. Also, the last parts of this trail often retain snow well into July. Avoid this hike on a hot day, as you'll be in the open about 95 percent of the time.

## GPS Trailhead Coordinates

UTM Zone (WGS84) 10T

Easting 555627

Northing 5063837

Latitude N 45.72585°

Longitude W 122.28513°

## IN BRIEF

There are several ways to reach the summit of Silver Star Mountain; this is the longest and toughest path to climb, and possibly the hardest to reach. But it is without question the most entertaining option, offering back-to-back excellent views, heaps of flowers, and few hikers, giving it an almost expeditionary feel.

## DESCRIPTION

*Epic.* That's the word that always comes to mind when I think of this hike. By the end of the (long, often hot) day, you'll feel like you've been on an adventure. And as you sit atop Silver Star, with all the slackers who came up one of the easy ways, you can tell them you ain't done nothin' if you ain't done Bluff Mountain Trail.

Speaking of those "easy" ways, one of them, Ed's Trail, is described in this book's Silver Star Mountain profile (hike 19, page 87). It's also a tedious drive, but the hike is easier than this one.

------------------------------------------

### *Directions* ———————————→

Take I-205 from Portland, driving 5 miles north of the Columbia River to take Exit 30B/Orchards. Turn right on WA 500 East, which turns into WA 503 in 0.9 miles (follow signs for Battle Ground). Continue 14.7 miles on WA 503, then make a right turn onto NE Rock Creek Road, which turns into Lucia Falls Road. Drive 8.5 miles on this road, then take a right onto NE Sunset Falls Road and follow it 7.4 miles to Sunset Campground. Turn right to go through the campground and across a bridge over the East Fork Lewis River, then leave the pavement, driving 9 bumpy miles on FS 41 to a big ridgetop parking area. The trailhead is on the right.

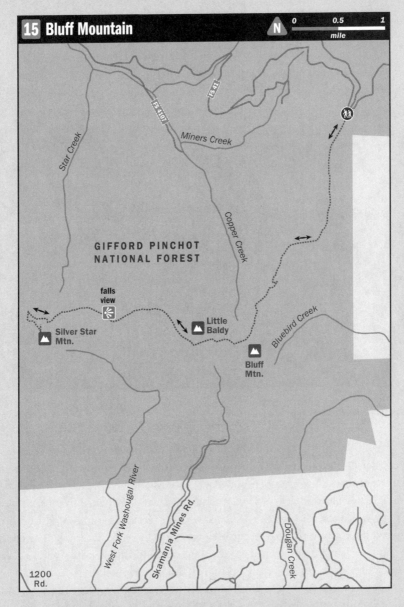

N

0    0.5    1
mile

FS 411

FS 4107

Star Creek

Miners Creek

Copper Creek

GIFFORD PINCHOT
NATIONAL FOREST

falls
view

Silver Star
Mtn.

Little
Baldy

Bluff
Mtn.

Bluebird Creek

West Fork Washougal River

Skamania Mines Rd.

Dougan Creek

1200
Rd.

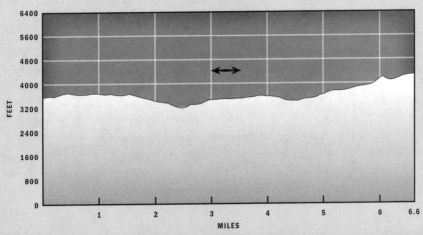

| FEET | | | | | | | |
|---|---|---|---|---|---|---|---|
| 6400 | | | | | | | |
| 5600 | | | | | | | |
| 4800 | | | | | | | |
| 4000 | | | | | | | |
| 3200 | | | | | | | |
| 2400 | | | | | | | |
| 1600 | | | | | | | |
| 800 | | | | | | | |
| 0 | 1 | 2 | 3 | 4 | 5 | 6 | 6.6 |

MILES

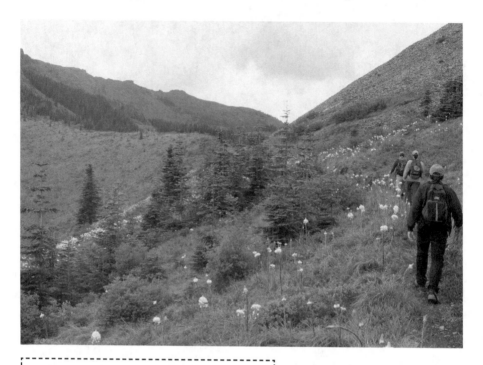

**Winding through the beargrass on Bluff Mountain Trail**

From the trailhead, Bluff Mountain Trail starts on an old jeep road along a ridge that looks and feels like it's way up in the alpine country of Mount Hood. That's because it's wide open and covered with flowers—but it's open because of a fire, not elevation. The 1902 Yacolt Burn was so intense that very few trees have grown back, though the 1960s saw some terracing and replanting.

Wander along this ridge, with views of other peaks and ridges swept clean by the fire, for 2.5 sun-baked miles, then descend into a notch where the road ends. Here, look for the trail taking off for the right (west) side of the ridge and passing under a series of dramatic cliffs (the north side of Bluff Mountain), with views of Little Baldy off to the right. You will probably have to skip over a couple of small creeks, which will be welcome sights on hot summer days.

At 3.5 miles, the trail climbs westward into a patch of forest notable for thickly packed, thin trees that seem like clones of one other. Emerging from this forest at 3.8 miles, you'll be greeted by a big view of your destination, the two-humped Silver Star Mountain, ahead. Having come this far and climbed through a forest to be greeted by this view, don't you feel like you're on an expedition? Silver Star looks bigger and more dramatic than other peaks, as its generally treeless east face rises beyond an impressive foreground.

Back out in the sun, continue south along the east side of Little Baldy, and in just under 5 miles you'll have a view of a big waterfall on Silver Star's flanks. At 5.3 miles, continue straight through an intersection with Trail 175, and you'll soon climb to the dramatic (perhaps nerve-wracking, for the acrophobic) ridges of Silver Star, which you wind along for almost a mile before descending into forest again just below the peak.

In these woods, your path intersects a road coming in from the right; this is the end of the Ed's Trail hike. Turn left on the road for a fairly steep climb (stay left again when the road splits) to a saddle between Silver Star's peaks. The higher one is on the left, and the view from here is as impressive as the one on the 6.6-mile hike you just did. On a clear day, you can see from the Three Sisters to Mount Rainier, and since you're on the highest peak in the immediate vicinity, there's a sense of being on a mountain throne.

The next rock to the south is Pyramid Rock. It's not impressive in and of itself, but in recent years there have been reports of at least one mountain goat hanging around there. So keep an eye out.

# 16 FALLS CREEK FALLS

### KEY AT-A-GLANCE INFORMATION

**LENGTH: 3.4 miles to the lower falls, 6.1 if you also visit the top of the falls**

**CONFIGURATION: Out-and-back or balloon**

**DIFFICULTY: Easy–moderate**

**SCENERY: Shady forest, a serene stream, and a big-time waterfall**

**EXPOSURE: Some cliff edges (easily avoided) at the end of the trail**

**TRAFFIC: Moderate on weekends, light otherwise**

**TRAIL SURFACE: Packed dirt**

**HIKING TIME: 2 hours to see the lower falls, 3.5 for the whole loop**

**DRIVING DISTANCE: 68 miles (1 hour 20 minutes) from Pioneer Square**

**SEASON: May–November**

**BEST TIME: May–June**

**BACKPACKING OPTIONS: One decent site at Upper Falls**

**ACCESS: No fee**

**WHEELCHAIR ACCESS: None**

**MAPS: Green Trails #397 (Wind River)**

**FACILITIES: Outhouse at the trailhead**

**INFO: Mount Adams Ranger District, (509) 395-3400**

## GPS Trailhead Coordinates

UTM Zone (WGS84) 10T

Easting 582221

Northing 5084105

Latitude  N 45.90560°

Longitude  W 121.93996°

## IN BRIEF

Looking for an easy trail to a spectacular destination? This is it. This 1.7-mile ramble gains about 700 feet—which you'll hardly notice on the way and will forget entirely when you reach one of the area's most impressive waterfalls. And if you're willing to put in a little more effort, you can visit the top of the falls.

## DESCRIPTION

The trail starts out flat through second-growth forest, passing huckleberry, Oregon grape, and Douglas fir. Not much to see here, but at least you don't have to work hard. A hundred yards in, ignore Trail 152 on the left and continue up 152A. If you're doing the loop, you'll see 152 later.

After a quarter mile, you'll traverse meadows with a view of an interesting rock formation to the left. Soon after this, you'll cross the creek in a narrow gorge; look for some cool, round, water-formed rock faces.

At 0.6 miles, now in an older forest, you'll pass a couple of impressive root balls in an area

*Directions* _____➤

Take I-84 from Portland, driving 37 miles east of I-205 to Exit 44/Cascade Locks. As soon as you enter town, make your first right to get on Bridge of the Gods, following a sign for Stevenson, Washington. Pay the $1 toll, cross the river, and make a right onto WA 14. Go 5.9 miles and turn left, following a sign for Carson, Washington. This is Wind River Road. Drive 14.5 miles on Wind River Road, then turn right (staying on Wind River Road) and go 0.8 miles. Make a right onto the gravel FS 3062. Drive 2 miles on this road, and make a right onto FS 057, following a sign for Lower Falls Creek Falls Trail. The trailhead is 0.5 miles ahead, at the end of the road.

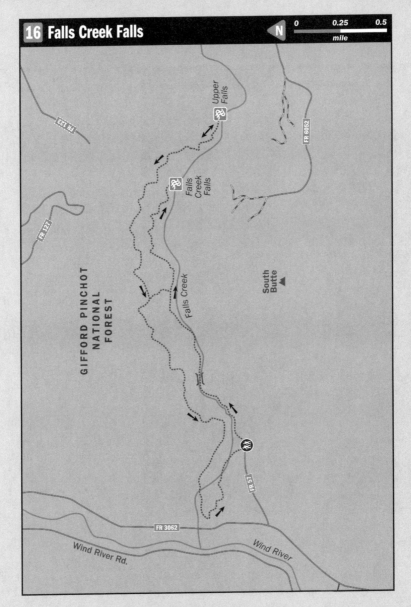

N

0        0.25        0.5
mile

FR 123

FR 127

GIFFORD PINCHOT NATIONAL FOREST

Upper Falls

FR 6052

Falls Creek Falls

Falls Creek

South Butte

FR 57

FR 3062

Wind River Rd.

Wind River

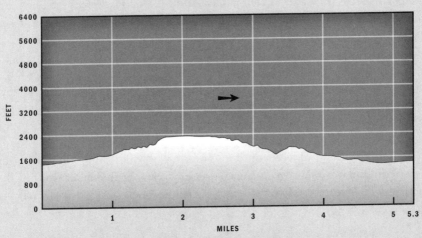

FEET

6400
5600
4800
4000
3200
2400
1600
800
0

1        2        3        4        5    5.3

MILES

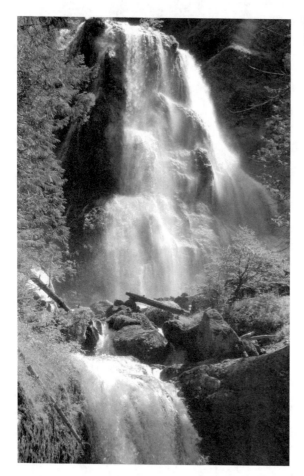

that might get treacherous when wet; a good slip could send you down toward the creek. At 0.75 miles, you pass nearly under a big Douglas fir; look for a dead one with countless woodpecker holes.

After hiking 1 mile almost effortlessly, you'll reach another junction with Trail 152; this is where the loop to the upper falls area takes off, but for now stay on the path you've been hiking. It may sound odd, but on this creek, Lower Falls is much more impressive than Upper Falls.

Over the next half mile, you'll pass a nice creekside picnic area on the right, cross a metal bridge over a lovely cascading creek, and go under a big rock formation on the left. By this time you should be hearing, and seeing through the trees, the main, lower falls.

When you arrive at the falls, in an area of large boulders that provide plenty of seating, you'll see two levels of falls plunging into a mossy bowl filled with maidenhair ferns. (In fact, there's a hidden, third level even higher, making for a total drop of 200 feet.) The whole scene seems like something straight out of *The Lord of the Rings;* one expects to see archers on the hill, guarding their sacred pool. It's particularly impressive in the early summer, when water flows are high.

Linger here a while, then on your way back consider taking the upper loop, recently maintained and signed by the Washington Trails Association. Follow the 152 steeply up through a draw to a junction at a sign. Turn right, following pointers for Road 165, and you'll climb another 0.5 miles—your last uphill for the day!

Right after the trail levels off, look for a social trail leading right 50 yards or so to the top of some cliffs. Here, you'll get a view of the upper third of the big falls, and down the canyon to some of the peaks of Trapper Creek Wilderness (hike 21, page 95).

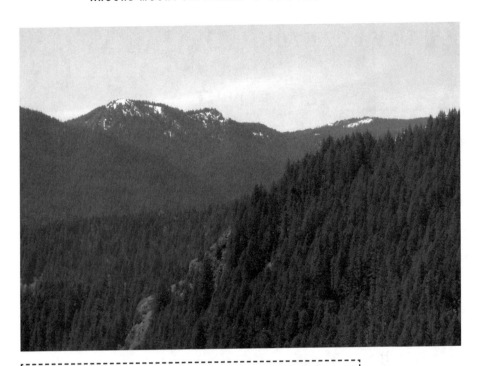

The peaks of Trapper Creek Wilderness, from Upper Falls Creek Falls Trail

Walk another five minutes and you're back at the creek, where a trail leads right and to another view. From this point, there's a sketchy path down toward the top of the falls; it can be done, but be *very* careful, and keep dogs leashed and kids nearby. Even if you don't go down there, you'll notice that you can't see the lower viewpoint from here—you're seeing a whole new section of falls.

There is a tiny bit of hiking left here, but it's just a few minutes to Upper Falls. Though the falls is only about six feet high, maybe, it does have a nice campsite where you can overnight or picnic before heading back.

When you do head back, stay with the 152 all the way down, just to see some new terrain. It is unspectacular but uncrowded. After 2 miles you'll cross Falls Creek on a bridge, turn left to walk half a mile along the water's edge, then reach the first junction you saw today, 100 yards from your car.

# 17  LAVA CANYON

## KEY AT-A-GLANCE INFORMATION

**LENGTH:** 1–6 miles

**CONFIGURATION:** Out-and-back, loop

**DIFFICULTY:** Easy for the upper section, difficult to do the whole thing

**SCENERY:** Waterfalls, canyon, geological wonders, suspension bridge

**EXPOSURE:** Mostly open; several sections are quite exposed. In fact, people have fallen to their deaths here; if it's rained or snowed recently, or if you don't like heights, stick to upper section.

**TRAFFIC:** Very heavy on summer weekends, heavy during the week, and moderate the rest of the season

**TRAIL SURFACE:** Paved, boardwalk, gravel, and a ladder

**HIKING TIME:** 30 minutes to do upper loop, 3 hours to do the whole thing

**DRIVING DISTANCE:** 85 miles (1 hour 40 minutes) from Pioneer Square

**SEASON:** June–October; call in June to make sure the road is snow-free

**BEST TIME:** June for water flow, October for fall colors

**ACCESS:** Northwest Forest Pass required

**WHEELCHAIR ACCESS:** There is a barrier-free trail in the upper section.

**MAPS:** USFS Mount St. Helens National Monument

**FACILITIES:** Toilets at the trailhead, but no water

**INFO:** Mount St. Helens National Volcanic Monument, (360) 449-7800

## GPS Trailhead Coordinates

UTM Zone (WGS84) 10T

Easting 570382

Northing 5112887

Latitude   N 46.16592°

Longitude  W 122.08832°

## IN BRIEF

An unparalleled look at geological forces at work, Lava Canyon is also a beautiful place to be, with several waterfalls, a dramatic bridge, some challenging hiking, and a short, barrier-free loop trail.

## DESCRIPTION

First, a little history, so you'll know what you're looking at here. In ancient times, a forest covered a deep valley. Then, 3,500 years ago, Mount St. Helens erupted, sending a massive mudflow down through the canyon, filling it with volcanic rock. Over the years, the river carved a path through the rock, forming a canyon with waterfalls, deep cuts, and towers of harder rock—Lava Canyon. Later mudflows covered all of that, and eventually forest grew back over the whole thing.

Then, on May 18, 1980, Mount St. Helens erupted again, melting 70 percent of its glaciers in an instant and sending millions of cubic feet of mud and rock blasting down the side of the mountain at about 45 miles an hour. That eruption cleaned out the forest and rock, exposing Lava Canyon for the first time in thousands of years. As you drove in, you got a glimpse of this 1980 mudflow (also

## Directions

Take I-5 from Portland, driving 21 miles north of the Columbia River to Exit 21/Woodland, then make a right onto WA 503 (Lewis River Road). Drive 23 miles, continuing straight to leave 503 for the 503 Spur. Ten miles ahead (3 miles past the town of Cougar), the 503 Spur turns into FS 90. Travel 3.5 miles on FS 90, then turn left onto FS 83, following a sign for Ape Cave and Lava Canyon. The Lava Canyon trailhead is 11.5 miles ahead, at the end of FS 83.

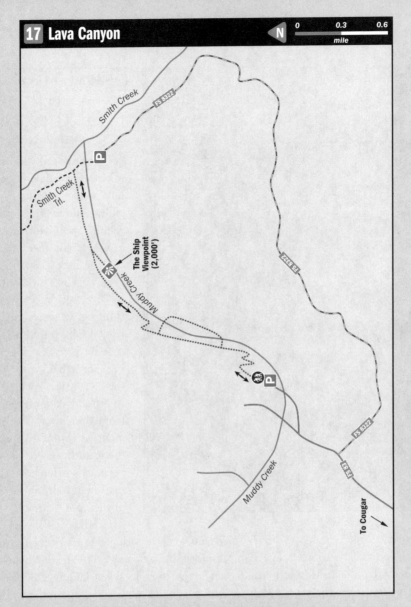

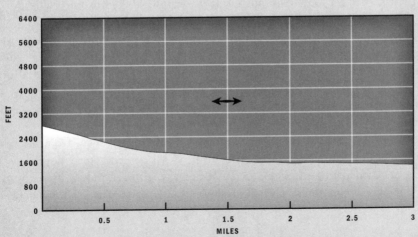

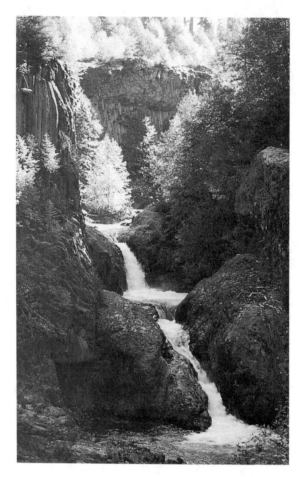

Waterfalls in Lava Canyon

known as a "lahar"); now go see what it gave us.

From the trailhead, take the paved path leading left, which, though officially barrier-free, would require some work to push a wheelchair through. You can see here that the trees around you survived the 1980 eruption, but everything below was wiped out. Also, look around for trees that have rocks embedded in them—that's how strong the eruption was, and this point is some 5 miles from the crater. The pavement will soon give way to boardwalk; two viewing platforms offer both information and dramatic views of the upper canyon.

Hike 0.4 miles to a junction with the loop trail. By now you've seen perhaps 15 warning signs telling you about various dangers and imploring you to stay on the trail. My favorite such sign is at this junction: "danger" is written in seven languages—and you have to get off the trail to read it! Anyway, be careful, and stay on the trail.

For the longer loop, continue straight for now; 100 yards on you'll have a nice view of a waterfall and the swirling pools above it. In 0.2 miles you'll come to the suspension bridge. Only 3 feet wide and 100 feet long, it was built by the same company that built the suspension bridge at Drift Creek Falls (hike 49, page 223). Kids, dogs, and people afraid of heights should not go beyond the suspension bridge, and everyone should be careful if it has rained recently. If you'd like to do only a 1.3-mile loop, cross the bridge and follow the trail back up to reach the first intersection after crossing another small bridge.

Otherwise, follow the trail downhill (and I do mean down) from the suspension bridge. In the next section of trail, you'll descend steep slopes, walk along unguarded ledges, cross a couple of creeks with no bridges (though one has a cable to hang onto), and climb down a 40-foot ladder. So if it has been raining, or you have small kids, or you're tired or nervous about heights, think twice before you go past the bridge.

After a steep half-mile descent that passes several beautiful waterfalls and an area where the river flows through a chute just a few feet wide, the trail mellows somewhat. After you've hiked a total of 1.1 miles, you'll climb down a ladder (be careful if your shoes are wet!) and then cross a mossy stream. The rock formation on your right is known as the Ship; it was one of the formations left standing thousands of years ago when the river cut a new course through the ancient canyon. The top of the Ship was the floor of the valley before 1980. There's a little perspective, eh?

It's worth the effort to get to the top of the Ship. A couple hundred yards past the ladder, an unsigned trail on the right leads 0.2 miles up it; it's pretty steep and includes rock steps and yet another (smaller) ladder, but there are late-summer huckleberries up there, and it's a heck of a place for a picnic, with an excellent view back up the canyon.

At this point, you've seen the best of the hike, so it's a good spot to turn around. But if you'd like to keep going, Lava Canyon Trail continues another 1.3 miles to the Smith Creek trailhead, losing 350 feet in elevation on the way. There's a bridge over the creek just 0.4 miles below the Ship trail that is worth visiting.

When you head back, cross the suspension bridge and take the loop hike back onto a pre-1980 lava flow. When you cross a small metal bridge, turn left, and you're 0.4 miles from your car.

# 18 LEWIS RIVER

 **KEY AT-A-GLANCE INFORMATION**

**LENGTH:** 5.2 miles
**CONFIGURATION:** Out-and-back
**DIFFICULTY:** Easy
**SCENERY:** Several waterfalls, a wild stream flowing through a wooded canyon, old-growth forest
**EXPOSURE:** Shady all the way
**TRAFFIC:** Heavy all summer long, especially on weekends
**TRAIL SURFACE:** Gravel at first, then packed dirt with some roots
**HIKING TIME:** 3 hours
**DRIVING DISTANCE:** 92 miles (2 hours 10 minutes) from Pioneer Square
**SEASON:** April–November; call ahead to see if the road is snow-free
**BEST TIME:** Early summer or fall
**BACKPACKING OPTIONS:** A few decent sites along the river
**ACCESS:** Northwest Forest Pass required
**WHEELCHAIR ACCESS:** Campground only
**MAPS:** Green Trails #365 (Lone Butte)
**FACILITIES:** Toilets at trailhead; May–October there's drinking water in campground
**INFO:** Mount St. Helens National Volcanic Monument, (360) 449-7800

## IN BRIEF

Here's a pleasant, mostly flat stroll along a beautiful river with three dramatic waterfalls. Chances are, they're unlike most falls you've seen. The long drive to the trailhead is worth it, especially if you get a campsite at the Lower Falls Recreation Area and make a night of it.

## DESCRIPTION

From the trailhead in the picnic area, follow a trail that starts just left of the restrooms. In 100 yards, turn right to reach several viewpoints above Lower Falls, one of the most dramatic falls around. The water looks like it's spilling off a shelf, and in fact it is—this is the edge of an ancient lava flow. Over the next stretch of trail, you're walking around the campground, so there are a lot of trails. Turning left will send you into the campground, but turning right will offer several opportunities to get down to the river. Once you're safely above the falls, there are some nice swimming spots.

About half a mile after you leave the campground area, look for a bridge (or,

## Directions

Take I-5 from Portland, driving 21 miles north of the Columbia River to Exit 21/Woodland. Make a right on WA 503 (Lewis River Road), which after 31 miles (2 miles past the town of Cougar) turns into FS 90. Continue 30 more miles on FS 90 (you'll have to turn right just past the Pine Creek Information Center to stay on FS 90) to reach the Lower Lewis River Falls Recreation Area. Take the first right off the entrance road for the trailhead. You may notice that a mile before the campground on FS 90 there's a Lewis River trailhead, just past a bridge. You can start there if you'd like, but it adds 3 miles to the round-trip hike without adding waterfalls.

GPS Trailhead
Coordinates

UTM Zone (WGS84) 10T
Easting 586514
Northing 5111845
Latitude   N  46.15469°
Longitude  W  121.87958°

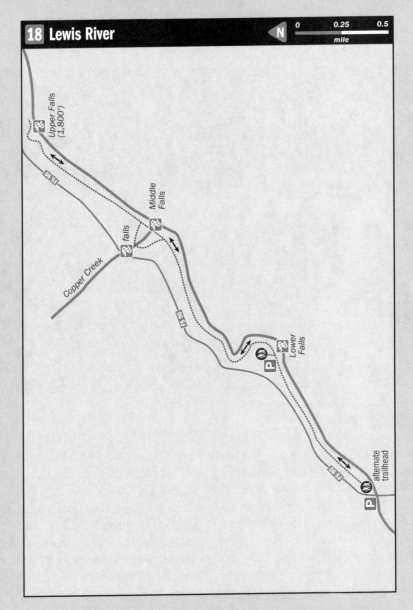

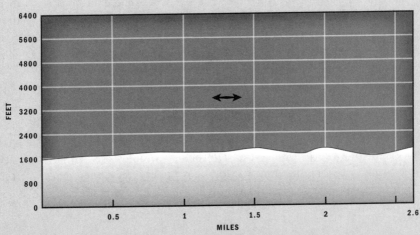

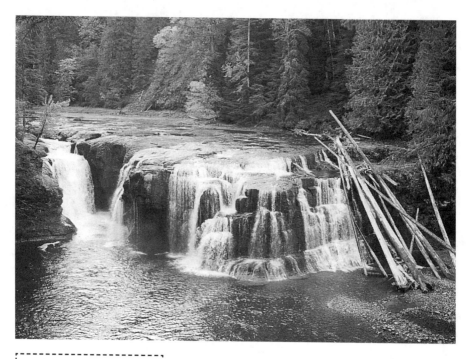

Lower Falls on the Lewis River

rather, half a bridge) across the river. According to the 1965 USGS map of the area, Lewis River Campground used to be on the far side of the river, so that bridge offered access from the campground to this trail.

Around 0.8 miles from the campground, you'll pass the top of a small water-fall, and then at 1.2 miles you'll cross another, larger falls, which looks like a waterslide into the Lewis River (don't try it). On the left, you may notice two trails leading up the hill, one just before Copper Creek and one just after. This is a half-mile scenic loop you can do on the way back, if you'd like. Just past the second of these trails, the main trail arrives at Middle Falls, another shelflike falls.

Back on the main trail, you'll soon pass under some enormous cliffs then descend into an area with some seriously large trees. There are western red cedars here that are close to six feet in diameter, and one Douglas fir on the left that must be ten feet in diameter. Just past this area you'll come to a campsite on the right, then the amphitheater of Upper Falls, which makes an 80-foot plunge. There are good logs and rocks in the sun here for picnicking or just lounging. A trail to the left leads 0.2 miles up the hill to a platform at the top of Upper Falls, a very worth-while side trip. Just above it there's a view of another falls above Upper Falls.

On the way back, just before Middle Falls, go ahead and take the "Copper Creek scenic byway." Just make the right before Middle Falls, climb briefly to another waterfall along the trail that follows Copper Creek, then make a left at the fork (the road is to the right) and you'll be back on the main trail, 1.5 miles from your car.

# SILVER STAR MOUNTAIN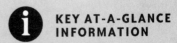

## IN BRIEF

You may be reading the directions to this one and thinking, "What a drive!" But when you're on Ed's Trail approaching Silver Star Mountain, you'll be thinking, "This is too beautiful and mountainous to be so close to town!" This flower-soaked traverse through rocky, alpine country is worth all the hassles of getting there.

## DESCRIPTION

Even the trailhead for this one is scenic, and, other than a few short stretches here and there, every foot of the trail is, too. From the trailhead, look for the path heading to the right, past a brown hiker's sign. Follow this pathway through several brushy switchbacks to an old jeep road, then head up that 150 yards to a wide gravel area with a nice view of Mount Hood through a notch in a ridge. Stop here, at the half-mile point, and catch your breath.

Where the road swings back to the right and heads uphill, look for Ed's Trail heading

---

## *Directions* ⟶

Take I-205 from Portland, driving 5 miles north of the Columbia River to Exit 30B/Orchards. Make a right on WA 500 East, which turns into WA 503 in 0.9 miles (follow signs for Battle Ground). Continue 14.7 miles on WA 503, then make a right on NE Rock Creek Road, which turns into Lucia Falls Road. Drive 8.5 miles on this road, take a right on NE Sunset Falls Road, follow it 2 miles, and turn right on NE Dole Valley Road. Go 2.4 miles on this road, and turn left on Road L 1100—you'll see "1100" on a tree, and a sign for Tarbell Picnic Area. On this road, continue straight at 2.2 miles, bear left (downhill) at 4.3 miles, then turn right (uphill) at 7.7 miles. The trailhead is 2.6 miles up, at the end of this narrow, bumpy road.

## KEY AT-A-GLANCE INFORMATION

**LENGTH:** 4.8 miles

**CONFIGURATION:** Balloon

**DIFFICULTY:** Moderate

**SCENERY:** Wildflowers, open ridgetops, rocky crags, a natural arch, several volcanoes

**EXPOSURE:** In the sun the whole time, with occasional stretches along rocky cliff edges and one brief section of semi-climbing

**TRAFFIC:** Moderate on weekends, light otherwise

**TRAIL SURFACE:** Dirt, rocks, some scrambling

**HIKING TIME:** 3 hours

**DRIVING DISTANCE:** 56 miles (1 hour 30 minutes) from Pioneer Square

**SEASON:** June–October

**BEST TIME:** July for flowers, October for cool temps

**BACKPACKING OPTIONS:** Poor

**ACCESS:** No fee

**WHEELCHAIR ACCESS:** None

**MAPS:** Green Trails #396 (Lookout Mountain) and #428 (Bridal Veil), though Ed's Trail isn't on either one

**FACILITIES:** None at trailhead; available in a campground along the way

**INFO:** Mount Adams Ranger District, (509) 395-3400

**SPECIAL COMMENTS:** The road to this one is not exactly smooth, but it passed my 1992 Nissan Sentra test.

---

GPS Trailhead
Coordinates

UTM Zone (WGS84) 10T

Easting 558960

Northing 5068391

Latitude N 45.76656°

Longitude W 122.24174°

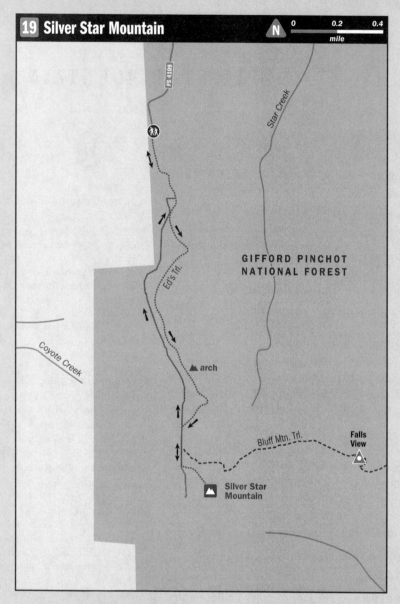

N

0        0.2        0.4
mile

FS 4109

Star Creek

GIFFORD PINCHOT
NATIONAL FOREST

Ed's Trl.

Coyote Creek

▲ arch

Bluff Mtn. Trl.

Falls
View

▲ Silver Star
Mountain

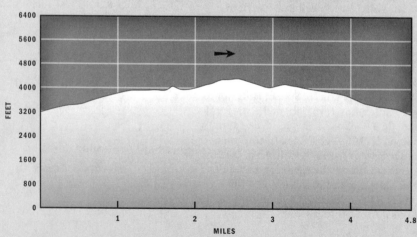

FEET

6400
5600
4800
4000
3200
2400
1600
800
0

1        2        3        4   4.8

MILES

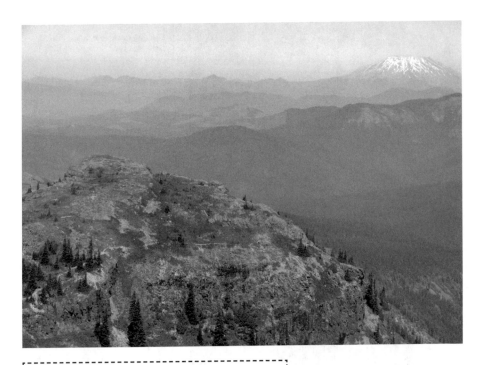

Mount St. Helens from the summit of Silver Star Mountain

left, along the ridge. We'll come back on the road, but it's better to follow Ed for now. Ed was Edward Robertson, a cofounder of the Chinook Trail Association, which built and maintains this trail. Ed must have been a lover of flowers and open country, because his trail is an amazing piece of work: an ambling, gentle climb along a ridge that looks as if it's thousands of feet higher than it really is. That's because in 1902, fires razed the forest, and very few trees have grown back—though more than 100 varieties of wildflowers and flowering shrubs have. So it's like you're getting a look at the decorated skeletons of the mountains, complete with bony spurs, cliffs, and rock formations normally covered by forest.

Climb toward some of these exposed formations, ascending 0.7 miles before the trail flattens out and starts a tour of the rocky ridgetop. At 1.5 miles, pass through a rock arch and beside a small, overhanging cave that offers just about the only shade around on a hot day. Soon the trail takes off up the ridge face, forcing you to almost climb in spots as you scramble up through the rocks to your first view of the two-humped Silver Star ahead. Dramatic, huh?

Now the trail descends through meadows and into the trees, then climbs again to a junction with the road you left behind. (This whole Ed's Trail was just a scenic, adventurous diversion.) Follow the road to the left, staying left at a junction a couple hundred yards up, and after 0.25 miles the road approaches a saddle between the two peaks. Head left for the big (shadeless) view at the official

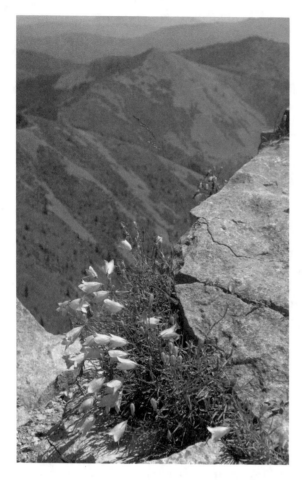

Looking east from Silver Star at
Little Baldy

summit, and enjoy views of the Columbia River Gorge, Mount Defiance (with radio towers), the back of Dog Mountain, Larch Mountain, the Portland area, and everything from Mount Jefferson to Mount Rainier. Look, also, for Bluff Mountain Trail (hike 15, page 72) along the narrow ridges to the east.

Silver Star Mountain got its name because, when seen from above, the ridges running out from the summit form a five-pointed star.

The next rock to the south is Pyramid Rock. It's not impressive in and of itself, but in recent years there have been reports of at least one mountain goat hanging around there. So keep an eye out.

On your way back to the car, enjoy some different scenery while avoiding a treacherous descent of Ed's Trail. Simply stay on the jeep road as it winds along the opposite side of the ridge. This will take you back to the far end of Ed's Trail, where you picked it up, and then to your car.

# SIOUXON CREEK  20

## IN BRIEF

An easy, pleasant stroll along a mountain stream, with old-growth forest and waterfalls all around, plus options that include a stream crossing and rugged climbing. What more could you want? Even the kids will like it; with supervision, they could go for a swim.

## DESCRIPTION

The only spectacular thing about this hike is how easy and scenic it is. There are no panoramic viewpoints, no exotic geological features, and no serious hiking challenges—unless you want them. It's just a beautiful river in a peaceful, lush, tree-filled canyon, with waterfalls all over the place and not too many hikers.

In fact, two mysteries have long intrigued me about this hike: One is why more people don't seem to know about it, and the other is why most people stop at Chinook Falls, when there are numerous beautiful spots farther up the creek, and the most amazing falls of all (Wildcat) just across it.

From the trailhead, there are several paths into the woods. Take any one and turn

### KEY AT-A-GLANCE INFORMATION

**LENGTH:** 10.8 miles along the creek, with side trips possible
**CONFIGURATION:** Out-and-back with an optional loop
**DIFFICULTY:** Easy–moderate along the creek, difficult to Siouxon Peak
**SCENERY:** Old-growth forest, waterfalls, pools in the river, mountaintop viewpoint
**EXPOSURE:** Shady all the way, optional creek wading, one set of slippery rocks
**TRAFFIC:** Moderate on summer weekends, light otherwise
**TRAIL SURFACE:** Packed dirt with some rocks and roots
**HIKING TIME:** 3–5 hours; more for the peak
**DRIVING DISTANCE:** 55 miles (1 hour 30 minutes) from Pioneer Square
**SEASON:** Year-round; muddy in winter and spring, with occasional snow
**BEST TIME:** Early summer or fall
**BACKPACKING OPTIONS:** Several good sites along the creek
**ACCESS:** Northwest Forest Pass required
**WHEELCHAIR ACCESS:** None
**MAPS:** Green Trails #396 (Lookout Mountain)
**FACILITIES:** None at trailhead; water on trail must be treated
**INFO:** Mount St. Helens National Volcanic Monument, (360) 449-7800

## Directions

Take I-205 from Portland, driving 5 miles north of the Columbia River to Exit 30B/Orchards. Make a right on WA 500, which turns into WA 503 in 0.9 miles (follow signs for Battle Ground). Continue 25 miles on WA 503, passing through the town of Amboy. Just past the Mount St. Helens National Volcanic Monument headquarters, make a right on NE Healy Road. Go 9 miles (note that Healy turns into FS 54 at 2.4 miles), then turn left (uphill) on FS 57. After 1.2 miles on FS 57, turn left on FS 5701. The trailhead is 3.6 miles ahead, at the end of the road.

### GPS Trailhead Coordinates

UTM Zone (WGS84) 10T
Easting 563772
Northing 5088452
Latitude   N 45.94668°
Longitude W 122.17721°

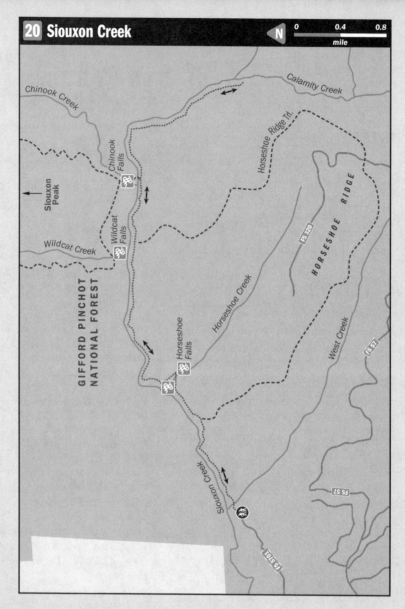

N

0        0.4        0.8
mile

Calamity Creek

Chinook Creek

Horseshoe Ridge Trl.

Siouxon Peak

Chinook Falls

Wildcat Falls

Wildcat Creek

HORSESHOE RIDGE

FS 320

Horseshoe Creek

GIFFORD PINCHOT
NATIONAL FOREST

Horseshoe Falls

West Creek

FS 57

Siouxon Creek

FS 57

FS 5701

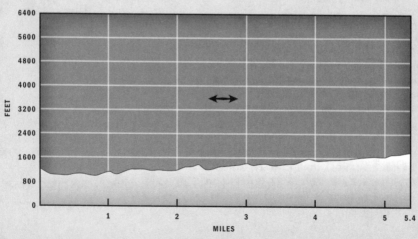

| FEET | | | | | |
|---|---|---|---|---|---|
| 6400 | | | | | |
| 5600 | | | | | |
| 4800 | | | | | |
| 4000 | | | | | |
| 3200 | | | | | |
| 2400 | | | | | |
| 1600 | | | | | |
| 800 | | | | | |
| 0 | 1 | 2 | 3 | 4 | 5  5.4 |

MILES

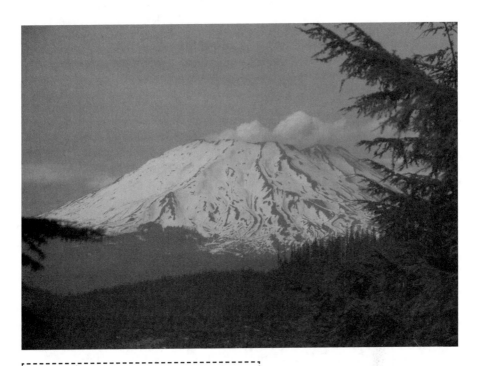

Mount St. Helens seen from the trail to Siouxon Peak

right when you reach the main trail. You'll walk downhill briefly, cross West Creek on a log bridge, then stroll over a small ridge to Siouxon Creek—and the first of many good campsites. At 0.9 miles you'll see, on the right, Horseshoe Ridge Trail, which makes a 7-mile, rugged, and solitary loop back to this trail. After 1.4 miles, your trail crosses Horseshoe Creek (so named because it drains a horseshoe-shaped ridge, of which you're crossing the open mouth). There will be a waterfall above and below you here; to get a view of the lower one, and visit a fine campsite, take a side trail to the left just after the bridge.

Over the next 0.3 miles you'll climb slightly to a viewpoint of Siouxon Falls, which could almost be called a really big rapids, as opposed to a classic falls. Then the trail traverses flat ground for half a mile, some 200 feet above the creek, before dropping to its side for half a mile. This is where some swimming might happen—just know that any dip will be brief, unless you're part polar bear.

At the 3-mile mark, you'll see two side trails in quick succession. The first, unmarked and on the left, leads down to the creek; this is one way to reach Wildcat Falls, but it involves a tricky crossing of Siouxon Creek that will be difficult for most people until late summer, at least. There's an easier way a little farther up. The second trail you'll see, heading up and to the right, is the second appearance of Horseshoe Ridge Trail.

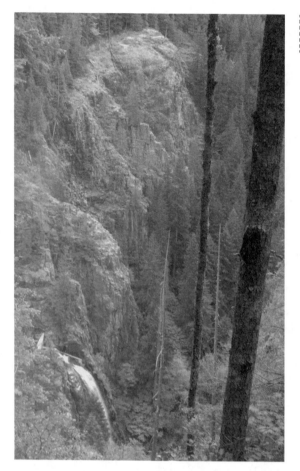

Go another 0.7 miles and you'll come to an unnamed creek on the right; careful here, as the rocks tend to be slick. There's also a nice bridge over Siouxon Creek, which at this point flows through a narrow gorge. Cross the bridge and go 0.3 miles to the beautiful, 50-foot Chinook Falls. There's also a good campsite along this trail.

Here, there are decisions to make. You could head back the way you came and, at just under 8 miles, call it a day. Or you could go visit Wildcat Falls by wading across Chinook Creek here and following an up-and-down trail to the left for half a mile to Wildcat Creek. Go up that creek from a junction, and after 0.2 miles you'll arrive at the base of the 100-foot beauty. The views are even more dramatic farther up the trail. And if you're *really* looking for some exercise, go another 3.5 miles (and about 3,000 feet) up this trail to Siouxon Peak, following a route that's well marked on the Green Trails map.

At the very least, from the bridge near Chinook Falls, go a little farther up Siouxon Creek. I have no idea why no other guidebook recommends this, because it's just as beautiful up there, requires no more effort, and passes several more waterfalls. There's another 1.7 miles of creekside trail, ending at a crossing of Calamity Creek (no bridge) and gaining only another 250 feet. Beyond Calamity Creek the trail climbs away from Siouxon, ending some 2 dull miles later on a road near Observation Peak and Sister Rocks.

# TRAPPER CREEK WILDERNESS  21

## IN BRIEF

This is like a secret hike. Most people have never heard of it, but everybody who goes there loves it. It's quiet and woodsy, with lots of creeks, two waterfalls, great campsites, and—if you want some elevation—a great view from Observation Peak.

## DESCRIPTION

I can't explain why so few people have heard of Trapper Creek. It's just over an hour from Portland, it's loaded with trails, and it couldn't be any prettier. If you're a fan of the forest, and especially if you don't mind climbing, this is the place to be. One section of the wilderness was actually set aside in the 1950s as a research area for old-growth Pacific silver firs. And up on the ridge, there are huckleberries—the big, blue, juicy kind—everywhere.

The wilderness covers a little more than 6,000 acres, and it's basically one U-shaped watershed, drained by Trapper Creek and its many tributaries. It's heavily forested with firs, hemlocks, cedars, and pines. Wildflowers are abundant in the spring and early summer, and

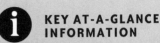

### KEY AT-A-GLANCE INFORMATION

**LENGTH:** 14.5 miles, but options abound

**CONFIGURATION:** Loop

**DIFFICULTY:** Easy–strenuous

**TRAFFIC:** Moderate on summer weekends, light otherwise

**SCENERY:** Magnificent forest, two waterfalls, a sweeping mountaintop view

**EXPOSURE:** A couple of lookouts, otherwise in the woods

**TRAFFIC:** Moderate on summer weekends, otherwise light

**TRAIL SURFACE:** Packed dirt, and rocks

**HIKING TIME:** 8 hours to do the big loop

**DRIVING DISTANCE:** 66 miles (1 hour 30 minutes) from Pioneer Square

**SEASON:** July–October to climb the ridge; lower elevations May–November

**BEST TIME:** September–October

**BACKPACKING OPTIONS:** Several nice sites

**ACCESS:** Northwest Forest Pass required

**WHEELCHAIR ACCESS:** None

**MAPS:** USFS Trapper Creek Wilderness

**FACILITIES:** None at trailhead; water everywhere, but it must be treated

**INFO:** Mount Adams Ranger District, (509) 395-3400

## Directions ⟶

Take I-84 from Portland, driving 37 miles east of I-205 to Exit 44/Cascade Locks. As soon as you enter Cascade Locks, make your first right to get on Bridge of the Gods, following a sign for Stevenson, Washington. Pay the $1 toll, cross the river, and turn right on WA 14. Go 5.8 miles and turn left, following a sign for Carson, Washington. This is Wind River Road. Drive 14.5 miles on this road, then continue straight, leaving Wind River Road and following a sign for Government Mineral Springs. Half a mile later, turn right on FS 5401; the trailhead is 0.4 miles ahead, at the end of the road.

## GPS Trailhead Coordinates

UTM Zone (WGS84) 10T

Easting 578462

Northing 5081467

Latitude  N 45.88230°

Longitude W 121.98884°

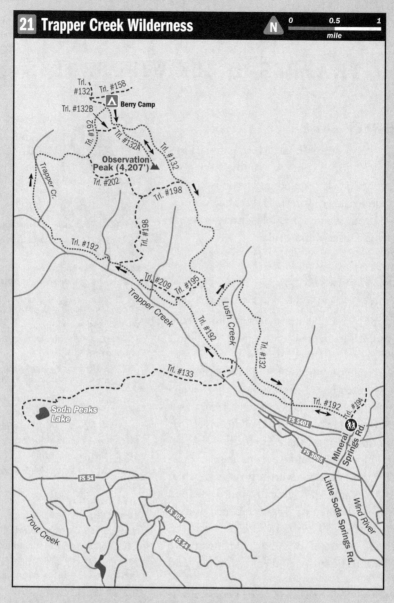

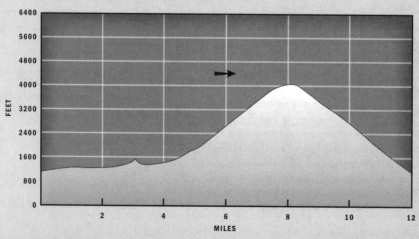

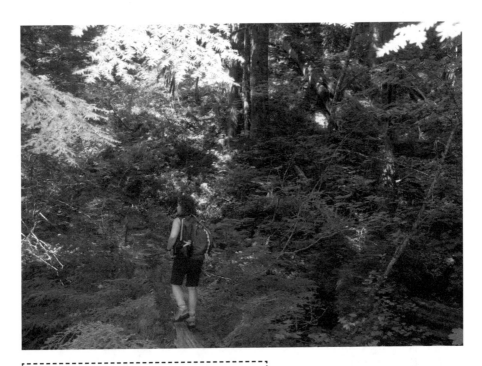

A one-log creek crossing in Trapper Creek Wilderness

the animals here include owls, black bears, cougars, and bobcats—though the only sign I've seen of any of those was the sound of an owl and some very fresh, berry-filled bear scat on the trail. You have virtually nothing to fear from a black bear; if you see one, you'll likely see its rump disappearing into the woods.

To explore this area, you have numerous options: casually wander the old-growth forest, climb to a seldom-visited lake, slog up the hill to the big view, or take one of several semi-maintained "adventure trails." Let this challenging 14.5-mile loop serve as an introduction, as it touches on all the other options, or plan for an overnight to break up the work a little.

From the trailhead, start into the woods on Trapper Creek Trail (192), which this loop follows 6 miles to its end. Right off the bat you'll intersect Dry Creek Trail (194), which runs about 4 miles north along Dry Creek. Half a mile out on 192, look for a rotting stump in the shape of an hourglass. Look, also, for such forest features as woodpecker holes in snags and new trees growing out of old stumps. Walk 0.9 miles, and you'll see Observation Trail (132) on the right; you'll be coming down this one if you do the big loop. For now, continue straight on 192—the forest gets even better as you get deeper into the canyon.

After another 0.7 leg-friendly miles, you'll cross Lush Creek and encounter Trail 133, Soda Peaks Trail, on the left. This leads to the one lake in the wilderness, Soda Peaks Lake; it's a climb of 2,500 feet in about 3 miles, and the trail doesn't loop back to this one. So unless you're looking for another hill to climb—or want to do some lakeside backpack camping—stay on 192, Trapper Creek Trail, to go up and around the end of a ridge, from which you'll get your first good views (or at least sounds) of Trapper Creek on the left.

About a mile later, barely climbing, you'll come to two trails: Big Slide Trail (195) and Deer Way Trail (209). Big Slide, like several other trails in the wilderness, was built and is maintained by the Mazamas, a Portland-based mountaineering club that has adopted this wilderness area. But before you go off on one of their trails, you should know a few things about Mazamas and their trails. For one thing—and I say this as a Mazama—there is an element in that crowd that uses the phrase "get your butt kicked" to mean "have a good time." Some of these trails were designed with that attitude: They're steep scrambles, without such niceties as switchbacks, and they can be tough to follow. And when a log falls across them, rather than cut the log away (like the Forest Service does), the Mazamas might cut a little notch in the top of it, to help you swing your leg over. So these trails are fun—and the Mazamas's signs are really cool—but they aren't what you would call "casual."

Deer Way Trail is basically an easy cutoff that avoids some elevation (plus scenery and campsites) for those in a hurry to get up the hill, so if that's your bag, take it. Otherwise, take Trapper Creek Trail, which dips down, for the first time, to almost touch Trapper Creek. Along the way, it passes Terrace Camp, a lovely spot with room for several tents. The trail continues steeply downhill, passing outrageous Douglas firs—some of which are on the ground, causing the trail to wind through them—and another campsite, even closer to the creek.

After a total of about 3 miles, the trail seems to disappear at a small side creek. In fact, it continues over a well-worn log, but there's a fun little side trip here, if you're up for it. Pick (and climb and crawl) your way up this creek a couple hundred feet or so, and you can get a view of a tall, hidden waterfall.

Continue 0.4 miles, passing the far end of the Deer Way cutoff, and next you'll cross Sunshine Trail (198) and its cool handmade sign. This Mazama masterpiece goes straight up about 2,000 feet in less than 2 miles. I've done it and wound up 80 percent lost and 110 percent exhausted; it's a "wonderful" butt-kicking.

Staying on Trapper Creek Trail, you'll have it pretty easy for another half mile, crossing Hidden Creek and a side trail to view Hidden Creek Falls. A trail on the left, at about 4 miles, leads to Rendezvous Flats, where you can enjoy some creekside loveliness; soon after, you'll pass a campsite at Cliff Creek. Then, if you'd like to, you can start climbing.

You'll put in about 1,700 feet in 2.5 miles, much of it in viewless switchbacks that are better for meditation than for any form of entertainment. There's a mighty nice bridge on the way, and about halfway up is a rocky ledge that makes a fine resting point with a view of a falls off to the left. And this ought to cheer you up: See that ridge over there, the really big one? Observation Peak is 600 feet higher than that.

When the climbing is done—you might notice a rare elevation sign saying 3,200 feet—you'll be in a dreamland forest. To my mind, there's nothing lovelier than a Northwest forest around 3,000 to 4,000 feet above sea level. And the crossing, at 3,300 feet, of Trapper Creek in a berry-filled basin is about as nice as it gets.

You'll cross one more Mazama trail, Rim Trail (202), before a trail (132B) to the right cuts off some distance to Observation Trail (132). Turn right here, then take another right on 132A in half a mile, and after just over a half mile of climbing you'll be at Observation Peak. Congratulations: you've now hiked 8 miles and gained a little more than 3,000 feet. Look for Mount St. Helens and its blast zone to the north; from there, around to the right, we have Mount Rainier, the Goat Rocks off on the horizon, and then Mount Adams, bigger than life. See if you can spot, well to the right of that, the meadow atop Dog Mountain—it's rare to see it from "behind"—and across from that the radio towers atop Mount Defiance, the highest point in the Columbia River Gorge. Right of that are Mounts Hood and Jefferson, and closer in are the two Soda Peaks, host to the aforementioned lake. Nice, huh?

Getting down from here is simple; just go back down the 132A trail you came up and turn right on Observation Trail (132). You can follow this trail 5 pretty boring miles to its end at the 192, a mile up from the parking lot, or you can test your knees going down a Mazama trail. Just turn right on either Sunshine Trail (198) or the much shorter Big Slide Trail (195), and don't blame me if you have a hard time walking the next day. Seriously, if you want to tackle one of these, go *up* them instead.

Either way you go, you'll come to Trapper Creek Trail; your car will be to the left.

## NEARBY ACTIVITIES

It's all about springs in this area. When you drive back down FS 5401 on your way out, take a right for Government Mineral Springs and follow signs to Iron Mike Well, for mineral water from an iron pump. Or, when you get back to Carson, go to Carson Hot Springs Resort, with its 1901 hotel and 1923 bathhouse and cabins. You can soak, get a massage, and then be wrapped in hot towels. A new hotel and golf course were in the works as this book went to press. Call (800) 607-3678 for details.

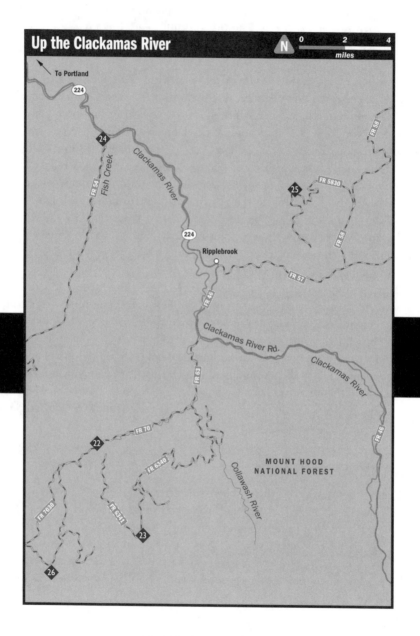

Up the Clackamas River

To Portland

224

24

FR 54 · Fish Creek · Clackamas River

224

Ripplebrook

FR 58

FR 5830

25

FR 58

FR 57

FR 46

Clackamas River Rd.

Clackamas River

FR 63

FR 70

22

FR 6340

FR 7020

FR 6341

Collawash River

MOUNT HOOD
NATIONAL FOREST

FR 46

23

26

N    0    2    4
          miles

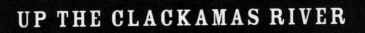

# UP THE CLACKAMAS RIVER

# 22 BAGBY HOT SPRINGS

## KEY AT-A-GLANCE INFORMATION

**LENGTH:** 3 miles round-trip to springs, 3.6 miles round-trip to Shower Creek
**CONFIGURATION:** Out-and-back
**DIFFICULTY:** Easy
**SCENERY:** Old-growth forest, a mountain stream, and wooden tubs of hot water
**EXPOSURE:** Shady all the way
**TRAFFIC:** Heavy
**TRAIL SURFACE:** Packed dirt and crushed rock with some muddy spots in winter and spring
**HIKING TIME:** 1 hour round-trip (not including time for a hot soak)
**DRIVING DISTANCE:** 74 miles (1 hour 35 minutes) from Pioneer Square
**SEASON:** March–November; sometimes open in winter, but call ahead for conditions
**BEST TIME:** Weekdays April–October
**BACKPACKING OPTIONS:** Several (crowded) sites just past the springs, many more up in the wilderness
**ACCESS:** Northwest Forest Pass required
**WHEELCHAIR ACCESS:** None
**MAPS:** USGS Bagby Hot Springs; USFS Bull of the Woods Wilderness
**FACILITIES:** Toilets but no water at the trailhead and the springs; stream water must be treated
**INFO:** Clackamas Ranger District office, (503) 630-6861
**SPECIAL COMMENTS:** Don't leave any valuables in your car at this trailhead.

## IN BRIEF

Unless you've got issues about being among naked people, this is one place you should absolutely visit; and even if you do dislike the disrobed, just avoid the bath houses. The hike isn't much of a challenge, but it's through sublime, ancient-growth forest. And the springs feature cedar-log tubs, some of them private. It can get rowdy on weekends (though alcohol is now banned at the springs), and there have been reports of car break-ins at the trailhead.

## DESCRIPTION

It seems everybody in the area knows about Bagby, even those who've never been there. Just the word seems to stand for something about life in the Pacific Northwest: soothing, relaxing, a retreat from the hustle and bustle, a journey back to the days of the ancient forest and natural elements.

Well, it's not just that. It can get a little crazy on weekends, and the chances you'll be the only one there are slim. On weekends you might have to wait to get your soak, unless you start early.

From the trailhead parking lot, start up the wide trail and cross the new, $200,000, 119-foot bridge over Nohorn Creek, named for an early pioneer in the area. The hiking

---

## GPS Trailhead Coordinates

UTM Zone (WGS84) 1oT
Easting 566395
Northing 4978642
Latitude N 44.95811°
Longitude W 122.15820°

## Directions

Take OR 224 from Portland, traveling 44 miles southeast of I-205, through the town of Estacada, to the Ranger Station at Ripplebrook. Turn right on FS 46. Drive 3.6 miles and make another right, onto FS 63. Travel 3.5 miles and turn right on FS 70. The trailhead is 6 miles ahead on the left.

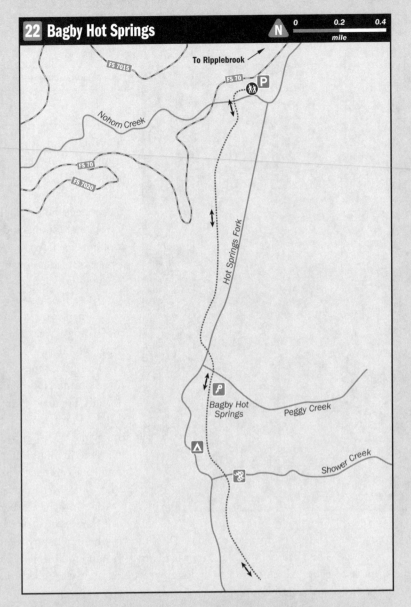

To Ripplebrook →

FS 7015

FS 70

P

Nohorn Creek

FS 70

FS 7020

Hot Springs Fork

P

Bagby Hot Springs

Peggy Creek

Shower Creek

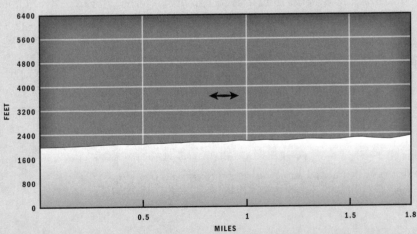

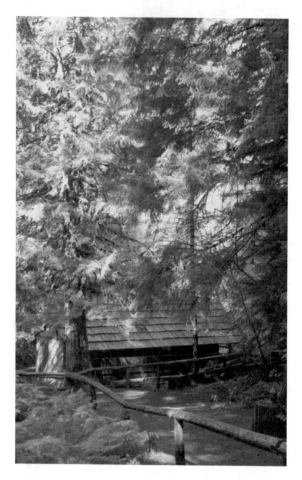

A bathhouse at Bagby Hot Springs

is pleasant, the river pools inviting, and the forest inspiring. You might notice some old metal loops tacked high in the trees; those once held telephone wires that connected fire lookouts back in the 1930s. Cross a bridge over Hot Springs Fork, and you're almost to the springs.

When you come to the springs area, the first thing you'll notice is the 1913 ranger cabin, which is listed on the National Register of Historic Places. It was a central communications station for those fire lookouts. I should mention that this cabin of 16-inch cedar logs was hand-built by one ranger, a certain Phil Putz, who first visited the area after walking 39 miles in one day. Do you think he was happy to arrive at the springs? The path behind the cabin leads to a monumental downed tree; check out the inside, which rotted away long before the giant was felled to keep it from squashing the bathhouses.

The bathhouse on the right has one big tub, with room for five or six adults. The one on the left has an open area with several tubs and five private rooms, each with a two-person log tub. The water comes out of the springs at 136°F and runs through a system of log flumes. To fill a tub, you just open up the valve and let the hot water in, then grab a bucket, fill it with cold water from a nearby tub, and get the temperature where you want it. Typically, a full tub needs four or five buckets of cold water to make it tolerable. As it cools off, just open up the valve and let some more hot water in. It's fantastic. Many bathers don't wear swimsuits, but outside the private rooms you're supposed to. The Forest Service seems to be paying more attention to this recently. It's also requested that, if people are waiting, you limit your soak to one hour.

Even if there's nobody around when you get to the springs, consider taking some time to explore farther up the trail before you soak. It's old growth all the way, up the Hot Springs Fork of the Collawash River, past Shower Creek and Spray Creek, and eventually into Bull of the Woods Wilderness. You should go at least as far as Shower Creek (0.3 miles past the springs and just 0.1 mile past a camping area on the right) to enjoy the 50-foot falls and a little wooden platform somebody built underneath it so that folks could take a shower.

Beyond that, the trail continues 6 miles and ascends 1,800 feet to reach Silver King Lake, in the heart of the wilderness. Trails fan out from that area to many other great locations.

Bagby is best avoided on weekend nights, when partiers sometimes take over the place. So unless you too are a yahoo, go on a weekday or early on the weekends.

# 23    BULL OF THE WOODS

GPS Trailhead
Coordinates

UTM Zone (WGS84) 10T

Easting 569774

Northing 4972196

Latitude   N 44.89977°

Longitude  W 122.11626°

## IN BRIEF

This is like two great hikes in one. Choose between an easy stroll through old-growth forest and rhododendrons to two beautiful lakes, and a more challenging climb to a fire lookout tower with a panoramic view. Either way it will introduce you to a magnificent wilderness area.

## DESCRIPTION

This trail has it all. Come in late June, as soon as the snow has cleared, and enjoy a mind-boggling display of rhododendrons among the old-growth forest on the way to Pansy Lake. (But bring bug repellent!)

Come in late summer and pick huckleberries up on the ridge. Or come in fall, when the ridge is awash in color and the mountains might see their first snow. Just make sure you get here.

The peak is the second-highest point in the 27,000-acre Bull of the Woods Wilderness, which boasts more than a dozen lakes bigger than an acre, 68 miles of hiking trails, and even the world-famous northern spotted

-------------------------------------------

*Directions* _____→

Take OR 224 from Portland, traveling 44 miles southeast of I-205, through the town of Estacada, to the Ranger Station at Ripplebrook. Bear right to take FS 46 and, 3.6 miles later, head right again to access FS 63. After 5.7 miles, turn right on FS 6340, following a sign for Bull of the Woods and Pansy Basin. At a junction 3.5 miles on, continue straight, still on FS 6340. Then, 4.4 miles past that junction (7.9 miles after FS 63), turn right on FS 6341, ignoring a sign to the left reading "Bull of the Woods Trail." The parking area is 3.6 miles ahead on the right.

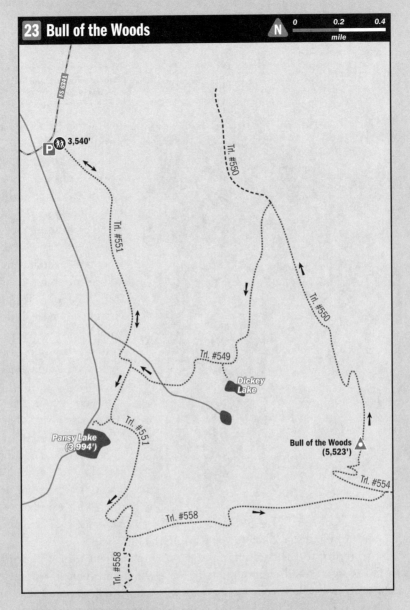

N

0    0.2    0.4

mile

FS 6341

P 🚶 3,540'

Trl. #551

Trl. #550

Trl. #550

Trl. #549

Dickey
Lake

Pansy Lake
(3,994')

Trl. #551

Bull of the Woods
(5,523')

Trl. #554

Trl. #558

Trl. #558

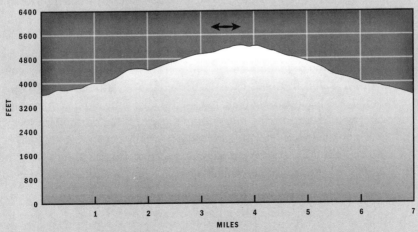

6400
5600
4800
4000
3200
2400
1600
800
0

FEET

1    2    3    4    5    6    7

MILES

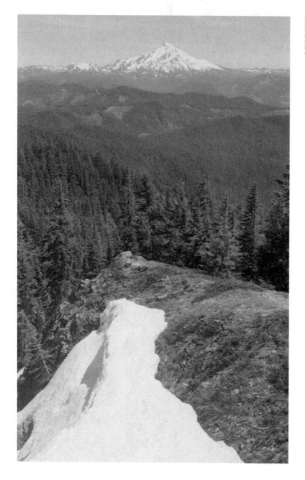

Mount Jefferson from Bull of the Woods lookout

owl, which you almost certainly won't see.

From the start, you're walking through a beautiful forest, on basically flat trail. In these 0.8 miles, you'll cross some nice little creeks and traverse gauntlets of rhododendrons before reaching a signed trail junction. Trail 549, coming down the hill from your left, is the return portion of the loop. Take a right here, following a sign for Pansy Lake.

Just before the lake, you'll pass a sign that says "Twin Lakes," but ignore it (for now) and continue straight to visit Pansy. There is a campsite on the right with excellent sitting rocks for picnicking or getting a quick rest and snack before you start up the hill.

Now, return to the trail and take what's now a right turn, following the Twin Lakes sign. You'll climb gradually for a while and then start a series of switchbacks. In just less than a mile from the lake, you'll gain 500 feet before you intersect Trail 558 in a saddle between Pansy Mountain and Bull of the Woods. Turn left onto 558.

While the switchbacks you just did were obviously steep, this trail is what I call "sneaky steep," which means that it doesn't look like much, but you'll feel the elevation gain. You're gaining about 700 feet in 1.1 miles, and since you're now going above 5,000 feet, you may start to feel the relative lack of oxygen. The forest in here is beautiful, though, and should take your mind off the climb. And if you're wondering why the moss doesn't grow on the bottom ten feet of the trunks, it's because that's how high the snow usually gets.

When you gain the top of the ridge and intersect Trail 554, turn left, and with one more push through some switchbacks you'll pop out at the top of Bull of the Woods, with its old Forest Service fire lookout tower. Walk up onto the deck and have a look around. You'll see Big Slide Lake below you, but Mount Jefferson, 20 miles away, dominates the view. On a clear day, you can see all the way from the Three Sisters on your right to Mount Rainier on your left. As the crow flies, it's about 175 miles from the Sisters to Rainier. Rest here and feel proud.

To continue the loop, find a trail junction in the trees on the opposite side of the watchtower from Mount Jefferson. This is Bull of the Woods Trail (550). Follow it to your right, along the ridge. You'll see occasional great views and many, many flowers over the next 1.1 miles, at which point you'll intersect Trail 549. Take 549 down and to the left, and you'll quickly lose elevation. Just past half a mile, peer through the trees on your left to see Dickey Lake—a lake spied through branches is always a magical sight. Also, look for a trail that leads down to the lake itself; it's just past a meadow on Trail 549.

After another half mile, most of it through a sea of rhododendrons, you'll get back to the trail where this whole thing started, Pansy Lake Trail (551). Turn right there, and you'll be back to the car in no time.

# 24 CLACKAMAS RIVER

## KEY AT-A-GLANCE INFORMATION

**LENGTH:** 7.8 miles one-way with a car shuttle, or 7.2 miles round-trip to Pup Creek Falls

**CONFIGURATION:** Out-and-back

**DIFFICULTY:** Moderate

**SCENERY:** Old-growth forest, a white-water river, and a few waterfalls

**EXPOSURE:** Shady all the way

**TRAFFIC:** Heavy on summer weekends, light–moderate otherwise

**TRAIL SURFACE:** Packed dirt, with roots and rocks

**HIKING TIME:** 4 hours for either option

**DRIVING DISTANCE:** 50 miles (1 hour) from Pioneer Square

**SEASON:** Year-round; muddy and possibly snowy in winter and spring

**BEST TIME:** Early summer–fall

**BACKPACKING OPTIONS:** One good site 2.5 miles in from Fish Creek

**ACCESS:** Northwest Forest Pass required at Fish Creek trailhead

**WHEELCHAIR ACCESS:** None

**MAPS:** Green Trails #492 (Fish Creek Mountain)

**FACILITIES:** Toilets at Fish Creek trailhead; water along the way must be treated.

**INFO:** Clackamas Ranger District, (503) 630-6861

## GPS Trailhead Coordinates

UTM Zone (WGS84) 10T

Easting 566750

Northing 5000800

Latitude N 45.15752°

Longitude W 122.15075°

## IN BRIEF

Convenient, not too tough, and not terribly long, Clackamas River Trail is a great way to stretch your legs and enjoy the scenery among old trees and along a beautiful river.

## DESCRIPTION

On that rare nice day in early spring—"nice" meaning it's not pouring—when you want to get out and do some hiking, here you'll find ferry slipper orchids and Clackamas lily in bloom. And if it's blazing hot in summer and you want to visit a cool, shady place . . . or it's autumn and you want to see the fall colors . . . whatever the time, it's always a nice day to go out and hike Clackamas River Trail. If you can bring a second car to stash at Indian Henry, it'll be that much better. Otherwise, you can do essentially the same distance and make a fine day of it.

From the trailhead, you'll start out in a flat section with the river a short distance to your left. After a half mile you'll come to a river-access point with moss-covered rocks and a sandy beach—perfect for chilling out or perhaps, if you've brought small kids, for turning around. Soon after, you'll come into

## *Directions*

Take OR 224 from Portland, traveling 33 miles southeast of I-205. Fifteen miles past the town of Estacada, just after crossing two bridges in quick succession, make a right on Fish Creek Road. Pass Fish Creek Campground, cross another bridge, and park in the parking lot on the right. The trail starts across the road on your left. To leave a car at the other end, drive another 7 miles on OR 224 and make a right into Indian Henry Campground. The trailhead is 0.5 miles up on the right.

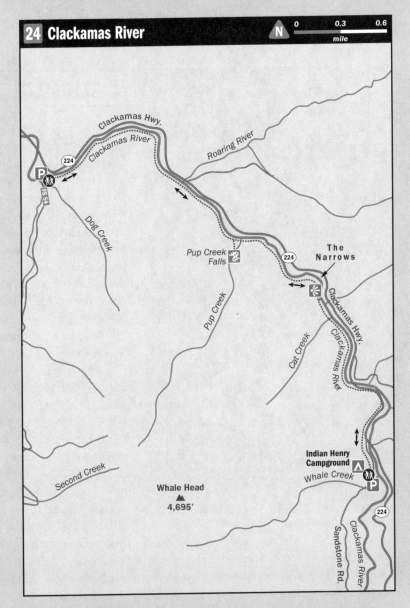

N 0 0.3 0.6
mile

Clackamas Hwy.

224

Clackamas River

P

FS 54

Dog Creek

Roaring River

Pup Creek Falls

Pup Creek

224

The Narrows

Clackamas Hwy.

Clackamas River

Cat Creek

Second Creek

Whale Head
▲
4,695'

Indian Henry Campground

Whale Creek

P

224

Sandstone Rd.

Clackamas River

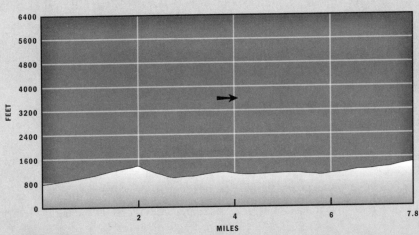

FEET

6400
5600
4800
4000
3200
2400
1600
800
0

2          4          6        7.8
MILES

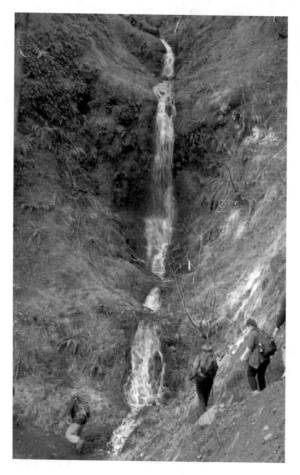

One of many side falls on Clackamas River Trail

the first exceptional old-growth forest, featuring five-foot-thick Douglas firs and even bigger western red cedars. In the next mile or so of trail, you'll do a little climbing and occasionally find yourself with some pretty serious drops to and views of the river to your left. Much of this early section burned in 2004, so you can check on how it's recovering.

If you're wondering about a good place to picnic or spend the night, you'll find it 2.5 miles up in a campsite. There's a stupendous western red cedar right by the water here and plenty of places to sit and gaze at the river. OR 224 is right across the river, by the way, but you'll hardly notice it. Again, if you've brought kids, think about turning around here, because in the next mile you'll go up, down, then up again (a couple hundred feet each time), and occasionally find the river a long 200 feet below you.

After you've hiked a total of 3.5 miles and descended the hill to find yourself under power lines, you'll come to Pup Creek, which the main trail crosses on a series of stepping stones. A side trail leads 0.1 mile up the creek to a view of beautiful Pup Creek Falls. If you didn't stash a car at Indian Henry, turn around here, and you'll have a 7.2-mile hike. If you did leave a second car there, keep on trucking.

In 0.9 miles a side trail will lead left to another beach—last chance to get to the river on this hike. Right after that you'll climb to a view up the Clackamas that includes the Narrows, a spectacular gouge in ancient lava. Down the other side of this hill, a side trail to the left will lead 0.1 mile to the Narrows themselves.

By the way, if you've seen some cables crossing the river in a few spots and wondered what that's about, they were put in by Portland General Electric

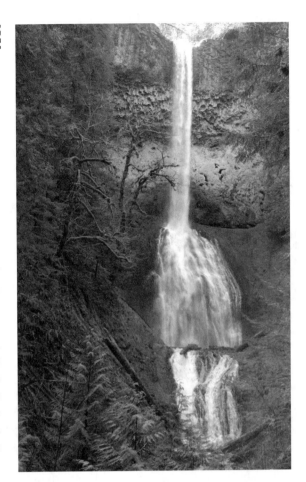

Pup Creek Falls

for cable-car access across the river to maintain their power lines.

In the last 3 miles to Indian Henry Campground, you'll cross several side creeks (the biggest one named Cat Creek), see numerous big cedars, get sprayed by a waterfall, and go under a cliff—in other words, enjoy a chorus of forest pleasures. About half a mile before the end, keep an eye out for a large stump on the left with a cable wrapped around it leading to another large stump. The Forest Service ties big stumps to keep them from rolling into the river and squashing people and boats on the water.

## NEARBY ACTIVITIES

If you haven't had enough riverside fun, stop by Promontory Park and its 350-acre North Fork Reservoir. The park has a marina, a campground with showers, and a store where you can get all your fishing supplies and licenses, rent boats, and enjoy an ice cream when you're done fishing. Small Fry Lake is for kiddie fishing only. Campsites are $16 per night and can be reserved at (503) 622-7229; for more info on the park and marina, call (503) 630-5152.

# 25 ROARING RIVER WILDERNESS

**KEY AT-A-GLANCE INFORMATION**

**LENGTH:** 1.4 miles round-trip to Shell-rock Lake, 5 miles to the Rock Lakes, 12.6 miles to do the whole thing

**CONFIGURATION:** Balloon

**DIFFICULTY:** Easy–difficult, depending on how far you go

**SCENERY:** Lakes, a meadow, forest, panoramic views

**EXPOSURE:** Shady most of the way, with a few open spots

**TRAFFIC:** Moderate on summer weekends, light otherwise

**TRAIL SURFACE:** Packed dirt, with roots and rocks

**HIKING TIME:** 1 hour to Shellrock Lake, 3 hours to Rock Lakes, 7 hours for the whole loop

**DRIVING DISTANCE:** 82 miles (2 hours 10 minutes) from Pioneer Square

**SEASON:** June–October

**BEST TIME:** August–October

**BACKPACKING OPTIONS:** Fantastic!

**ACCESS:** No fee

**WHEELCHAIR ACCESS:** None

**MAPS:** Green Trails #492 (Fish Creek Mountain) and #493 (High Rock)

**FACILITIES:** Nearby at Hideaway Lake Campground; none at trailhead; water on trail should be treated

**INFO:** Clackamas Ranger District, (503) 630-6861

## IN BRIEF

Seven lakes, a flower-filled meadow, late-summer huckleberries, and dramatic views await on this loop hike, which is part of the new Roaring River Wilderness, designated in 2009. Whether you go 1 mile or 12, beauty awaits here. Just bring mosquito repellent if you come in the early summer.

## DESCRIPTION

It used to be that you could drive to Frazier Turnaround, knocking some 3.6 miles off this hike. And, technically, you still can. But I can no longer, in good conscience, send people down that road—I've been cursed for doing so—and besides, hiking in this new way adds two lakes and some lovely forest to the experience.

Consider camping at Hideaway Lake before you do this hike; start early in the morning to beat the crowds, and you can go for a swim when you get back in the heat of the afternoon.

At the Shellrock Lake trailhead, you may at first wonder why you're here. Hiking through a clearcut for half a mile doesn't exactly scream "wilderness," but there are plenty of beautiful flowers, and at least the trail is nearly flat. The reward for your patience is big, beautiful Shellrock Lake, with

## GPS Trailhead Coordinates

UTM Zone (WGS84) 10T

Easting 580964

Northing 4997540

Latitude N 45.12669°

Longitude W 121.97046°

## Directions ───────►

Take OR 224 from Portland, traveling 44 miles southeast of I-205, through the town of Estacada, to the Ranger Station at Ripplebrook. Half a mile past the Ranger Station, turn left onto FS 57. Drive 7.6 miles on FS 57, and turn left onto FS 58. Go 3 miles and turn left onto FS 5830 and follow it 5.7 miles to the trailhead, on the right just past Hideaway Lake Campground.

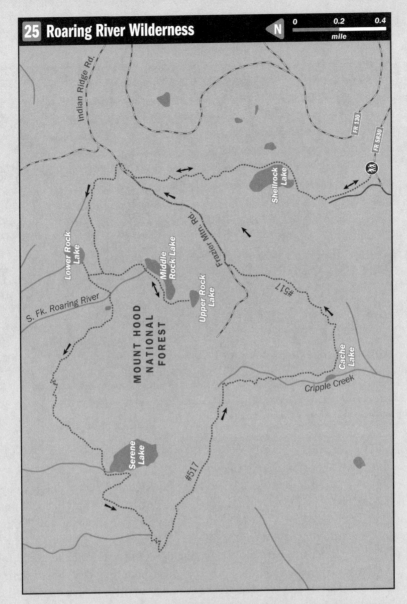

N

0        0.2        0.4
mile

Indian Ridge Rd.

FR 130

FR 5830

Shellrock
Lake

Lower Rock
Lake

Frazier Mtn. Rd.

Middle
Rock Lake

Upper Rock
Lake

#517

S. Fk. Roaring River

MOUNT HOOD
NATIONAL
FOREST

Cache
Lake

Cripple Creek

Serene
Lake

#517

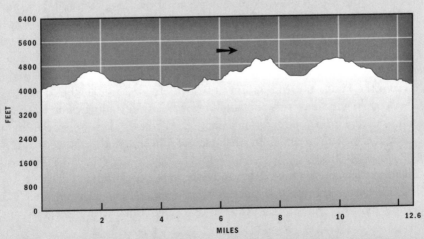

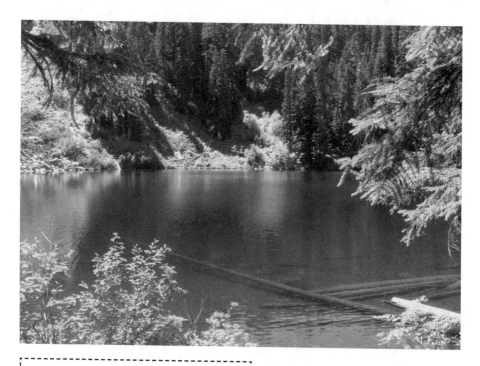

Upper Rock Lake, where a sweet campsite awaits

campsites galore and stocked trout—a fine, easy destination if you have kids or just don't care about putting in the miles.

To keep going, circle the lake on the right side and follow the trail up the hill. It gets rocky in places, and mildly steep, until 1 mile past the lake, where you'll hit Trail 517. Turn right (downhill) here, and in a moment you'll arrive at Frazier Turnaround, the old trailhead.

Look for Serene Lake Trail (512) going downhill and to the left, and follow it 0.8 miles to a junction. The loop keeps going here, but you should definitely go left a flat quarter mile to Middle Rock Lake, with campsites on both shores. Turn right, cross the creek, walk to the far end of the lake, then follow a short trail up the hill to Upper Rock Lake, the smallest of the three—and host to a single, private, dreamy campsite. That trail gets a little brushy and can be tough to follow in early summer. The loop to Middle and Upper Rock Lakes adds just over 1 mile to your day.

From the main trail (if you did not turn left for Middle Rock Lake), go another couple hundred yards and you'll come to a trail leading right, to Lower Rock Lake, which has one inferior campsite. All these lakes are stocked with trout, by the way, so if you're into fishing, get a license and bring your rod. If you've got small kids, or you feel done for the day, you are now 3 miles from your car. But for an even nicer lake, and then some, keep going.

You'll put in another 0.7 miles going downhill, then turn up (steeply at times) for most of a mile to gain the top of a ridge, thick with bear grass. Just over the top of the hill (now 4.3 miles from the trailhead), you'll come to Serene Lake and several side trails leading left, to campsites. Serene Lake is just what its name implies; anglers pull 15-inch trout from its deep, cold, green water, and the same boulders, grassy shallows, downed trees, and thickly vegetated shoreline that hide the fish also make for outstanding scenery for humans. This is the finest lake of the loop. Follow the right-hand shoreline to continue our hike.

If you're camping, there are several excellent spots, one with a picnic table (who put *that* there?) at the trail junction, one at the far end on a point that sticks out into the lake, and another on the left side. There's also a huge boulder about 100 yards along the shoreline from the trail junction—an awesome spot to jump into the (very cold) lake. There's a decent trail all the way around the lake, but you'll have to cross a couple of rockslides to make the circuit.

Beyond Serene Lake, the trail climbs about 600 feet in 1 mile to the top of a ridge and a junction with Grouse Point Trail (517). Turn left here, climb a small hill, and in 0.7 miles you'll reach a clearcut, which was put in for helicopters to drop off firefighters. Not a romantic history, but there's a cliff with a sublime view back down to Serene Lake, and out to Mounts St. Helens, Rainier, Adams, and Hood. The two bare peaks to the right are the Signal Buttes. Also, as you look north toward Hood, you're seeing an area of about 8 miles, as the crow flies, with only one road and two trails to break it up.

The trail now drops 700 feet in a mile, and when you get to the flower-filled Cache Meadow, you'll find an intersection. The right-hand trail leads out to another road; another heads into the meadow, where you can see the lily-filled Cache Lake to the left. To continue the loop, turn left and go 200 yards to the site of an old shelter. From here, you can cross the seasonal creek on your right and go 0.2 miles to Cripple Creek Lake, yet another mountain beauty with a couple of campsites. They're everywhere!

A minute past the shelter site, turn left to stay on Trail 517 and take it uphill 1 mile (you'll get all of that 700 feet back!) until you come to an abandoned road. Turn right, and in a mile you'll be back at the trail leading down to Shellrock Lake and your car. Just keep an eye out, in the clear areas along the road, for a view back to Mount Jefferson. That makes this a seven-lake, five-volcano hike!

# 26 WHETSTONE MOUNTAIN

 **KEY AT-A-GLANCE INFORMATION**

**LENGTH:** 4.8 miles

**CONFIGURATION:** Out-and-back

**DIFFICULTY:** Moderate

**SCENERY:** Old-growth forest on the way up, a sweeping mountain view up top

**EXPOSURE:** Shady all the way, some steep slopes in sidehill sections

**TRAFFIC:** Moderate on summer weekends, light otherwise

**TRAIL SURFACE:** Some rock at the very top

**HIKING TIME:** 3 hours

**DRIVING DISTANCE:** 74 miles (2 hours) from Pioneer Square

**SEASON:** June–October

**BEST TIME:** June for rhododendrons, October for fall colors

**BACKPACKING OPTIONS:** Not good

**ACCESS:** No fee

**WHEELCHAIR ACCESS:** None

**MAPS:** USGS Bagby Hot Springs, USFS Bull of the Woods Wilderness

**FACILITIES:** None at trailhead; closest are at Bagby Hot Springs trailhead along the hike

**INFO:** Clackamas Ranger District, (503) 630-6861

**SPECIAL COMMENTS:** Consider doing this one as part of an overnight trip to the area, as it's a lot of driving for not much hiking.

## GPS Trailhead Coordinates

UTM Zone (WGS84) 10T

Easting 562987

Northing 4969424

Latitude N 44.87545°

Longitude W 122.20256°

## IN BRIEF

It's a long, tedious drive. And it isn't much of a hike, if you're looking for a ton of exercise. But, my goodness, what a view you get from Whetstone Mountain! And for what it's worth, you can do an up-close comparison of clearcut and old-growth forests.

## DESCRIPTION

Whetstone Mountain got its name in pioneer days because of a rock prevalent in the area and useful for sharpening knives. The peak hosted a fire lookout tower for many years, but both it and the useful rock are gone. What's left, though, is an easy-to-reach viewpoint that rivals anything around there.

You can actually see your destination from the large and wide trailhead, which sits in the middle of a clearcut. Whetstone is the forested ridge right in front of you; a little to the left, you can see the flat-topped Battle Ax Mountain in the distance (hike 27, page 124). To reach Whetstone, you will head toward it, swing to the left, gain that ridge you see, then ascend the other side to the tiny, rocky summit.

---

### Directions

Take OR 224 from Portland, driving 44 miles southeast of I-205, through the town of Estacada, to the Ranger Station at Ripplebrook. Turn right on FS 46, drive 3.6 miles, and make another right, on FS 63. Travel 3.5 miles on FS 63, turn right on FS 70, and go 9.6 miles (keep right at an unmarked junction around 8 miles) before turning left on FS 7030. Continue 5.7 miles on FS 7030, turn right on FS 7020, then go 0.6 miles to Spur Road 028, on the left. The trailhead is at the end of that road, 0.1 mile ahead.

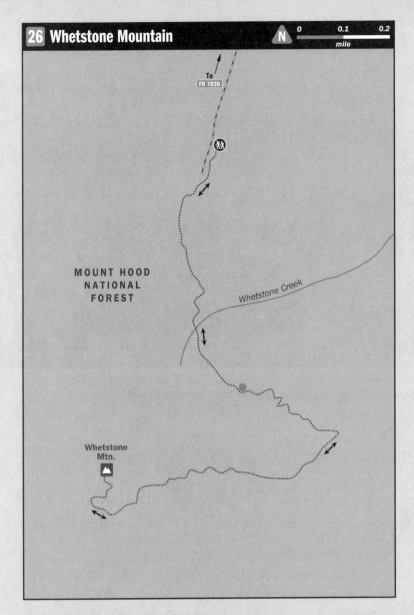

MOUNT HOOD
NATIONAL
FOREST

To
FR 7030

Whetstone Creek

Whetstone
Mtn.

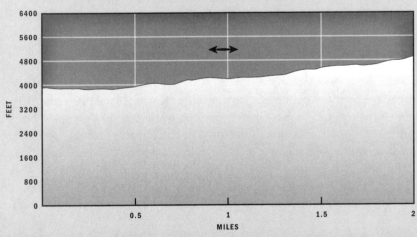

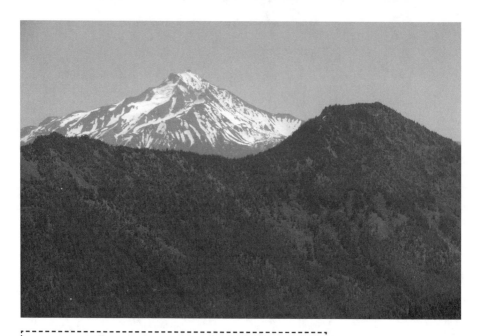

Mount Jefferson and Battle Ax Mountain, from Whetstone Mountain

When you start out hiking downhill, don't be concerned; that's the right trail. You'll descend about 0.25 miles, passing rhododendrons (which bloom in late June) and huckleberries (ripe in mid-August). This area was cut around 1980 and then replanted, so you get a chance to see how it's recovering. It's when you enter Bull of the Woods Wilderness, about 0.2 miles in, that you'll see the amazing difference between cut and uncut forest. You'll get a bigger-picture view of this later.

Where you start uphill, about 0.3 miles in, look for a meadow on the right with a spring, then cross a couple of its outlets. Just past half a mile, you'll reach the base of a rockslide, with a pond on your left, then hike a few switchbacks—one with a nice view of Mount Hood on the left—as you get up onto the ridge.

At the ridgeline, just over a mile into the hike, your path intersects Trail 3369. You've been on Trail 546, and if you're wondering, you've gone from three digits to four because you've just hiked from Mount Hood National Forest to Willamette National Forest. Here, turn right and start a slowly rising traverse along the north side of the ridge, enjoying occasional views down and to the left into Opal Creek Wilderness. There are a couple of sections in here where you'll be walking on a sidehill section of trail with a fairly steep drop to the left, but the good news is that, in August, you'll also be walking through Huckleberry Heaven.

When you've gone about a mile since the turn, you'll make another right turn, this time up the short, steep trail to the rocky summit; going left here would take you 3.5 miles down to an intersection early in the Opal Creek trip (hike 29, page 134). Gaining Whetstone's summit requires a few steps on rocky terrain,

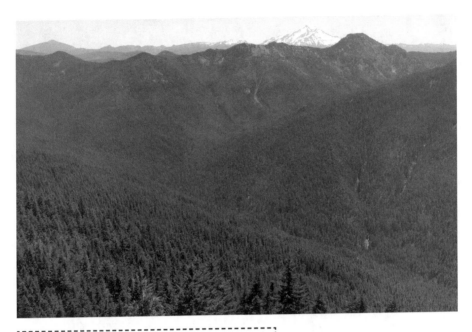

Opal Creek drainage and Mount Jefferson from the peak.

but nothing challenging. Besides, when you get there, the summit is so small, and so high relative to its surroundings, you may feel like you're airborne.

Catch your breath, then let's do the visual tour. The easy way to start is to find Mount Hood, to the northeast. Left of that is Mount Adams, and left of *that* is Mount Rainier. To the right of Hood, and seemingly at your feet, there's a ridge going east toward the (unseen from here) Silver King Lake, in the heart of Bull of the Woods and at the top of the Bagby Hot Springs trip (hike 22, page 102). The right side of that ridge is the drainage for Battle Ax Creek, which joins Opal Creek at Jawbone Flats, almost directly beneath you.

In the distance to the east is the knob-topped Olallie Butte, and to the right of that is Mount Jefferson, 25 miles away but seemingly right behind Battle Ax, which is 5 miles away. Still moving right, look for crumbly Three-Fingered Jack; the next pointy one to the right is Mount Washington, followed by the tiny-looking Coffin Mountain and then the Three Sisters, Broken Top, and, way out there, Diamond Peak, just north of Crater Lake. Near as I can figure, the straight-line distance from Diamond to Rainier is about 225 miles.

Quite a view, eh? Worth the drive? Thought so. If you're looking for some backpacking options, there's nothing good on this trail, but Bull of the Woods is filled with lakes, trails, and campsites; just turn left instead of right at the intersection on the ridge. But if you're thinking of a car shuttle to Opal Creek, consider this: you could hike from this trailhead to that one in less than 6 miles, but the drive via FS 46 is more than 60 miles!

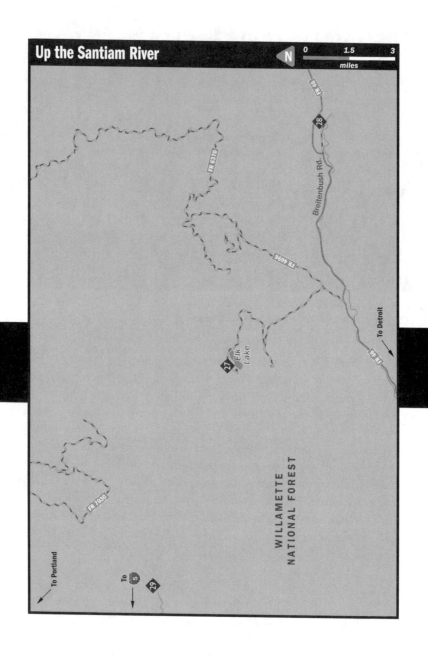

# Up the Santiam River

N

0     1.5     3

miles

FR 48

28

Breitenbush Rd.

FR 6370

FR 4696

To Detroit

FR 46

Elk Lake

27

FR 7030

WILLAMETTE NATIONAL FOREST

To Portland

To 5

29

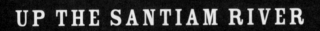

UP THE SANTIAM RIVER

# 27 BATTLE AX MOUNTAIN

## KEY AT-A-GLANCE INFORMATION

**LENGTH:** 5.1 miles round-trip from the trailhead, 6.5 from the campground

**CONFIGURATION:** Loop

**DIFFICULTY:** Strenuous

**SCENERY:** Forest, rock formations, mountain vistas

**EXPOSURE:** Lots of time in the open, some rocky slopes and sidehills

**TRAFFIC:** Light

**TRAIL SURFACE:** Rocky in places

**HIKING TIME:** 4 hours

**DRIVING DISTANCE:** 102 miles (2 hours) from Pioneer Square

**SEASON:** June–October

**BEST TIME:** August–September

**BACKPACKING OPTIONS:** Plenty in the vicinity, though limited on this trail; [see end of profile]

**ACCESS:** No fee

**WHEELCHAIR ACCESS:** None

**MAPS:** USGS Bull of the Woods Wilderness

**FACILITIES:** Restrooms (but no drinkable water) at nearby Elk Lake Campground

**INFO:** Detroit Ranger District, (503) 854-3366

**SPECIAL COMMENTS:** The road to this trailhead is pretty bumpy; call ahead for current conditions.

## GPS Trailhead Coordinates

UTM Zone (WGS84) 10T

Easting 569183

Northing 4963904

Latitude  N 44.82519°

Longitude W 122.12487°

## IN BRIEF

It's a long drive, and a bumpy road. And parts of the hike up are rather dull. So why hike Battle Ax? Three reasons: one of the greatest views among all the hikes in this whole book, few fellow hikers, and easy access to a fantastic, lake-filled wilderness area.

## DESCRIPTION

Okay, let's start with the road, because there's a chance that when you mentioned Battle Ax Mountain or Elk Lake to friends, they told you some horror story about having their teeth rattled out of their heads while driving up there. First, the road has been worked on quite a bit in the last few years, and second, I got my 1992 Nissan Sentra up there with no problem in 2009. Sure, I was going 5 miles an hour at times, but I made it just fine. Just drive around the bigger potholes and rocks, and you'll be okay. And while you're up there, consider spending the night at the campground, which

## Directions

Take I-5 south from Portland, driving 45 miles to Exit 253/Detroit Lake. Follow OR 22 east 49 miles to the town of Detroit, then turn left onto FS 46, following signs for Breitenbush Hot Springs. After 4.4 miles, turn left on FS 4696; note that from here on, many intersections have no signs. Go 0.8 miles on FS 4696 and turn left on FS 4697, following it 2.2 miles to a T-intersection, where you'll turn right. Drive 1.8 miles and make a left. This is where the road gets rough(er). Follow it 2.1 miles to another left, and then 0.3 miles to a fork just above the campground. Go right (on an even bumpier road) 0.4 miles to reach the trailhead, on the right; or make a left and go 0.3 miles to park in the campground.

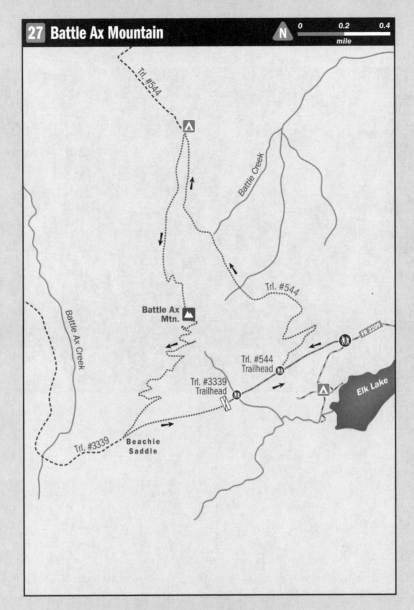

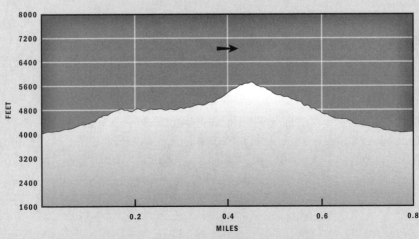

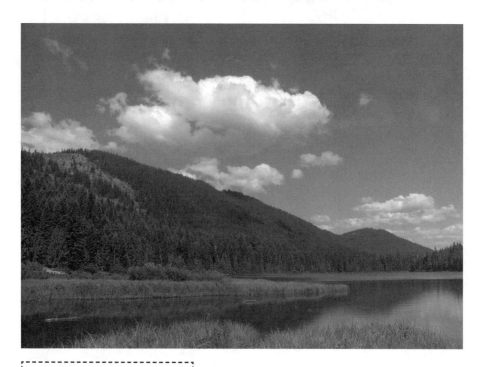

Elk Lake, seen from the campground

is free (when this book went to press, anyway) but has a reputation for a little weekend rowdiness.

Now, the hike. If you drive to the trailhead, you'll knock 1.4 miles off your walk, and I'll describe it as if you did that. (If you're parked at the campground, just walk back up to the fork and go left to reach the trailhead.) It isn't too exciting at first, winding up Bagby Trail 544 through thick forest. The initial 0.6 miles gains 500 feet to reach a pair of small ponds, and 0.2 miles past them it flattens out to start a 1-mile traverse along the northeast side of Battle Ax. So, at this point, you're actually walking away from the peak, which will be visible over your left shoulder.

Halfway across this traverse, you'll enter an impressive rockslide where, if you give a shout, you'll notice that the sound really bounces around. The far end of this slide offers a great view back to Battle Ax; and don't worry, you're not going up that side of it. You'll next cross a series of brushy, spring-fed forks of Battle Creek, with views north into the heart of Bull of the Woods Wilderness.

When you're 1.8 miles from the trailhead, the trail intersects Battle Ax Trail heading up and to the left. You'll also see, on the right, one of the more pitiful campsites of your life. It's a nice place for a rest or snack before you start climbing, but if you're looking to camp overnight, check the backpacking options below.

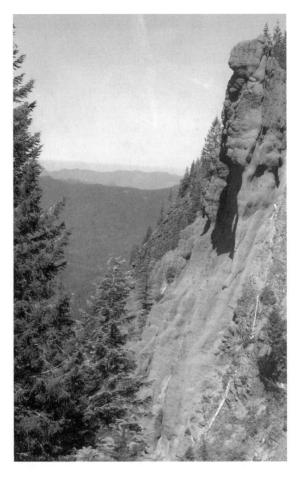

While you're resting and snacking, perhaps you'd like to know where Battle Ax got its name. One theory is pretty simple: it's shaped like an ax. Another theory is that an old woodsman named it for a brand of chewing tobacco that was popular in the 1890s and that he chewed a lot of it while exploring the area. I say we go with that theory.

To get up Battle Ax, take the trail from this junction, and soon you'll be climbing and in the sun, as the forest thins out and you approach 5,000 feet in elevation. Another rockslide offers a view southeast to Mount Jefferson, as does a rocky bowl 0.3 miles up. After half a mile of climbing, you'll cross over the ridge, and then your view will be west, down Battle Ax Creek—not to be confused with Battle Creek (on the other side)—and into the Opal Creek Wilderness.

Now you'll switchback up 0.6 miles, gaining a final 600 feet to put you at the north end of the broad, flat summit. There are remnants of the old fire lookout, and a 1947 benchmark from the U.S. Coast and Geodetic Survey, which hasn't been an independent agency since 1970.

A big rock at the southern end of the peak offers a great view back down to Elk Lake, 1,800 feet below. Otherwise, you can see from Mount Hood to the Three Sisters. Try to spot the distinctive Coffin Mountain, and Whetstone Mountain (hike 26, page 118), which is on the far side of Opal Creek Wilderness (hike 29, page 134).

Now you're heading down to the saddle between Elk Lake and Battle Ax Creek. Take the trail that heads to the right (when looking at the lake) from near the southern end of the summit, and descend a series of rocky, dusty, sun-drenched switchbacks. (This is why you came up the other way!) Some of this trail is also mildly exposed on steep, rocky sidehills—nothing life-threatening, but a fall would ruin your day.

A little less than a mile downhill, you'll pass some neat rock formations. Check out Mount Beachie, across the way. It looks like somebody took a saw to the summit, cut out a rectangular chunk, and planted a tree in it. You can go up there later, if you want.

A mile and a half below the summit, you'll come to Beachie Saddle and an old road that is now Battle Ax Trail (3339), to your right; this leads 4 miles down to Jawbone Flats in the middle of Opal Creek Wilderness. So, the walk from Elk Lake to Jawbone Flats on the trail is about 5.5 miles; the drive is 46 miles. (I think these things are fascinating.) Above you is Mount Beachie, with a well-shot-up sign marking the start of that 1.5-mile, 800-foot climb.

To get to your car, head left and down the gravel road, which is at times a trail and at times something less than that. You'll pass the trailhead for 3339—imagine driving there!—0.2 miles before our original trailhead, which is 0.7 miles from the campground and the lake you now deserve to jump into.

**BACKPACKING OPTIONS:** Since you're at the corner of two wilderness areas, why not use this simple hike as a way into the backcountry? There are more options—and a dozen lakes at least an acre in size—in Bull of the Woods. From the campsite at the junction above, it's about 3 miles (*descending* 800 feet!) to Twin Lakes, which is right in the middle of the wilderness. Get a map and go for it; with a long car shuttle, you could even end the hike at Bagby Hot Springs!

# BREITENBUSH HOT SPRINGS AREA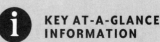

## IN BRIEF

With its combination of old-growth majesty and New Age spirituality and wellness, the area around Breitenbush Hot Springs is one of the most peaceful and inspiring places in Oregon. The trails are plentiful and (mostly) easy, the surroundings are sublime, and the water is hot.

## DESCRIPTION

Like a refuge of tranquility amid a sea of logging operations, the area along the South Fork of the Breitenbush River is often described with words like peaceful, magical, and special. The resort is itself a draw—with its pools, tubs, well-being programs, massage, and other healing arts—but easy, pleasant walks through the forest and along the river beckon.

One option is to simply go register for a day pass at the hot-springs resort (see details below) and start your hike at the Spotted Owl trailhead, across from the resort parking lot. After 1.1 miles on that trail, you'll come to a junction with Cliff Trail. Turn right on Cliff Trail and climb 0.5 fairly steep miles, including some semi-exposed sections along a cliff,

---

## Directions

Take I-5 from Portland, driving 35 miles south of I-205 to Exit 253/Stayton/Detroit Lake. Turn left (east) on OR 22 and follow it 49 miles to Detroit. Turn left on FS 46. For the trailheads on FS 4685, travel 12.2 miles, make a right on FS 4685, and go a half mile to the trailhead, on the right. The trailhead nearest the gorge is another 1.6 miles up the road. For the hot springs, from Detroit go 10 miles on FS 46 and make a right onto a one-lane bridge just past Cleator Bend Campground. Over the next 1.2 miles, keep left at three junctions.

### KEY AT-A-GLANCE INFORMATION

**LENGTH:** 1–8 miles
**CONFIGURATION:** Out-and-back, or one-way with a car shuttle
**DIFFICULTY:** Easy–strenuous
**SCENERY:** Ancient forest, river, a narrow gorge, a mountain viewpoint
**EXPOSURE:** Shady all the way
**TRAFFIC:** Moderate–light
**TRAIL SURFACE:** Packed dirt, a few roots
**HIKING TIME:** 30 minutes–5 hours
**DRIVING DISTANCE:** 103 miles (2 hours) from Pioneer Square
**SEASON:** Year-round, but even lower elevations could be snowy in winter
**BEST TIME:** October, for fall colors and fewer crowds
**BACKPACKING OPTIONS:** A few options along the South Breitenbush
**ACCESS:** Northwest Forest Pass to park on FS 4685, day-use fee to park at hot springs
**WHEELCHAIR ACCESS:** None
**MAPS:** USGS Breitenbush Hot Springs; free maps at resort office
**FACILITIES:** None at the trailhead; all available at the hot springs
**INFO:** Breitenbush Hot Springs, (503) 854-3320; Detroit Ranger District, (503) 854-3366
**SPECIAL COMMENTS:** If you're not using the resort facilities, park at a parking area just outside their gate.

---

### GPS Trailhead Coordinates

UTM Zone (WGS84) 10T
Easting 581648
Northing 4959277
Latitude N 44.78223°
Longitude W 121.96796°

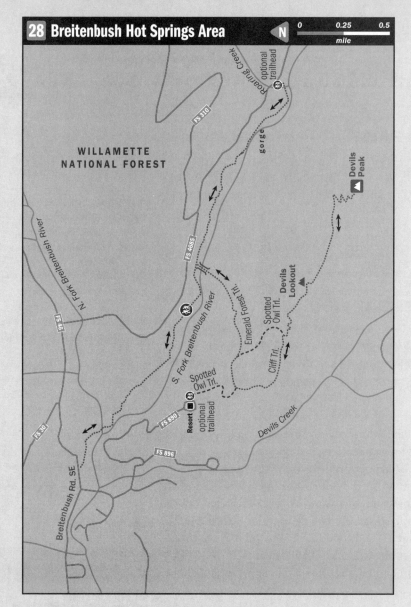

N

0        0.25        0.5

mile

WILLAMETTE
NATIONAL FOREST

Roaring Creek

optional
trailhead

gorge

Devils
Peak

FS 310

N. Fork Breitenbush River

FS 4685

Devils
Lookout

Emerald Forest Trl.

Spotted
Owl Trl.

S. Fork Breitenbush River

FS 46

Cliff Trl.

Spotted
Owl Trl.

Resort
optional
trailhead

FS 890

Devils Creek

FS 30

FS 896

Breitenbush Rd. SE

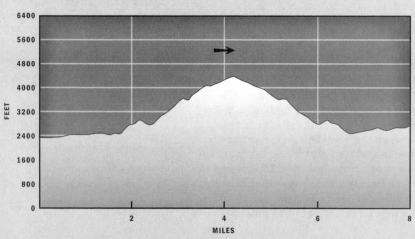

| FEET | | | | | |
|---|---|---|---|---|---|
| 6400 | | | | | |
| 5600 | | | | | |
| 4800 | | | | | |
| 4000 | | | | | |
| 3200 | | | | | |
| 2400 | | | | | |
| 1600 | | | | | |
| 800 | | | | | |
| 0 | | 2 | 4 | 6 | 8 |

MILES

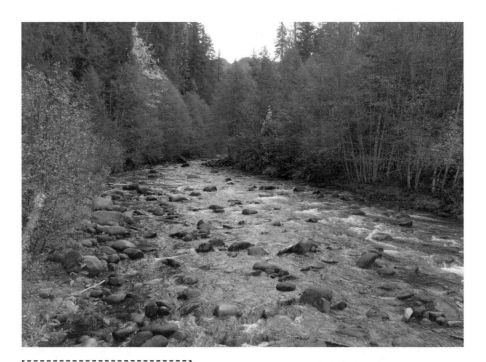

South Fork of the Breitenbush River

to an intersection with Devils Ridge Trail, which climbs steeply to Devils Lookout and Devils Peak. Staying on Spotted Owl Trail, you'll come to Emerald Forest Trail in a half mile at a junction that we'll describe below. The hot springs also has a hiking map, so you can just ignore my directions and take a spiritual walkabout, if you prefer.

For the shortest hike in the area, walk about a mile to see Breitenbush Gorge, a 100-yard-long, 40-foot-deep chasm that the river rips through. From the upper trailhead on Road 4685, start downhill and, after a couple of minutes, turn right on Gorge Trail. Cross Roaring Creek and, after 0.3 miles, you'll pass through an open area where lots of trees were blown down by a storm on Thanksgiving Day in 1999. To find the gorge from this area, look for two parallel logs pointing downhill between a big cedar and a root ball with ferns and hemlock saplings. The unsigned trail drops 100 feet or so to a viewpoint; here the gorge has several big logs lying across it. A little trail heading left and under some logs leads to a view of the upper part of the gorge.

Our most recommended hike starts at the lower parking area on FS 4685. From there, walk 0.1 mile downhill and turn left onto South Breitenbush Gorge National Recreation Trail. You will only hear the river at this point, so for views you'll have to "settle" for the big Douglas firs, hemlocks, and western red cedars towering over you and the clover-like oxalis and early-summer wildflowers. Rhododendrons bloom here in June.

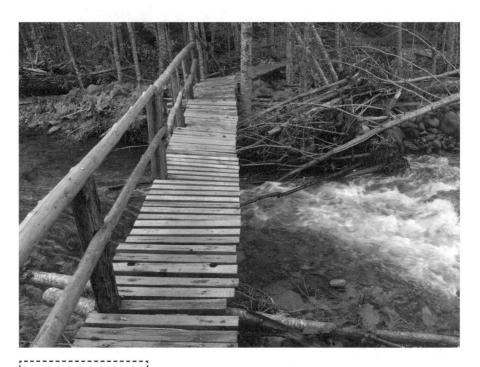

Bridge over Roaring Creek

After 0.7 miles, you'll come to a descending trail on the right, signed Emerald Forest. Take the Emerald Forest Trail 0.1 mile downhill to the South Breitenbush, which hikers used to cross on a bridge. (If you opt to continue straight and bypass the Emerald Forest Trail, it's a 1-mile flat hike to the gorge.) The same 1999 storm rolled this one-log bridge over on its side, officially closing it. But subsequent storms blew several more trees down over the river, and someone added a helpful handrail to one of these logs. (If you care, this is where the author photo was taken.) Cross it, and on the other side climb half a mile on Emerald Forest Trail through as pretty a forest as you'll ever see.

When you've gone 0.8 miles past the bridge, your path intersects Tree Trail and Devils Ridge Trail. Along the way, you may notice a sign referring to the Neotropical Migratory Bird Conservation Program, which was a program of small grants that improved habitats for birds in Central and South America; many of those birds come here for the summer. Make a right, toward Spotted Owl Trail, if you want to return to the hot springs. But if you're looking for some serious exercise and a spectacular view, turn left onto Devils Ridge Trail, which soon becomes frighteningly steep in its 0.25-mile climb to Cliff Trail. From this intersection, you can turn right and loop back, again toward Spotted Owl Trail, passing steep cliffs about 0.2 miles out. Or you can turn left and keep doing the horribly steep thing—it's 700 feet (in 0.5 miles!) to Devils Lookout and 1,500 feet (in 1.5 miles) to Devils Peak.

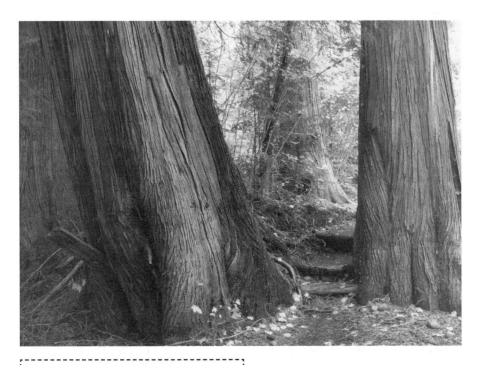

Western red cedars along the South Breitenbush

Like I said, there are a lot of options around here, but all of them are beautiful, and all of them are close to the hot springs.

## NEARBY ACTIVITIES

Breitenbush Hot Springs is open from 9 a.m. to 6 p.m. to day-use visitors, but it often fills. Advance reservations are required, so plan ahead: you'll have access to the pools, steam room, and daily well-being programs for a sliding-scale fee (that is, one based on your ability to pay) that ranges from $13 to $26. Lunch and dinner (all vegetarian) are $11 each. Overnight rates, depending on time of year, range from $54 for a tent site to $115 for a cabin with a bathroom. For more information, visit their Web site at **www.breitenbush.com.**

# 29 OPAL CREEK WILDERNESS

## KEY AT-A-GLANCE INFORMATION

**LENGTH:** 7 miles round-trip to Opal Pool, 10 miles round-trip to Cedar Flats, 13 miles to see it all

**CONFIGURATION:** Out-and-back

**DIFFICULTY:** Easy–moderate

**SCENERY:** Uncut forest, clear-water pools, historic mining structures

**EXPOSURE:** Shady

**TRAFFIC:** Heavy on summer weekends, moderate otherwise

**TRAIL SURFACE:** Packed road for 3.1 miles; otherwise dirt, roots, rocks

**HIKING TIME:** 2.5 hours to Opal Pool, 5 hours to Cedar Flats, 6 hours to see it all

**DRIVING DISTANCE:** 92 miles (2 hours) from Pioneer Square

**SEASON:** April–November

**BEST TIME:** August–September

**BACKPACKING OPTIONS:** Plentiful

**ACCESS:** Required Northwest Forest Pass can be purchased at trailhead

**WHEELCHAIR ACCESS:** None

**MAPS:** USFS Opal Creek Wilderness

**FACILITIES:** Outhouses at trailhead, composting toilet in meadow at Jaw-bone Flats

**INFO:** Opal Creek Ancient Forest Center, (503) 892-2782 or www.opalcreek.org

## IN BRIEF

Opal Creek's history stretches from ancient times to a modern-day legislative showdown, but its value can hardly be measured. It is an almost completely preserved sample of what the Northwest used to be, a place that hasn't been logged and where the water runs clear. The largest such low-elevation area in the state, it doesn't require that you work hard to see most of it.

## DESCRIPTION

For thousands of years, the Santiam Indians had their summer camp at the confluence of what we now call Opal Creek and Battle Ax Creek. Other tribes would come here to trade such items as fish from the Pacific Ocean and obsidian from east of the Cascades. In the 1850s, pioneers arrived and started mining for silver and gold. Not much of either was found, but there were enough other minerals to keep mining alive here until the early 1980s. A mining town was built at the confluence in the 1920s, and it came to be known as Jaw-bone Flats; the story has it that while the men were out mining, the women were back there "jaw-boning." A sawmill was also built nearby, but it burned in the 1940s. In 1992 the mining

## GPS Trailhead Coordinates

UTM Zone (WGS84) 10T

Easting 557979

Northing 4967627

Latitude N 44.85970°

Longitude W 122.26616°

## Directions

Take I-5 from Portland, driving 35 miles south of I-205 to Exit 253/Stayton/Detroit Lake. Turn left (east) onto OR 22 and follow it 22.5 miles, then turn left onto North Fork Road, following a sign for Elkhorn. In just over 15 miles, the pavement will end; beware that beyond this there are some large potholes. Keep left at both junctions; the trailhead is at the end of the road, 5.6 miles after you leave the pavement.

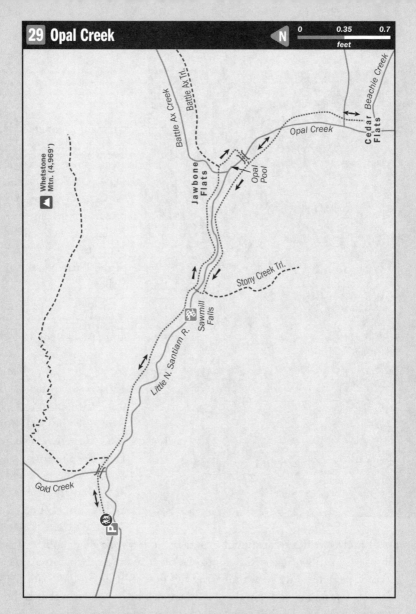

Battle Ax Creek

Battle Ax Trl.

Beachie Creek

Opal Creek

**Cedar Flats**

Whetstone Mtn. (4,969')

**Jawbone Flats**

Opal Pool

Stony Creek Trl.

Sawmill Falls

*Little N. Santiam R.*

Gold Creek

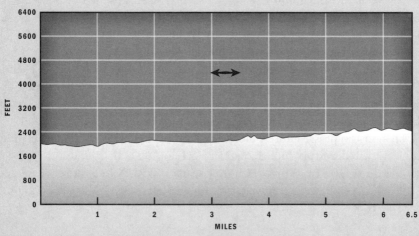

| FEET | | | | | | | | |
|---|---|---|---|---|---|---|---|---|
| 6400 | | | | | | | | |
| 5600 | | | | | | | | |
| 4800 | | | | | | | | |
| 4000 | | | | | | | | |
| 3200 | | | | | | | | |
| 2400 | | | | | | | | |
| 1600 | | | | | | | | |
| 800 | | | | | | | | |
| 0 | 1 | 2 | 3 | 4 | 5 | 6 | 6.5 | |

**MILES**

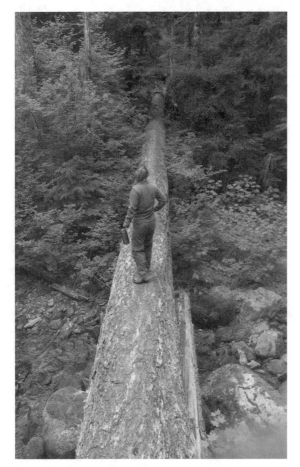

Crossing Beachie Creek on a giant log

company donated 4,000 acres of land to a nonprofit group now known as the Opal Creek Ancient Forest Center, asking that it be preserved. Meanwhile, the Forest Service announced plans to log 15,000 acres of the Little North Santiam Valley.

This is when Opal Creek became world-famous; a massive effort was launched to save it from the saw. National TV crews visited, a book was written, and the fight went all the way to the U.S. Congress, where in 1998 the 35,000-acre Opal Creek Wilderness and Scenic Recreation Area was finally established. Today the Opal Creek Ancient Forest Center operates educational programs at Jawbone Flats, and a Y-shaped system of easy trails brings visitors into the magical land of what used to be.

From the gate, start by walking slightly downhill on an old road. Most of the big trees are still ahead, but there is a Douglas fir on the right that is thought to be between 700 and 1,000 years old; a side trail leads to the tree at about 0.2 miles. There's a rustic outhouse at 0.3 miles, just before a high bridge crosses Gold Creek; 0.1 mile past that, you'll see Whetstone Mountain Trail (3369) on the left. This 3.5-mile trail climbs 3,000 feet to a superb view from atop Whetstone Mountain, but if you want to see that, it's much easier to do the Whetstone Mountain hike listed elsewhere in this book (hike 26, page 118). About 0.2 miles past that trailhead, you'll cross a series of "half bridges"; keep an eye out for an old mining shaft on the left just past them.

The most impressive forest along the road occurs between 1 and 1.5 miles out, where you'll find six-foot-thick Douglas firs. At a wide spot in the road 1.5 miles out, look for a trail to the right that leads 100 yards to a rocky viewpoint. At 1.9 miles, you'll see a tiny waterfall on the left, flowing between exposed cedar tree roots.

At 2 miles, you'll see a trail on the right leading into an area filled with old mining equipment and the burned-out remains of the sawmill's steel and masonry boiler. Behind the one building still standing is a trail leading 100 feet to a falls; it's known as either Sawmill Falls or *Cascadia de los Niños* ("Waterfall of the Children"), depending on who you ask. Look for a log stuck on the rocks high up on the left. That should give you an idea how high the water gets here.

Just past the sawmill site, you'll come to a fork. From here, head straight ahead on the road to reach a river access point on the right 0.2 miles farther on; Jawbone Flats is 1.2 miles past that. There, you'll find several cabins from the 1920s and 1930s (some can be rented overnight!), and two built since a fire in 1999. (They were both constructed largely of wood cut and milled right on the site.) To reach the local highlight, Opal Pool, from here, take the road straight through the camp, following signs to make a right-hand turn and pass a collection of old vehicles that includes, oddly, a U.S. Navy fire truck. The pool is 0.1 mile past the cars.

Back at the first fork in the road, a right turn will take you across a bridge and then left, onto Opal Creek Trail proper. Along this trail, several side trails lead left to the Little North Santiam; you'll also pass several sweet campsites on the left, down by the river. Continue 1.4 miles to a sign directing you to the sublime Opal Pool on the left. In summer you may see people jumping off the rocks into the amazingly clear, cold water. You're now looking at Opal Creek itself, probably the clearest water you'll ever see, and the best bet in Oregon for a stream you can drink from. I have ingested several gallons of Opal Creek and never gotten sick; take that for what it's worth and make your own decisions.

A quarter mile past Opal Pool, a bridge offers a glimpse into the crystal-clear waters—when this book was written, the bridge was closed because storm damage had brought it below Forest Service standards. There was a slim chance it would be fixed by summer 2010; more likely, it will be ready in 2011. While it's technically closed because it's missing one of two rails, folks still cross it. Call ahead if you're concerned about this.

Another mile up—a total of 5 miles from the gate—the trail more or less ends at Cedar Flats, where Beachie Creek flows into Opal Creek from the left, and three 1,000-year-old cedars frame the trail. There's also good camping in this area.

I say "more or less ends" because the trail beyond there is not maintained, but it is possible, even recommended, to go off exploring. Look for a big log over Beachie Creek and then just go with it. Sometimes there's a trail; sometimes there are logs to walk on; sometimes there are logs to climb over. If a trail dead-ends near a log, hop up on it, walk a ways, and look around; you just might find some more trail. I can't give any specifics (not that I'm unwilling—I just can't explain it), but there is at least one more waterfall and one more pool like Opal Pool up there. Some folks just wander up the creek itself, but that can be dangerous.

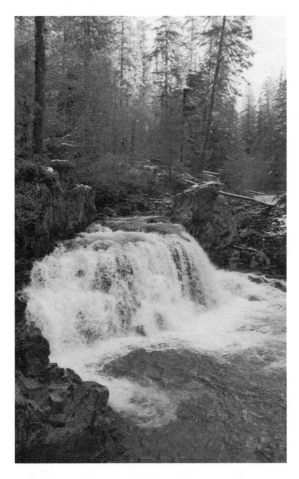

There are long-term plans to relocate the trail and build a new 4-mile section up to Opal Lake. There are also plans to connect Opal Creek Trail with Little North Santiam Trail, which currently ends several miles down that river. None of that work had begun when this book was written, but one day you may be able to hike from the Elkhorn recreation area (back on Little North Santiam Road) to Opal Lake, 17 miles one-way.

And Opal Creek has still more to offer. From Jawbone Flats, look for an old road that goes up Battle Ax Creek; follow it to a trail heading down toward the creek, and you might be able to locate old train tracks related to the mining operations. From the start of Opal Creek Trail, near the bridge, another trail leads up Stony Creek to a hidden waterfall. There's even a trail that branches off Whetstone Mountain Trail, heading up Gold Creek; beyond Whetstone Mountain it's 14 miles down to Bagby Hot Springs. The Ancient Forest Center has an excellent map that covers all of this.

Basically, it's hiker heaven. Get some friends together, rent a cabin in Jawbone Flats for the weekend, and go for it.

## NEARBY ACTIVITIES

A mile back on OR 22, you may have noticed the Gingerbread House. It will be on your left as you head home. Stop in there for some fresh, warm gingerbread with ice cream after the hike, and your day will be complete.

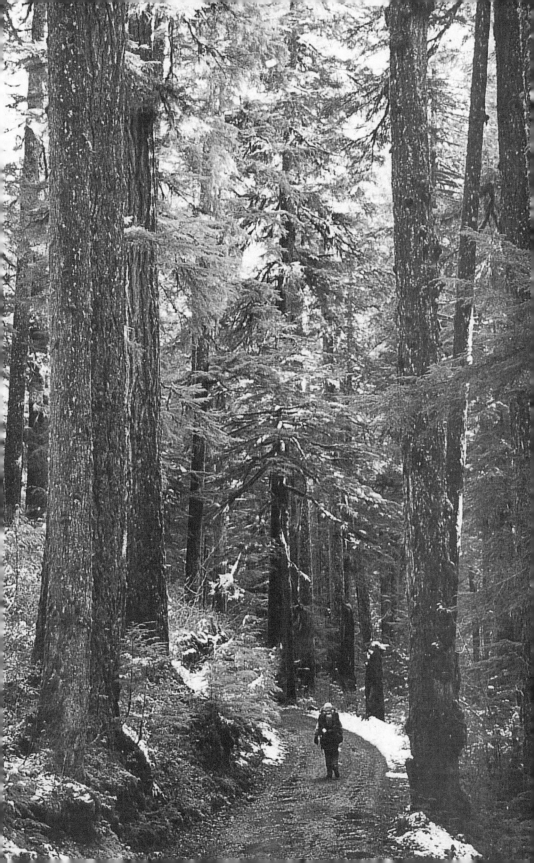

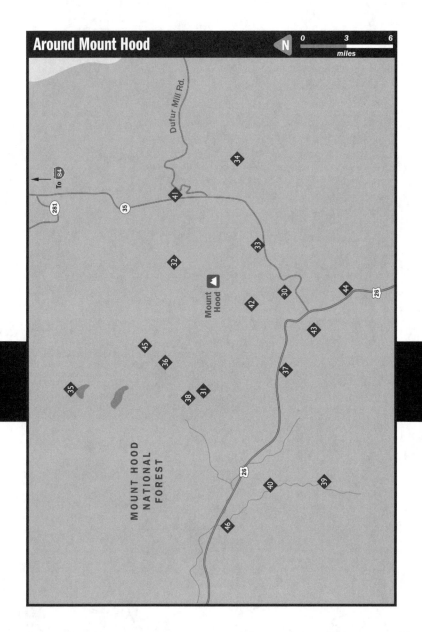

**Around Mount Hood**

N

0    3    6
miles

To 84

281

35

Dufur Mill Rd.

34

41

33

32

Mount Hood

30

44

26

42

43

45

36

37

35

38    31

MOUNT HOOD NATIONAL FOREST

26

40

39

46

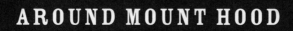

# AROUND MOUNT HOOD

# 30 BARLOW PASS

## KEY AT-A-GLANCE INFORMATION

**LENGTH:** Up to 10 miles, or 5 miles with car shuttle

**CONFIGURATION:** Out-and-back, or one-way with shuttle

**DIFFICULTY:** Moderate

**SCENERY:** Forest, meadows, views of Mount Hood, two river canyons

**EXPOSURE:** Forest on the way up, open on top

**TRAFFIC:** Light

**TRAIL SURFACE:** Packed dirt, with some roots

**HIKING TIME:** 3.5 hours one-way

**DRIVING DISTANCE:** 62 miles (1 hour 30 minutes) from Pioneer Square

**SEASON:** Late June–October

**BEST TIME:** August–September

**BACKPACKING OPTIONS:** One good creekside site along the way

**ACCESS:** Northwest Forest Pass required

**WHEELCHAIR ACCESS:** None

**MAPS:** USFS Mount Hood Wilderness; Green Trails #462 (Mount Hood)

**FACILITIES:** None; water must be treated

**INFO:** Hood River Ranger District, (541) 352-6002

**SPECIAL COMMENTS:** Consider doing this hike as a one-way, 5-mile trek with a second car parked at Timberline Lodge.

## IN BRIEF

There's a great view of Mount Hood at the top, and a one-way car-shuttle option that ends at Timberline Lodge, but this convenient, not-too-tough hike is all about the forest, traversing some of the finest high-elevation old-growth around and ending at an Oregon landmark.

## DESCRIPTION

There are more-spectacular hikes in the Mount Hood area, but none offers the combination of solitude and old-growth beauty that this one does. It's also perfect for a picnic, or just a dose of sunshine, in a high-altitude meadow with Mount Hood towering above. You can do the one-way option with a shuttle, possibly combining this with the Twin Lakes trip (hike 44, page 199), and wind up at Timberline Lodge.

From the trailhead, walk across Forest Service 3531 and into the woods on the PCT (2000). Stop to admire the relief map of the PCT in Oregon, and contemplate some of the distances on there. People who hike the whole PCT in five or six months average about 20 miles a day! You'll get in 4 to 5 miles today—a distance most PCT long-haul hikers fly through, with dreams of showers

### GPS Trailhead Coordinates

UTM Zone (WGS84) 10T

Easting 603070

Northing 5015062

Latitude  N 45.28150°

Longitude  W 121.68581°

### *Directions* ⟶

**Take US 26 from Portland, driving 51 miles east of I-205, then turn north on OR 35, following signs for Hood River. Drive 2.5 miles on OR 35, make a right onto FS 3531, and follow signs for Barlow Pass and the PCT. The trailhead is 0.2 miles ahead on FS 3531.**

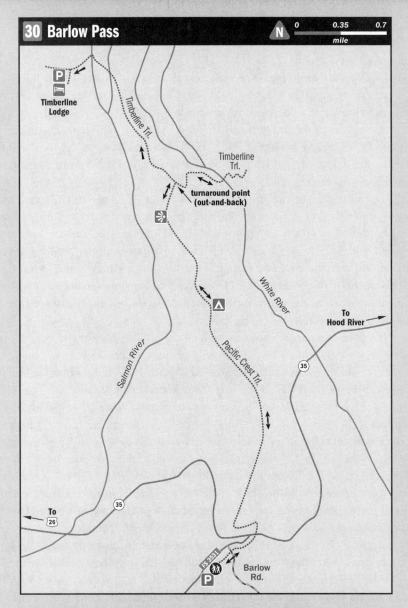

N

| 0 | 0.35 | 0.7 |

*mile*

Timberline
Lodge

Timberline Trl.

Timberline
Trl.

turnaround point
(out-and-back)

White River

To
Hood River

35

Salmon River

Pacific Crest Trl.

To
26

35

FS 3531

Barlow
Rd.

P

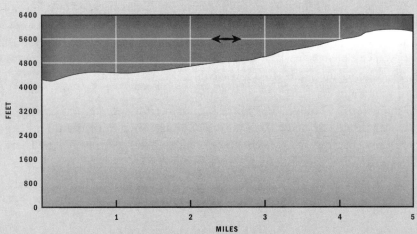

and food up at the lodge. Note that on the USGS Mount Hood South map, which was created in 1962, this trail is still labeled as Oregon Skyline Trail, an old path that mostly got swallowed up when the PCT was created.

At the sign, take the left-most fork of the trails before you, walking north on the PCT toward Mount Hood. You'll take a few steps across the historic Barlow Road and, after 0.1 mile, *carefully* cross OR 35. The trail continues in a small draw on the far side.

The first part of the trail isn't too exciting; in fact, after 0.5 miles you'll traverse a fairly recent clearcut. But right after that you enter a glorious stand of mostly noble fir, with its long, straight, branchless trunks. In early summer the ground will be blanketed with wildflowers. In late summer, you'll see several species of huckleberries, and in fall, red-and-orange vine maple. If you're quiet, especially early in the day, you'll hear birds and possibly see deer or elk. It's just a pleasant place to be, and the trail's altitude gain (less than 400 feet per mile) is entirely manageable.

If you're wondering about those blue diamonds up on the trees early in the hike, they mark winter trails for cross-country skiers and snowshoers. Their height should give you a sense of how much snow falls in these parts. The white diamonds mark the PCT all the way from Mexico to Canada.

At the 2-mile mark, you'll enter a more diverse forest that includes firs and hemlocks, then cross a creek beside a small campsite at 2.7 miles. A little more than 3 miles into the hike, you'll reach an overlook of Salmon River Canyon and the headwater of the Salmon River. The Salmon is the only river in the lower 48 states classified as a Wild and Scenic River from its headwater to its mouth, and here you're looking at its headwater. The river flows from a glacier above Timberline Ski Area, snaking its way down to the Sandy River along US 26. Two hikes along the lower Salmon—Salmon River Trail and Wildwood Recreation Area—are described elsewhere in this book (hikes 40 and 46, pages 182 and 208).

Just past here, the forest will start to open up; in August, you'll see meadows filled with wildflowers, especially the spectacular beargrass, which looks like a giant cotton swab. In a few minutes, your trail intersects Timberline Trail in just such a meadow, with Mount Hood rising above you. Relax here, if you'd like, and then turn around; or continue 0.3 miles left on Timberline Trail to reach a spectacular lookout with views of the White River Canyon, hundreds of feet deep.

If you've opted to park a car up at Timberline and are doing a one-way hike, keep going up Timberline Trail (which, at this point, is also the PCT) toward the mountain. It's 1.25 miles to the lodge—700 feet up—so it's not too much more work. However, most of the climbing is along the first part of the trail, which is also, at points, as sandy as a beach. So it can get arduous. And if there's any rough weather around, it will be up here, so bring a coat. There's nothing to stop the wind this high on the mountain.

You first go along the edge of the White River Canyon and then through meadows and across the tiny Salmon River. This crossing has no bridge but is manageable. Look for views south to Mount Jefferson, some 45 miles away, and a sign on the PCT with mileages to Canada and Mexico. You'll also encounter Mountaineer Trail, which loops up to the Silcox Hut then back down to Timberline Trail west of the lodge, in a section that's part of the Timberline Lodge trip (hike 42, page 190). When you get close to the lodge, trails will go every which way, so just aim for the hot chocolate and finish the hike with style.

It's possible to hike just the upper part of this walk from Timberline Lodge—especially recommended if you have kids with you. This shorter option is an easy, scenic alternative with very little elevation gain; if you go to the White River Canyon overlook, it's about 1 mile round-trip.

## NEARBY ACTIVITIES

If you've got some clearance on your vehicle, you can drive Barlow Road for miles, eventually making your way to The Dalles—though the road improves dramatically a long way before The Dalles.

# 31 BURNT LAKE-ZIGZAG MOUNTAIN

## KEY AT-A-GLANCE INFORMATION

**LENGTH:** 6.8 miles round-trip to the lake, 9.4 miles to the hilltop

**CONFIGURATION:** Out-and-back

**DIFFICULTY:** Easy along the creek, moderate to the lake, strenuous to the mountain

**SCENERY:** Shady creekside forest, a lovely mountain lake, a spectacular summit view

**EXPOSURE:** Some ridgetop walking near the top

**TRAFFIC:** Heavy on summer weekends, moderate otherwise

**TRAIL SURFACE:** Packed dirt, some rocks

**HIKING TIME:** 5.5 hours to do it all

**DRIVING DISTANCE:** 54 miles (1 hour 20 minutes) from Pioneer Square

**SEASON:** June–October, though there will be some snow higher up in early summer

**BEST TIME:** July–September

**BACKPACKING OPTIONS:** Great sites at the lake

**ACCESS:** Northwest Forest Pass required

**WHEELCHAIR ACCESS:** None

**MAPS:** Green Trails #461 (Government Camp)

**FACILITIES:** None at the trailhead; stop in Zigzag on the way

**INFO:** Zigzag Ranger District, (503) 622-3191

## GPS Trailhead Coordinates

UTM Zone (WGS84) 10T

Easting 592231

Northing 5024973

Latitude N 45.37220°

Longitude W 121.82213°

## IN BRIEF

This is really three hikes in one: a cool, shady amble along a creek, a steady climb to a beautiful lake with a view of Mount Hood, and a strenuous climb to an old lookout site with an impressive view of Mount Hood.

## DESCRIPTION

Burnt Lake Trail (772) starts off in an area where there's no lake and no evidence anything has ever burned. It's all cool, moist, and shady as you wind your way up through a young forest with a branch of Lost Creek off to your right. If that name sounds familiar, it's because there are enough things called "Lost" in Oregon (not to mention things called Salmon, Elk, and Huckleberry) to fill a whole hiking book.

Walk 0.25 miles and, just past a big cedar on the right, the forest gets a little more interesting. At just under half a mile there's an unmarked trail to the left leading to a clifftop view toward the main stem of Lost Creek. On the main trail, you'll get your first glimpse of actual water around 1 mile out, and at just under 2 miles you'll hop across a tiny creek.

Continue climbing ever so gently for half a mile, past some old burned-out snags, and look for a trail dipping left to a picnic site by

## Directions

Take US 26 from Portland, driving 36 miles east of I-205 to Zigzag. Turn left (north) onto Lolo Pass Road, which is 0.6 miles past milepost 41. Go 4.2 miles and turn right on FS 1825, which is 0.1 mile past a Mount Hood National Forest sign and is marked "campgrounds and trailheads." Stay right at 0.7 miles, cross a bridge, and, 2 miles later, just past Lost Creek Campground, turn left onto a gravel road, continuing 1.3 miles to the trailhead.

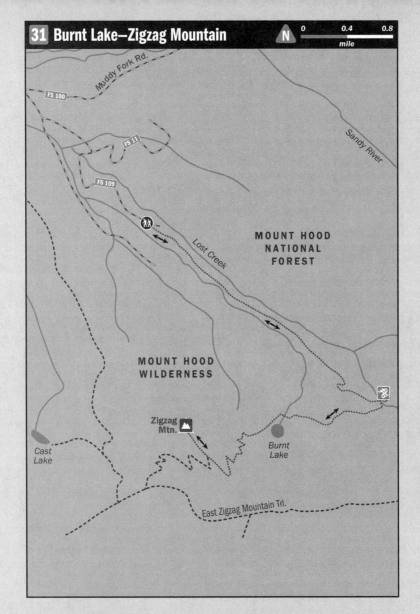

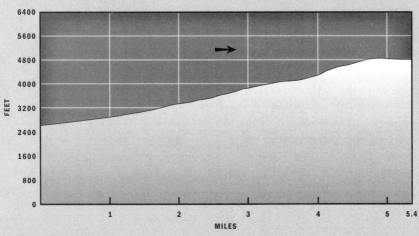

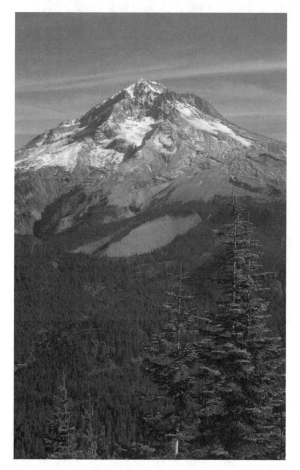

Mount Hood from Zigzag Mountain

a small waterfall. You have now found the main branch of Lost Creek, and a good place (2.3 miles out) to turn around if you're tired or have little kids in tow.

Soon you'll make a switchback to the right and climb 1 mile, passing several small creeks, some of them in open areas that offer views back along the valley you've been coming up. You'll see Mount Hood over your right shoulder, but the real views start just after you cross Burnt Lake's outlet creek and arrive at the shores of this local wonder.

You'll immediately realize that lots of folks come up here; even if it's not crowded when you arrive, you'll notice trails leading all over the place. If you're camping, you must stick to designated spots and not make wood fires. If you're just up for the day, linger a bit, explore the trail around the lake, take a swim, and soak in the rays and the views of Hood. Turn back here, and you have a 6.8-mile day.

To reach the lookout, which is another 1.3 miles and 800 feet up, continue right on the trail as it leads away from the lake, following a pointer toward Zigzag Mountain Trail (775). Cross a marshy area, then switchback up and out of the lake basin, intersecting the 775 after 0.8 miles. Turn right here, and it's quite a steep quarter-mile climb to a viewpoint of Hood where rhododendrons surround you. After the trail levels, continue straight through another junction and push up the final 0.3 steep miles to the rocky summit.

From the top, your view runs from two-humped Rainier in the north to Mount Jefferson in the south, with Olallie Butte just to the left of it. To the left of Mount Hood, between it and Mount Adams, look for an open stretch alongside a ridge, bisected by a trail; that's Bald Mountain and a section of Timberline Trail, which you can visit on the McNeil Point trip (hike 36, page 168). The valley below that is that of the Muddy Fork of the Sandy River, which starts at Sandy Glacier, clearly visible from here, left of the summit. To the right, beyond Zigzag Glacier, you can see dramatic Zigzag Canyon, which you can visit on the Timberline Lodge trip (hike 42, page 190), and beyond that are two buildings that are part of Timberline Lodge, alongside Palmer Glacier.

So it's a two-creek, one-lake, four-volcano, three-glacier day, and yet there are still more trails up here to explore. The trail you took to the summit, Zigzag Mountain Trail, continues west over the summit toward Cast Lake and a veritable noodle bowl of trails, including the continuation of Burnt Lake Trail (772), which you left behind at the junction just below this summit. So you could make a loop out of all that, or even head for the lookout atop the west end of Zigzag Mountain—if, for some reason, what you've already done isn't enough for you.

# 32  COOPER SPUR

## KEY AT-A-GLANCE INFORMATION

**LENGTH:** 7.5 miles

**CONFIGURATION:** Balloon

**DIFFICULTY:** Strenuous

**SCENERY:** Old-growth forest, glaciers, wide panoramas, the upper reaches of Mount Hood

**EXPOSURE:** Mostly out in the open, with plenty of wind

**TRAFFIC:** Moderate on summer weekends, light otherwise

**TRAIL SURFACE:** Packed dirt, roots, sand, rocks

**HIKING TIME:** 4.5 hours

**DRIVING DISTANCE:** 88 miles (2 hours 15 minutes) from Pioneer Square

**SEASON:** July–mid-October

**BEST TIME:** August–September

**BACKPACKING OPTIONS:** One good site at the shelter; camping not allowed in Tilly Jane Historic Area

**ACCESS:** Northwest Forest Pass required

**WHEELCHAIR ACCESS:** None

**MAPS:** USGS Mount Hood North; USFS Mount Hood Wilderness; Green Trails #462 (Mount Hood)

**FACILITIES:** Outhouse and water at trailhead

**INFO:** Hood River Ranger District, (541) 352-6002

**SPECIAL COMMENTS:** No matter the forecast, bring warm clothing. Weather at this altitude can change quickly.

## GPS Trailhead Coordinates

UTM Zone (WGS84) 10T

Easting 605085

Northing 5028368

Latitude  N 45.40094°

Longitude  W 121.65730°

## IN BRIEF

Though it's not the toughest, this is the highest hiking trail in this book—right up into the realm of the mountain climber. You'll be in the world of rock and snow, and you won't even wear yourself out getting there—well, not completely. You'll also get to see the oldest buildings on Mount Hood and the results of a massive landslide and a recent forest fire.

*Note:* The area around the trailhead burned in 2008, and access was restricted in 2009. Call the Ranger Station to make sure you can do the hike you want to do.

## DESCRIPTION

If you want to get way, way up there, this is your hike. In the days before Timberline Lodge and the road to it were built, Cooper Spur was the standard climbing route to Mount Hood's 11,239-foot summit, and people still climb it that way today.

The whole area, in fact, is historically significant. Just up a hill from the trailhead, and at the end of the road, is Cloud Cap Inn. Built in 1889 by two prominent Portland families as a recreation destination, it's the oldest building on Mount Hood. The hotel

## Directions

Take US 26 from Portland, driving 51 miles east of I-205; turn north on OR 35, following signs for Hood River. Continue 17 miles on OR 35, then turn left at a sign for Cooper Spur Ski Area. Drive 2.4 miles, turn left, and follow another sign for Cooper Spur Ski Area. In 1.4 miles, continue straight, leaving the pavement. Go 8.3 winding miles to a T-junction and turn right. The trailhead is half a mile ahead on the right, in Cloud Cap Saddle Campground.

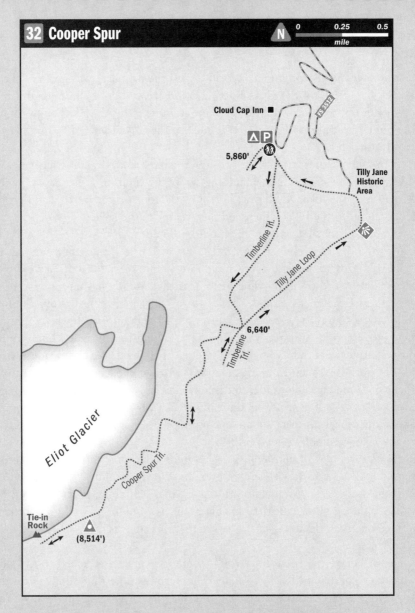

Cloud Cap Inn

5,860'

Tilly Jane
Historic
Area

FS 3512

Timberline Trl.

Tilly Jane Loop

6,640'

Timberline
Trl.

Eliot Glacier

Cooper Spur Trl.

Tie-in
Rock

(8,514')

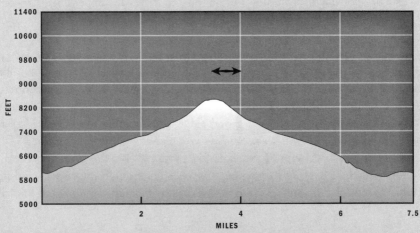

FEET

11400
10600
9800
9000
8200
7400
6600
5800
5000

MILES
2    4    6    7.5

venture never took off, and by World War II the property was given to the Forest Service. In 1956 the Crag Rats, a Hood River–based climbing and rescue organization, took it over, and they maintain it to this day. Although officially the public isn't allowed in, if you're nice to the folks there, they might let you pop in for a bit.

In 2008 a forest fire swept through this area, and dramatic measures were taken to save the buildings, including wrapping them in a protective material. As you start the hike, you'll get to see how the forest is recovering, and probably feel grateful to the folks who saved the area's historic legacy.

More history later; now, for the hike. The trail starts at the far end of the campground. Take Timberline Trail (600) to the left and enter a rare, snow-zone, old-growth forest, where mountain hemlock and Pacific silver firs get bigger than you'd think possible in an area that usually has ten feet of snow by the end of December. Walk 1.2 miles to reach a junction just above the forest; following a sign for Cooper Spur, turn uphill—and get used to the climbing.

Just a couple hundred yards up, back among the twisted whitebark pines on your right, sits the Cooper Spur shelter at the end of a small side trail. But for our purposes, keep climbing. The trail will switchback through the sand and rocks on a manageable grade, and Eliot Glacier will gradually come into view to the right. You'll hear it pop and rumble as it carves the side of the mountain, and if you're lucky, especially on late-summer afternoons, you'll see big pieces of it calving and tumbling downhill.

After 2 miles of climbing, you'll come to the top of the ridge, where you should look for a rock with some impressive carvings. "July 17, 1910," is carved into the stone here, commemorating a Japanese climbing party's ascent. Since you've climbed all the altitude at this point, you might as well go another 0.2 miles along the ridgetop—just be aware that this ridge is thin, rocky, and usually windswept.

Just before the snow line, you'll come to a plaque attached to the side of what they call Tie-in Rock, so named because it's here that climbers tie themselves to one another to venture out onto the glacier. Do not, under any circumstances (short of having ropes and crampons and relevant experience), go out onto the glacier. Be satisfied with being at the top of your local hiking world, and relax among the sheltering rocks to take in the view.

From left to right, with Mount Hood behind you, you can see Eliot Glacier, and, way off in the distance, the bare face of Table Mountain in the Columbia River Gorge, Mount St. Helens, Mount Rainier, Mount Adams, Elk Meadows, and Gnarl Ridge at your feet. Lookout Mountain is on a ridge to the east; there's a building below you on a Mount Hood ridge, which is the top of a ski lift at Mount Hood Meadows Ski Area. Now do you feel like you're way up there?

Now look up at Mount Hood. The Cooper Spur climbing route begins on the snowfield right in front of you and proceeds up through the rocks, tending slightly to your left. As climbers like to say, it's not as steep as it looks. Look for a prominent rock called the Chimney, just below the summit, and Pulpit Rock more to your right. The Crag Rats say that whenever somebody falls on the Cooper Spur climbing route, they generally wind up within about 200 feet of the same falling spot down below at the top of Eliot Glacier.

When you've descended to the junction where you originally turned right, continue straight, leaving Timberline Trail for Tilly Jane Loop. Hike 0.6 miles, and you'll come to an overlook of a large, bare bowl on your right. That's what was left behind by the Polallie Slide, a massive debris flow and flood in December 1980 that wiped out parts of OR 35.

A short distance on, you'll find yourself at some old buildings. This is part of the 1,400-acre Tilly Jane Historic Area. This area, by the way, is immensely popular with cross-country skiers and snowshoers, who come up a 2.7-mile trail from Cooper Spur Ski Area and spend the night here. And if you're wondering about that name, Tilly Jane was the nickname of the matriarch of the Ladd family, one of the builders of Cloud Cap Inn.

To get back to your car, just put Mount Hood on your left and follow the trail half a mile back to the trailhead.

## NEARBY ACTIVITIES

When you get back to OR 35, go north (left) and indulge yourself at some of the berry and fruit stands in the Hood River Valley. Some let you pick your own. See **www.hoodriverfruitloop.com** for details.

# 33 ELK MEADOWS

## KEY AT-A-GLANCE INFORMATION

**LENGTH: 2 miles to Newton Creek, 5.5 miles to Elk Meadows, 10.8 miles to see it all**

**CONFIGURATION: Out-and-back with optional loops**

**DIFFICULTY: Moderate to Elk Meadows, strenuous to Gnarl Ridge**

**SCENERY: Meadows, mountain streams, extreme close-ups of Mount Hood, a fire-recovery area**

**EXPOSURE: In and out of the trees with two bridgeless creek crossings**

**TRAFFIC: Moderate on summer weekends, light otherwise**

**TRAIL SURFACE: Dirt, some roots and rocky areas**

**HIKING TIME: 3.5 hours to Elk Meadows, 6 hours for the whole loop**

**DRIVING DISTANCE: 69 miles (1 hour 30 minutes) from Pioneer Square**

**SEASON: July–October**

**BEST TIME: August–September**

**BACKPACKING OPTIONS: Several good ones**

**ACCESS: Northwest Forest Pass required**

**WHEELCHAIR ACCESS: None**

**MAPS: USFS Mount Hood Wilderness; Green Trails #462 (Mount Hood)**

**FACILITIES: Outhouse at trailhead; water on trail must be treated**

**INFO: Hood River Ranger District, (541) 352-6002**

## IN BRIEF

One of the most spectacular sights in the Mount Hood area, sprawling and flower-filled Elk Meadows is relatively easy to reach. And beyond it lies Gnarl Ridge, with its awesome close-up view of the mountain.

*Note:* This makes an excellent snowshoe or ski trip, but you'll have to start at the Clark Creek Sno-Park on OR 35. The Green Trails map shows winter trails.

## DESCRIPTION

If I were to tell you there's a place where you can skip along through meadows and over creeks, picking berries all the way, and wind up in a flower-filled wonderland with a snow-covered peak above it, and if you wanted, you could climb up through more meadows to a rocky point with a huge view of everything around, right up where the water blasts out from under the glaciers . . . you'd be interested in that, right?

That's this hike. And if all you're doing is going to Elk Meadows, there's only one moderate hill between you and your destination. In fact, you and the kids could walk a flat mile, see two mountain streams, and have a ball. And you could do the whole thing in an easy day, without even driving on gravel!

## GPS Trailhead Coordinates

UTM Zone (WGS84) 10T

Easting 606937

Northing 5019766

Latitude N 45.32325°

Longitude W 121.63550°

## Directions

**Take US 26 from Portland, driving 51 miles east of I-205. Turn north on OR 35, following signs for Hood River. Drive 7 miles and turn left at the second entrance for the Mount Hood Meadows Ski Area (the one for the Nordic Center). The trailhead is half a mile ahead on the right.**

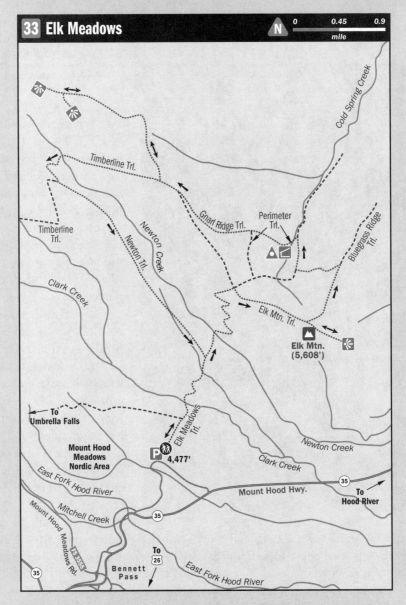

N

0    0.45    0.9
mile

Cold Spring Creek

Timberline Trl.

Timberline Trl.

Newton Creek

Newton Trl.

Clark Creek

Gnarl Ridge Trl.

Perimeter Trl.

Bluegrass Ridge Trl.

Elk Mtn. Trl.

Elk Mtn. (5,608')

To Umbrella Falls

Mount Hood Meadows Nordic Area

Elk Meadows Trl.

4,477'

Newton Creek

Clark Creek

East Fork Hood River

Mount Hood Hwy.

35

To Hood River

Mitchell Creek

35

Mount Hood Meadows Rd.

FS 3555

35

To 26

Bennett Pass

East Fork Hood River

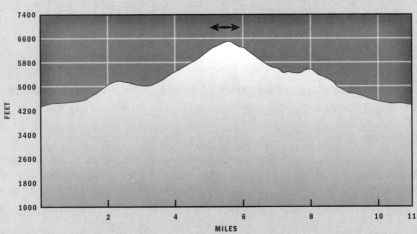

7400
6600
5800
5000
4200
3400
2600
1800
1000

FEET

2    4    6    8    10    11

MILES

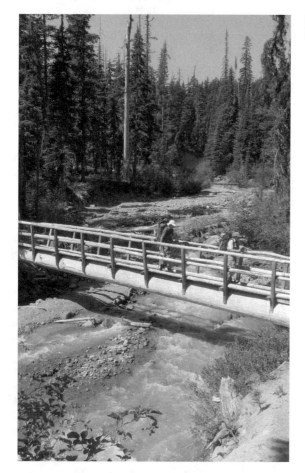

The bridge over Clark Creek

From the trailhead, you'll follow a flat path through moss-draped forest, pocket meadows with wildflowers, and huckleberries that ripen in late August. You may notice that some of these meadows aren't entirely natural (they're filled with stumps); that's because they are actually Nordic ski runs, part of the Mount Hood Meadows ski resort.

After hiking 0.5 miles you'll cross Clark Creek on a bridge, which skiers and snowshoers can attest is a lot more interesting with about two feet of snow on it. There is also a campsite at this crossing, but better ones await.

Keep going straight (ignoring trails leading left), and after another 0.6 miles you'll cross Newton Creek—on logs, one hopes. If you're early in the season and the logs aren't in place yet, this crossing (and a later one) might be tricky.

While we're here, a few words about the names of these creeks. They both flow from Newton Clark Glacier. What many people don't realize is that Newton Clark was just one guy, a teacher and surveyor who moved from South Dakota to Hood River Valley in 1877 and lived until 1918. There's also a county in South Dakota named for him.

Safely across Newton Creek, you are at the hill. Hike 0.8 miles to gain almost 700 feet in a series of long switchbacks; consider this the price of admission to Elk Meadows. Just over the top, you'll come to a four-way intersection. For Elk Meadows, go straight and you'll be there in just a few minutes. For a side trip to Elk Mountain, turn right, into an area that burned in 2006.

The trail to Elk Mountain is not spectacular in and of itself, but it's quiet and woodsy and leads to a nice view east across OR 35 to Mount Jefferson to the south. To get to the lookout, climb 0.6 miles and continue straight through the junction with Bluegrass Ridge Trail (647). The lookout is 0.3 miles ahead.

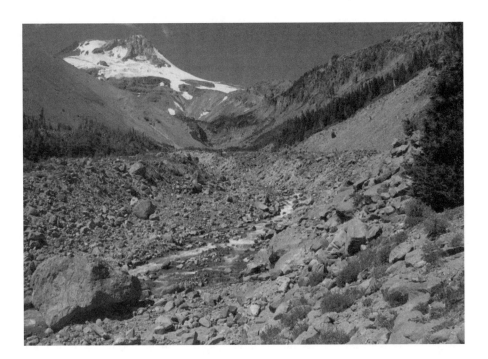

Mount Hood from the upper Newton Creek crossing

When you come back, take Bluegrass Ridge Trail (it would now be a right turn) and follow it half a mile along the ridgetop—through the heart of the burned area—before turning left, at a large stone cairn, and plunging 0.4 miles down Bluegrass Tie Trail (647B) to Elk Meadows.

Elk Meadows is almost unbelievable. It's basically a circular area of meadows about half a mile in diameter, with islands of trees throughout and streams crisscrossing it. For the good of the flowers and grass, resist the temptation to go meadow stomping, but by all means find a log or rock on the perimeter and have a rest. To complete a loop around the meadows, or to explore the other loop on this hike, follow the trail to the right.

When you come to a sign for Polallie Campground (at 2.5 miles), stay left on the perimeter trail, and 0.1 mile later you'll come to another trail leading left. Take it and continue straight, out into the middle of the meadows, where a stone shelter hosts backpackers most summer nights (there are also some tent sites behind the shelter in the woods).

On the way back from the shelter, take a left onto Gnarl Ridge Trail and start climbing along the side of the meadow, passing a couple more campsites along the way. In about half a mile you'll come to a junction with Perimeter Trail. To return to your car, turn left here, finish the loop around the meadows, and then turn right at the junction with Elk Meadows Trail. But to climb a little toward Mount Hood, stay straight here on Gnarl Ridge Trail.

After a little more than a mile of gradual climbing, you'll join Trail 652, and

0.3 miles past that reach Timberline Trail (600). Here you have another choice to make: turn left to start back toward the car, or turn right to climb another 900 feet in 1.5 miles to the top of Gnarl Ridge. That trail leads through more meadows and an ever-thinner forest, with views of Mount Adams to your right, and Lookout Mountain (hike 34, page 159) behind you. You can also clearly see the whole of Bluegrass Ridge, the scene of that 2006 fire.

The gravelly viewpoint of Gnarl Ridge offers one of the finer vistas around. The glaciers of Hood loom above you, with the headwater of Newton Creek bursting out from under them, and across the way you can make out a ski-lift building on the resort. Mount Jefferson and the Three Sisters are out beyond that. A short trail leads up to Lamberson Butte (6,633 feet), the official summit of the ridge.

Keep wandering up Timberline Trail—it's out in the open for quite a while now and leads just a couple miles over to Cooper Spur—or head back down to the junction and turn right. A gradual descent will bring you back to another crossing of Newton Creek, where again (one hopes) logs will help you across. On the far side, pass another fine campsite next to a spring creek, climb about a third of a mile, then turn left at the ridgetop onto Newton Creek Trail (646). Two miles down that heavily huckleberried trail, your path intersects the trail you started all this wandering on—Elk Meadows. Turn right to hike less than a mile back to the trailhead.

## NEARBY ACTIVITIES

For a little piece of Oregon history, pay your respects at the Pioneer Woman's Grave, off OR 35 just north of its intersection with US 26. Workers building the old Mount Hood Loop Highway found the woman buried beneath a crude marker; her remains have since been moved twice, and to this day people lay crosses or flowers on the pile of rocks marking her grave.

# LOOKOUT MOUNTAIN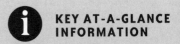

## IN BRIEF

One of the easternmost points in this book, Lookout Mountain is also one of the widest and most wonderful viewpoints, stretching from south of the Three Sisters all the way to Mount Rainier, and including desert, lake, and river.

## DESCRIPTION

First, for the "studly" out-and-back route, which is a whole lot more work but comes with a lot of benefits. From the Gumjuwac trailhead on OR 35, the first couple of miles are relentlessly uphill. You'll gain 1,400 feet in 2 miles, then catch a little break over the last half mile to Gumjuwac Saddle. At the top of the real climbing, around 2 miles up, there's a wonderful rocky viewpoint back toward Mount Hood—basically the first thing you'll see, other than trees.

At Gumjuwac Saddle, you'll encounter several trails. Gumjuwac Trail crosses FS 3550 and drops down the other side of the ridge

------------------------------------------

## *Directions* ⟶

Take US 26 from Portland, driving 51 miles east of I-205. Turn north on OR 35, following signs for Hood River. For the longer hike on Gumju-wac Trail, go 10.5 miles on OR 35 and park on the right, just after the road crosses the East Fork of Hood River. To drive to High Prairie for the shorter loop, go 2.5 miles farther on OR 35 and make a right on FS 44. Drive 3.7 miles, and turn right (following a sign for High Prairie) onto the gravel FS 4410. Over the next 4.6 miles, dur-ing which the road occasionally rides like a washboard, take the larger, more uphill road at all the junctions. At a sign for Badger Lake on the right, follow FS 4410 around to the left; the parking area is 100 yards ahead.

---

### (i) KEY AT-A-GLANCE INFORMATION

**LENGTH:** 2.2 miles for the loop (starting from High Prairie, 9.2 for the out-and-back (starting at OR 35)

**CONFIGURATION:** Out-and-back, or loop

**DIFFICULTY:** Easy loop, strenuous out-and-back

**SCENERY:** Meadows, forest, and one of the great vistas in Oregon

**EXPOSURE:** Shady, exposed rock at the top

**TRAFFIC:** Moderate on weekends, light otherwise

**TRAIL SURFACE:** Packed dirt, and rock

**HIKING TIME:** 1 hour for the loop, 5 for the out-and-back

**DRIVING DISTANCE:** 60 miles (1 hour 30 minutes) from Pioneer Square

**SEASON:** July–October

**BEST TIME:** August–September

**BACKPACKING OPTIONS:** Not great, some sites around Senecal Spring

**ACCESS:** Northwest Forest Pass required at both trailheads

**WHEELCHAIR ACCESS:** None

**MAPS:** Green Trails #462 (Mount Hood); USGS Badger Lake

**FACILITIES:** Outhouse at High Prairie; two springs on the way up from Gumju-wac and one more near the summit

**INFO:** Barlow Ranger District, (541) 467-2291

--------------------------------

### GPS Trailhead Coordinates

UTM Zone (WGS84) 10T

Easting 615671

Northing 5021917

Latitude   N 45.34122°

Longitude W 121.52359°

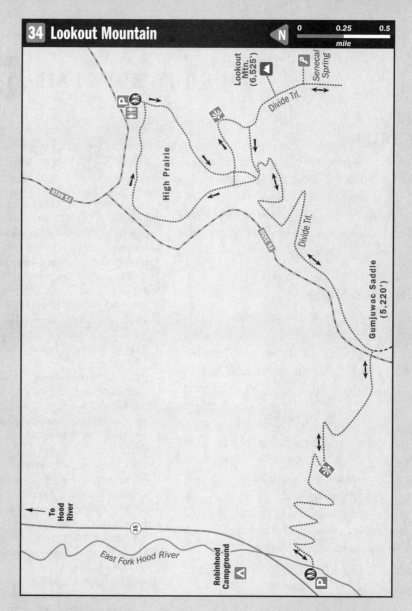

N

0        0.25        0.5
mile

Lookout Mtn. (6,525')

Senecal Spring

Divide Trl.

High Prairie

FS 4410

FS 3550

Divide Trl.

Gumjuwac Saddle (5,220')

To Hood River

35

East Fork Hood River

Robinhood Campground

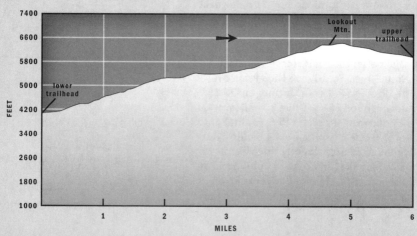

lower trailhead

Lookout Mtn.

upper trailhead

7400

6600

5800

5000

4200

3400

2600

1800

1000

FEET

1        2        3        4        5        6

MILES

into Badger Creek Wilderness. Coming in from the right is Gunsight Trail, popular with mountain bikers because it's 4.5 miles along the ridge with very little elevation change. In case you're thinking of driving FS 3550 to this point, you'd better have some clearance. But if you insist, turn right at the Badger Lake sign mentioned in the directions to High Prairie (see Directions) and then bounce about 3 miles to the saddle.

And if you're wondering about the name "Gumjuwac," it comes from a sheepherder, Jack. Apparently, Jack liked gum shoes, hence Gum Shoe Jack. Somehow that became "Gumjuwac" over the years. This is explained in what's left of the sign at the Saddle; that sign also refers to Mount Hood Loop Highway, which hasn't existed for decades.

To keep going to Lookout Mountain, simply walk across FS 3550 and start walking to your left, on Divide Trail (458). You'll encounter a lovely spring half a mile up; on this stretch you'll also have a view of Lookout Mountain straight ahead. And you'll see why this trail is called Divide Trail. Technically, it splits two watersheds—Hood River from the Dalles—but it also exhibits the amazing contrast between east and west. Coming up Gumjuwac Trail, it was all shady, with a view of glacier-covered Mount Hood; but on this side you'll encounter meadows, flowers, and views of the desert. As you climb with Hood on your left, look for views over your right shoulder to Badger Lake. Watch for wildlife, too; I once saw two falcons chasing each other around here, and I scared up an owl in the woods.

Keep climbing, and just below the summit, continue straight (and uphill) when the High Prairie Loop (493) cuts down to the left. This will put you on a rocky outcrop with an amazing view; many people stop here, but it's not the top of Lookout Mountain. To get there, put Mount Hood behind you and keep going, staying on Divide Trail. You'll walk along a rocky ridge looking down into the Badger Creek drainage; keep right where an old road goes left, then climb a short way to a trail leading left, to the wide-open summit and the foundation of an old fire lookout. For a description of the view, see below.

There's one more spring up here that's worth visiting. To reach Senecal Spring (named for a Forest Service ranger from the turn of the 20th century), take Divide Trail 0.2 miles past the summit and turn left on a trail that's barely visible and whose sign is often lying on the ground. The (very cold) spring is a quarter mile below Divide Trail.

Now, if you're more into driving up long hills than walking up them, here's High Prairie Loop. There are many trails on Lookout Mountain, some of which are not on maps. So take our map with you and remember that just about all these trails go to the same two places: Lookout Mountain and the trailhead.

From the parking area on FS 4410, walk straight across 4410 and up the wide path—so well worn it's practically paved—into the meadows. The fields of

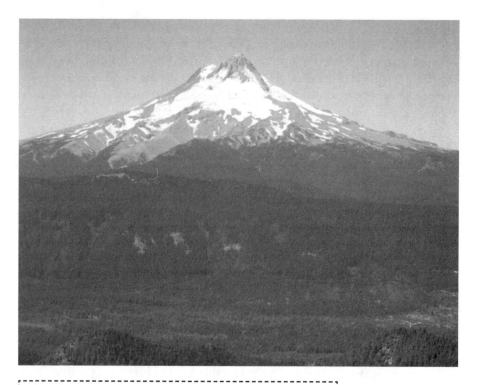

Mount Hood from the first viewpoint on the way up Lookout Mountain

daisies and lupine might make you want to stop there, but it's worth it to keep going. The trail you see immediately on your right, labeled for horses, is High Prairie Loop (493), which heads back to the trailhead. Ignore it for now.

Follow the wide trail ahead 0.7 miles until, in an area of reddish rock, it splits into three. The faint path through the trees on the right is a cutoff to the return portion of Loop Trail; ignore it. The path straight ahead (and up the hill) is a cutoff to Divide Trail. If you stay on the wide trail, you'll loop around to the left to a point with a fine view east of the Cascades, out into the Oregon High Desert. The road then loops back around to the right and intersects Divide Trail (458). Turn left on Divide Trail, climb a short way, and follow a narrow trail to the left to reach the summit. Like Gumjuwac Trail, this approach is listed on our elevation profile.

The view from Lookout Mountain's 6,500-foot summit is one that you just can't get from the western side of the Cascades, or for that matter from most points in the Cascades. From left to right, on a clear day, you can see Diamond Peak, the Three Sisters, Jefferson, Hood (absolutely huge just 7 miles across the way), St. Helens, Rainier, and Adams. From Diamond Peak to Rainier, as the crow flies, it is about 225 miles. You can also see, if you look closely, a stretch of the Columbia River to the northeast.

If you came up from Gumjuwac, you might as well see some new country on the way back by completing High Prairie Loop. To do this, when you're on Lookout Mountain walk toward Mount Hood on Divide Trail. At 0.3 miles, take the signed Loop Trail to your right and follow it as it crosses the face of Lookout Mountain and dives into the woods. Walk 0.7 miles, then turn right at a sign and walk back through the meadows to rejoin the wide, packed trail you started on just above FS 4410.

# 35 LOST LAKE

## GPS Trailhead Coordinates

UTM Zone (WGS84) 10T

Easting 592211

Northing 5038809

Latitude  N 45.49672°

Longitude  W 121.81979°

## IN BRIEF

This is like a resort area, with boats for rent, picnic tables with grills, a campground, and a beautiful lake stocked with trout. It's also a lovely walk around the natural, 240-acre lake, including an interpretive, barrier-free old-growth trail and one of the most photographed views of Mount Hood. All this, and there are two optional longer hikes, one of them to a fine lookout point.

## DESCRIPTION

Whether you're looking for a pleasant family campout or a good day of hiking, Lost Lake has what you need; that's why there are often so many people there. But, as is always the case, their number decreases in direct proportion to how far you walk.

For the 3.3-mile trail around the lake, start in front of the newly renovated general store. Walk to the boat dock and turn right. The first quarter mile of this trail, which parallels the road, is dotted with lakeside picnic

## *Directions*

Take I-84 from Portland, driving 55 miles east of I-205 to Exit 62/W Hood River. Make a right at the end of the off ramp, then immediately turn right again, onto Country Club Road, following signs for several wineries. At the end of Country Club Road, 3 miles on, turn left at a stop sign onto Barrett Drive. Continue 1.3 miles and turn right on Tucker Road, the second stop sign you'll come to on Barrett Drive. Go 2 miles up Tucker and turn right on Dee Highway, where a sign says "Parkdale." Drive 6.5 miles on Dee Highway, then turn right again onto FS 13, following signs for Lost Lake. The resort is 14 miles ahead at the end of the road. Just keep following the Lost Lake signs.

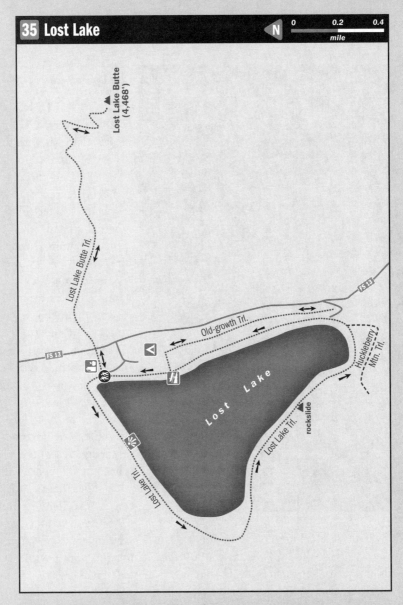

N

0        0.2        0.4
mile

Lost Lake Butte
(4,468')

Lost Lake Butte Trl.

FS 13

FS 13

Old-growth Trl.

Huckleberry Mtn. Trl.

Lost Lake

Lost Lake Trl.

rockslide

Lost Lake Trl.

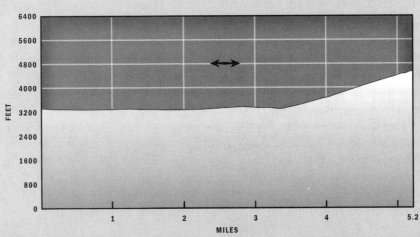

FEET

6400
5600
4800
4000
3200
2400
1600
800
0

1        2        3        4        5.2

MILES

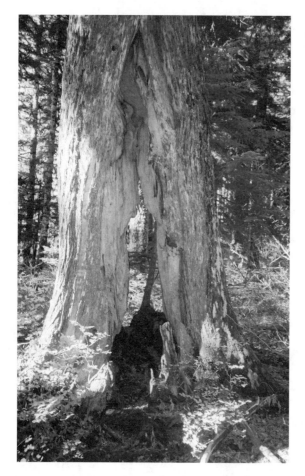

tables. Soon you'll come to a platform with a killer view of Mount Hood.

Beyond the platform, the trail leaves the road, and you start to feel like you're actually out in the woods. In late summer, your progress will be slowed by plump, ripe huckleberries; you can pick a handful or two, then choose a little beach off the trail, sit on a log, and peacefully enjoy your lunch. Keep an eye out for signs identifying tree species.

After just less than a mile, you'll come to a marshy area where the trail becomes a boardwalk. At 1.6 miles there's a rockslide with excellent swimming. After you've hiked another mile, you'll see Huckleberry Mountain Trail (617) leading right 2.5 miles to an intersection with the PCT. Along its 900-foot climb, this trail passes between Devils Pulpit and Preachers Peak—but nowhere near Huckleberry Mountain. Go figure. If you really want some exercise, hike about 4.5 miles south on the PCT to Buck Peak. If you're backpacking, the best site is at Salvation Spring, just north (right) on the PCT from where you join it.

Back at Lost Lake's shore, just past Huckleberry Mountain Trail, veer right from Lakeshore Trail, then stay left as you approach a group of buildings. This will put you on a road; Old Growth Trail (657) begins 100 yards ahead on a boardwalk and immediately passes between two of the largest cedars you are ever likely to see—both in the neighborhood of 12 feet in diameter.

This trail is a great one for the kids because it's not too long and includes educational signs explaining the roles that nurse logs, the forest canopy, the weather, and pileated woodpeckers and other animals play in a forest's life. Some of these trees are hundreds of years old and more than 200 feet tall. When the boardwalk runs out, continue another 0.3 miles, follow a trail through the campground down to the lake, and turn right to get back to your car.

To climb Lost Lake Butte for a view of, as the resort's hiking map puts it, "pretty near everything worth seeing," start in the general store's parking area. Walk back up the road and, at the turnoff for the main exit, look for a sign and a trail heading into the woods. You'll come to an unsigned trail intersection; turn right and uphill here. A hundred yards later, you'll cross another road; aim for a sign that says "Lost Lake Butte Trailhead." It can get confusing in here, but when in doubt, keep going uphill. It's a steady climb of 1,300 feet in 2 miles to an old fire lookout. Mount Hood, of course, is the dominant view to the south, but you can also see as far north as Mount Rainier (but not Mount Baker, as the resort map claims). Then just come back down the way you went up and get yourself a cool drink or ice cream in the store as a reward for all your effort. Constant access to refreshments is one of the great things about Lost Lake.

*Note:* A one-day fishing license (required for those age 14 and up) costs $12; for ages 14 to 17, it's $6.75.

# 36  MCNEIL POINT — Amazing!
## tough hike but worth it.

## KEY AT-A-GLANCE INFORMATION

**LENGTH: 9.2 miles**

**CONFIGURATION: Out-and-back**

**DIFFICULTY: Easy to Bald Mountain viewpoint, strenuous to McNeil Point**

**SCENERY: Old-growth forest, meadows, rugged mountainside**

**EXPOSURE: Shady, with a few stretches on rock and snow**

**TRAFFIC: Moderate on summer weekends, light otherwise**

**TRAIL SURFACE: Packed dirt with roots, a few small stream crossings, some rocks and snow**

**HIKING TIME: 5.5 hours**

**DRIVING DISTANCE: 58 miles (1 hour 30 minutes) from Pioneer Square**

**SEASON: July–October**

**BEST TIME: August–September**

**BACKPACKING OPTIONS: Excellent**

**ACCESS: Northwest Forest Pass required**

**WHEELCHAIR ACCESS: None**

**MAPS: USFS Mount Hood Wilderness**

**FACILITIES: None at trailhead; water on trail must be treated**

**INFO: Zigzag Ranger District, (503) 622-3191**

**SPECIAL COMMENTS: No matter what the weather is when you start, bring warm clothing if you're going to McNeil Point. It's above the tree line, and weather changes quickly up there.**

## IN BRIEF

You don't have to do this whole trail to make it worthwhile; it opens with a great view, passes through a cathedral forest to wildflower meadows and alpine ponds, then gets up close and personal with Mount Hood. But if you do go all the way up, you can see the trickle that is the source of the Sandy River and hear glaciers pop and rumble.

## DESCRIPTION

This is a honey of a hike! You start out on Top Spur Trail, which climbs gradually for half a mile to a veritable highway interchange of trails. First you'll reach the PCT; turn right on that. Hike 100 feet to a four-way junction with Timberline Trail. From here, the PCT leads down 2.2 miles to Ramona Falls Trail (hike 38, page 175).

To simply head for McNeil Point, follow Timberline Trail (600) uphill and to the left. But it's well worth it to see the magnificent view from the open side (not actually the top) of Bald Mountain, a mere 0.4 miles the other way on Timberline Trail. Head out there to take in the sweeping view of Mount Hood and the Muddy Fork of the Sandy River. Then keep going, toward Mount Hood, and look for a faint cutoff trail that goes over the ridge

## GPS Trailhead Coordinates

UTM Zone (WGS84) 10T

Easting 595032

Northing 5028926

Latitude  N 45.40740°

Longitude  W 121.78560°

## Directions

**Take US 26 from Portland, driving 36 miles east of I-205 to Zigzag, and turn left onto Lolo Pass Road at the Zigzag Store. Go 10.6 miles to Lolo Pass and make a right onto the paved FS 1828, which is the first right at the pass. Go 3.1 miles and turn left onto the gravel FS 118. The trailhead is 1.2 miles ahead on the right.**

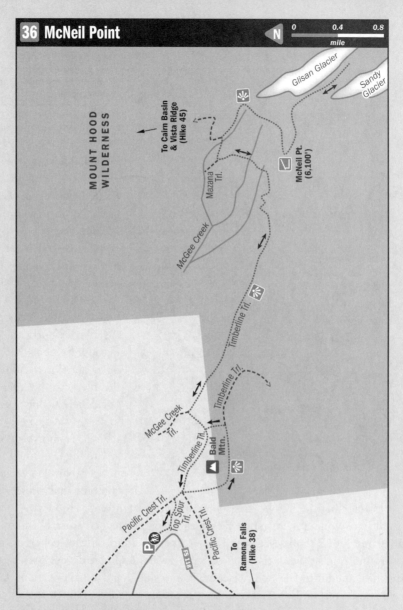

MOUNT HOOD WILDERNESS

N

0    0.4    0.8
mile

Glisan Glacier

Sandy Glacier

To Cairn Basin & Vista Ridge (Hike 45)

McNeil Pt. (6,100')

Mazana Trl.

McGee Creek

Timberline Trl.

Timberline Trl.

McGee Creek Trl.

Timberline Trl.

Bald Mtn.

Pacific Crest Trl.

Top Spur Trl.

Pacific Crest Trl.

To Ramona Falls (Hike 38)

P

FS 118

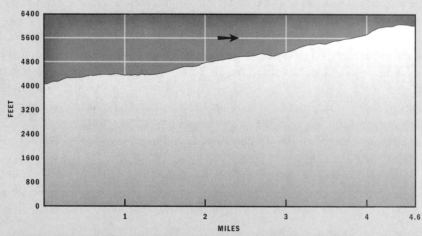

FEET

6400
5600
4800
4000
3200
2400
1600
800
0

1    2    3    4    4.6

MILES

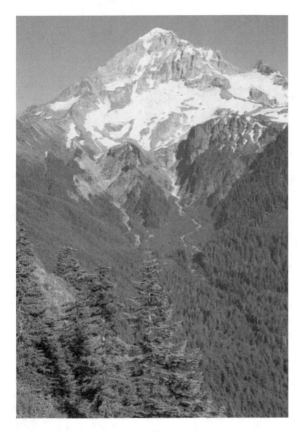

to your left, just before the PCT heads back into the woods. The cutoff extends about 100 yards over the ridge and back to Timberline Trail; turn right for McNeil Point.

This stretch of Timberline Trail is in a true cathedral forest—the tall, straight trees, mostly hemlocks, have no branches in their lower portions, creating a forest scene that's both open and lofty. Adding to the pleasure are the many huckleberry bushes that make up the ground cover; their juicy morsels are ripe in late August. You'll hardly notice that you've started climbing in earnest.

On Timberline Trail, at the first big view of Mount Hood you come to (you'll have gone 2.3 miles), look for the large, unnamed waterfall across the valley on Hood's flank. At 3.5 miles, you'll cross a fork of McGee Creek and, if it's around August, be in the land of wildflowers. Lupines, daisies, pasque flowers, lilies, and butterflies will welcome you to the high country. Just a bit farther are a couple of ponds, which make ideal places to stop for lunch and also host some fine campsites. You can skip and frolic in this area and call it a day, or keep going to the higher country.

At about 3.8 miles, just after Mazama Trail has come in from the left, you'll reach a tiny stream flowing out of a flower-filled bowl with a snowfield at the top. A minute past that, look for a trail heading up the ridge to the right. If you just want more meadows without more climbing, stay on the main trail as it swings to the left, negotiate a stream crossing that can be mildly dangerous in high water, and connect with the outer reaches of the Vista Ridge trip (hike 45, page 203) for Cairn Basin and Eden Park. If you're set on McNeil Point, turn right and climb the ridge.

About 0.5 miles up, the trail crosses a rockslide and (in most years) a snowfield. Be careful on both these terrains; they aren't steep, but remember that even big rocks move, and that even packed snow is slippery. The trail keeps

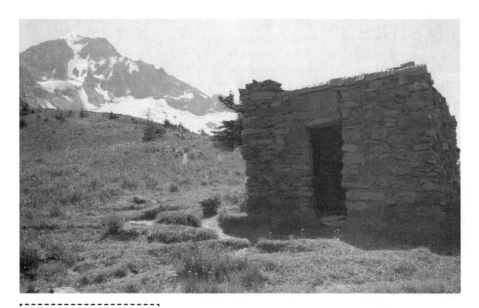

The shelter at McNeil Point

ascending the ridge face, crossing more small patches of snow. At a junction near the top, head right for the easiest route or left to stay higher and try your skills at glissading down a small snowfield.

One mile from the turnoff at the creek, you'll reach the 1930s-era stone shelter at McNeil Point. From here the view is stupendous: Mount Hood soaring above you, the valley of the Muddy Fork of the Sandy stretching out below you, the other Cascade volcanoes beyond. As you look at Mount Hood, the sprawling glacier on your right is Sandy Glacier, and the trickle coming out the bottom of it is the beginning of the Sandy River, which flows into the Columbia down at Troutdale.

Also, as you look at Mount Hood, you'll notice more trail above you, heading into the Really High Country. It's not on any maps, but if you follow it you will (a) soon run out of breath as you approach 7,000 feet in elevation with virtually no switchbacks, and (b) find yourself on a narrow, rocky ridge between the Sandy (on your right) and Glisan (on your left) glaciers.

I sat up there one day listening to the glaciers pop and moan as they slid slowly but relentlessly down the face of the mountain. You might even see massive boulders tumbling down the slope; you can certainly pick out their trails on the snow. At all costs, be careful up there, and most definitely resist the temptation to hop onto the snow.

You may hear or see reports of another, more direct trail between McNeil Point and Timberline Trail, connecting with the latter at a point west of the ponds. The word from many hikers, including this one, is to avoid that trail. It's steep, rocky, difficult, and unnecessary. The one described here is easier and more scenic.

# 37 MIRROR LAKE

**KEY AT-A-GLANCE INFORMATION**

**LENGTH:** 2.8 miles to the lake, 6.4 miles to the top of the ridge

**CONFIGURATION:** Out-and-back

**DIFFICULTY:** Easy to the lake, moderate to the ridge

**SCENERY:** Rhododendrons; deep forest; a small, placid lake; a big view

**EXPOSURE:** Shady on the way up, open at the lake, wide open atop the ridge

**TRAFFIC:** Heavy all summer, insane on weekends

**TRAIL SURFACE:** Packed dirt, rocks

**HIKING TIME:** 2 hours to the lake, 3.5 hours to the ridgetop

**DRIVING DISTANCE:** 52 miles (1 hour 15 minutes) from Pioneer Square

**SEASON:** Late June–October

**BEST TIME:** August–September

**BACKPACKING OPTIONS:** A few sites at the lake

**ACCESS:** Northwest Forest Pass required

**WHEELCHAIR ACCESS:** None

**MAPS:** Mount Hood Wilderness; Green Trails #461 (Government Camp); USGS Government Camp

**FACILITIES:** Sometimes a portable outhouse at the trailhead

**INFO:** Zigzag Ranger District, (503) 622-3191

## IN BRIEF

You can go a short way on this hike and join the weekend throngs at a lovely little lake that has a great view of Mount Hood. Or you can put in a little more effort and leave the crowds behind to claim an even better view at the top of, believe it or not, Tom, Dick, and Harry Mountain.

## DESCRIPTION

When you come around the corner on US 26 and see 75 cars parked on the side of the road, know that it's not a fair: it's the Mirror Lake trailhead. The interest in this trail is well justified, so think about starting early or going on a weekday to have a decent chance for some quiet time.

The lower portions of the trail to Mirror Lake have rhododendrons that will bloom pink in late June, and the upper portions are cool and shady, keeping you from warming up too much as you head up the hill. But it isn't even much of a hill, gaining less than 700 feet in 1.4 well-graded miles. Just below the lake, you'll come to the outlet creek and a trail junction. You can go either way to loop 0.4 miles around the lake, but if you're headed up the ridge, bear right. The lake itself is a beauty. The beaches are on the right side, the

---

GPS Trailhead
Coordinates

UTM Zone (WGS84) 10T

Easting 594687

Northing 5017749

Latitude  N 45.30686°

Longitude  W 121.79216°

*Directions*

**Take US 26 from Portland, driving 45 miles east of I-205. Park at the trailhead, on the right. It's half a mile past the historic marker for the Laurel Hill Chute, which is also on the right.**

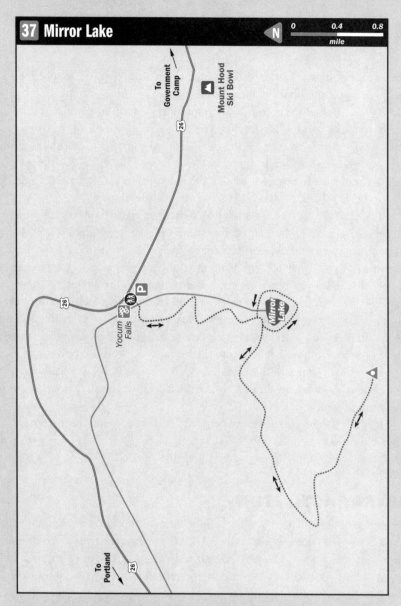

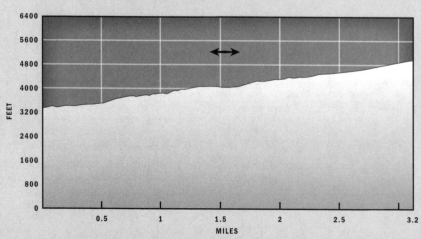

campsites are on the left, and the view of Mount Hood you're looking for is at the far end, on the boardwalk in a marshy area.

To get to the top of Tom, Dick, and Harry Mountain, walk to the far right side of the lake (as you face it when you arrive), and follow a trail that goes right and steadily climbs the face of the ridge. Your destination is actually right above you, but you have to walk almost 2 miles to get there. As for the mountain's name, it indicates the three peaks on the ridge—not, as some would suggest, the fact that every Tom, Dick, and Harry hikes this trail.

The trail is really just two lengthy switchbacks, each one almost a mile long. It's time to turn left when you get to some very odd, large piles of rocks, which no one has ever been able to explain to me. The forest opens up a little more here and, as you approach the summit, the trail gets a smidgen steeper. When you reach a rocky area (neither steep nor dangerous), you're almost there.

The view from atop this ridge is really something, considering how close you still are to the car. For starters, look at how pitifully small Mirror Lake is—and how far down there. It never ceases to amaze me how quickly one gains elevation when hiking. Right across the highway is Mount Hood, in all its glory. Mount Adams is actually blocked by it. To the left is Mount St. Helens. What looks like a shoulder on St. Helens is in fact Mount Rainier, some 100 miles to the north of you.

In case you're still feeling energetic, resist the temptation to explore the other two peaks on this ridge—Tom and Dick, as it were. They're offlimits because they are home to protected peregrine falcons.

## NEARBY ACTIVITIES

The easternmost peak of Tom, Dick, and Harry Mountain is the summit of Mount Hood Ski Bowl, which, in the summer, is like a constant carnival. You can bungee jump, ride the alpine slide, play minigolf, drive go-carts, take a trip in a helicopter, or ride the chairlift to the top of the hill and hike or mountain bike down. The entrance is 1 mile east on US 26.

# RAMONA FALLS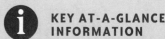

## IN BRIEF

This trail is immensely popular, and it's no wonder. It's a fairly easy hike to a uniquely beautiful falls, with plenty of room for a picnic when you get there. There's even a side trip that takes you up onto a shoulder of Mount Hood.

## DESCRIPTION

This hike starts on a trail that looks like a highway; that's because it's basically flat and thousands of people make the trek to Ramona Falls every year. Walk 0.2 miles and cross Sandy River Trail, a connector from Riley Horse Camp. Continue on Trail 797 toward Ramona Falls, pausing to admire a very large, cracked boulder near the junction.

A short walk rewards you with a nice view of Mount Hood up the main stem of the Sandy River. You will also see the results of a massive flood event that occurred in November 2007. The deep cut you see here didn't exist before that flood, and the trail has been moved in a few places to replace sections that

## *Directions* ⟶

Take US 26 from Portland, driving 36 miles east of I-205 to Zigzag. Turn left (north) onto Lolo Pass Road, which is 0.6 miles past milepost 41. Go 4.2 miles and make a right onto FS 1825, which is 0.1 mile past a Mount Hood National Forest sign and is marked "campgrounds and trailheads." Stay right at 0.7 miles, cross a bridge, and continue another 1.7 miles to turn left onto Spur Road 100, which leads 0.5 miles to the trailhead. Note that this intersection is occasionally without signs, so trust the odometer. Going right at this last fork would take you 0.3 miles to Lost Creek Campground, which has water and toilets.

### KEY AT-A-GLANCE INFORMATION

**LENGTH:** 7.1 miles to the falls, 15.4 up Yocum Ridge
**CONFIGURATION:** Balloon
**DIFFICULTY:** Easy
**SCENERY:** A pleasant stream, a historic cabin, a one-of-a-kind waterfall, and maybe a trip to the high country
**EXPOSURE:** In the woods all the way, with occasional open spots
**TRAFFIC:** Heavy use, especially on summer weekends
**TRAIL SURFACE:** Packed dirt
**HIKING TIME:** 3.5 hours
**DRIVING DISTANCE:** 53 miles (1 hour 10 minutes) from Pioneer Square
**SEASON:** May–October
**BEST TIME:** July–September
**BACKPACKING OPTIONS:** Campsites very near the falls and up on Yocum Ridge
**ACCESS:** Northwest Forest Pass required
**WHEELCHAIR ACCESS:** None
**MAPS:** USFS Mount Hood Wilderness; Green Trails #461 (Government Camp); USGS Bull Run Lake
**FACILITIES:** None at trailhead; campground with water and toilets less than a mile away
**INFO:** Zigzag Ranger District, (503) 622-3191
**SPECIAL COMMENTS:** Hiking bridge over the Sandy is in place only from mid-May to mid-October. Call ahead or check online.

- - - - - - - - - - - - - - - - - - - - - - - - - - - - - -

GPS Trailhead
Coordinates
UTM Zone (WGS84) 1oT
Easting 591514
Northing 5026541
Latitude N 45.38640°
Longitude W 121.83100°

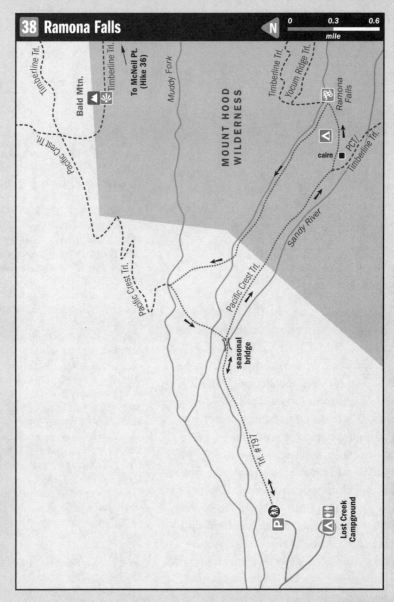

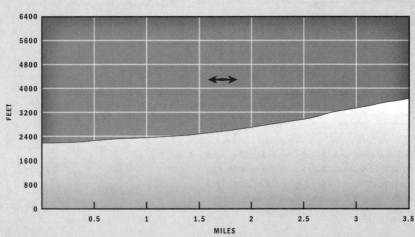

are probably now down in the Columbia River. In fact, at one point about a mile up, you can see the trail reappearing on the far edge of a big bend in the gorge; that gives you some perspective, huh?

At 1.2 miles, you'll reach the Sandy River crossing. The bridge here is in place from mid-May to mid-October; there are generally signs at the trailhead alerting you to its status, but call ahead, if you like. In the fall, the river can often be crossed without the bridge—if there hasn't been much rain.

After crossing the river, follow the ribbons across the new debris flow, eventually putting in a quarter mile to reach the junction with the PCT, which here is making its way around the west side of Mount Hood. This is also where your loop starts, so for now, turn right (south) onto the PCT and continue your gradual climb over moss-covered ground and under some very large rhododendrons. A mile past the junction, you'll reach the top of a bluff from which the Sandy, below you to the right, is more audible. Keep an eye out for eroded cliffs across the way, which offer a cross-section of Mount Hood's volcanic deposits. Those deposits are much older than the ones you just left.

When you're 1.5 miles past the junction (and 3 miles from the car), the PCT dips to the right and toward the river; follow it for a little scenic side trip. At the bottom of a short descent, you'll reach a campsite near the Sandy's shore. The PCT crosses the Sandy here and starts a long climb toward Timberline Lodge, and it's worth walking out to the crossing to stand on the 2007 debris and catch some cool views up the canyon toward Hood and some big-time waterfalls. Follow pink ribbons if you get confused.

Back at the far end of the campsite, look for log steps leading up the hill to a 1935 ranger station, built to keep hikers out of the protected Bull Run watershed. The rangers are long gone, but hikers can spend the night here. The leaky cabin is lousy with mice and has been boarded up for years, but there are some tent sites nearby, and a nice view of Sandy River Canyon about 100 yards uphill.

Follow the PCT back up the hill to Ramona Falls Loop, turn right, and in 0.2 miles you'll come to a horse gate protecting the entrance to the falls area. From here, you can descend to the left to find campsites; camping is not allowed at the falls itself. Pass through the gate and enter the falls area.

Ramona Falls is a perfect example of how a tiny stream can make a heck of a waterfall. These falls are best compared to one of those pyramids of Champagne glasses; as the water cascades over broken columns of basalt, it spreads across a 120-foot-wide expanse, the force of the water sending a cool, misty spray into the open air. No wonder so many people come here with kids and dogs and picnic supplies! Just beware of the gray jays that haunt the area; they'll take food right out of your hands if you're not careful.

There's a nice story, by the way, behind the naming of Ramona Falls. In 1933 a Forest Service employee came across the falls while scouting the area for a trail; at the time, he was courting his future wife and named the falls after a popular romantic song of the time called "Ramona."

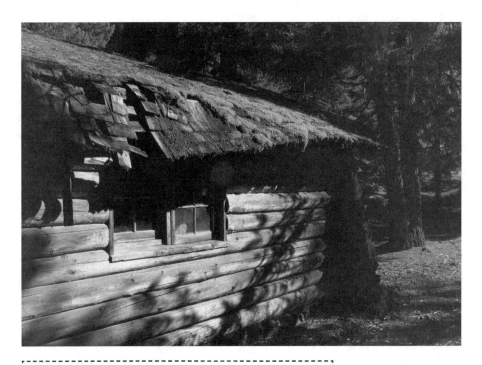

The historic Sandy River Guard Station, near Ramona Falls on the PCT

Continue over the bridge to reach a junction at the far end. To head back to the car, go straight. Or, if you're looking for an adventure, make a right on Timberline Trail, which goes 42 miles around Mount Hood. You can follow this trail 5 or so miles around the headwaters of the Sandy River's Muddy Fork to wind up on the flanks of Bald Mountain (also part of the McNeil Point hike (hike 36, page 168). That trail, though, has suffered over the years from mudslides and washouts, despite crews working to keep it open. Best to call the ranger district ahead of time to check on conditions before heading this way.

What you can still do is put in just over half a mile on Timberline Trail and then head up Yocum Ridge Trail (771), an occasionally steep affair that gains 2,100 feet in 4.1 miles. The reward for that effort is an amazing bit of alpine splendor, far enough from any trailhead that it receives relatively few visitors—certainly compared to Vista Ridge or McNeil Point.

To complete the much simpler loop back to the parking lot from Ramona Falls, follow the trail straight ahead and down Ramona Creek, perhaps singing a romantic tune as you go. It's a gentle 1.6-mile descent, featuring several log-bridge crossings of the creek, with views of fantastic rock walls on the right. See if you can spot a little section of "underground" creek as well.

Leave the PCT when it turns right for a hiker's bridge across the creek; continuing straight ahead on Trail 797, go through a fence 0.1 mile later, then turn left and walk half a mile back to where your loop started. Backtrack across the Sandy to your car, which is 2 miles down from where you hit the PCT.

# SALMON BUTTE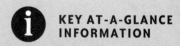

## IN BRIEF

This easy-to-get-to trail offers a mellow climb through old-growth forest and giant rhododendrons to a viewpoint that takes in Mount Hood, Mount Jefferson, and the heart of the Salmon–Huckleberry Wilderness. And when the rhodies are blooming, it's a treat!

## DESCRIPTION

This trail is so well graded that you'll hardly notice you're going uphill, except for catching occasional views down the valley or up toward the peak. Other trails might climb a similar elevation in half the distance, but they'll leave you more tired. So this is a perfect way to get on top of something without spending the whole day or wearing yourself out.

The trail starts out through an area that was clearcut 30 years ago, so there's not much in the way of old trees, but soon you get into not only the hemlocks and moss-draped Douglas firs, but also some very large rhododendrons that will bloom in late June. At 1.3 miles, you'll reach an area at the end of a ridge with a view to the top of the butte and some nice rocks to sit on. Just less than 2 miles up, a trail to the right at a switchback leads to a steep, wildflower-filled meadow with a perfect rock to stand on for a photo

### KEY AT-A-GLANCE INFORMATION

**LENGTH:** 8.4 miles

**CONFIGURATION:** Out-and-back

**DIFFICULTY:** Moderate

**SCENERY:** Pleasant forest on the way up, panoramic view on top

**EXPOSURE:** Shady with occasional open spots, then wide open on top

**TRAFFIC:** Moderate on summer weekends, light otherwise

**TRAIL SURFACE:** Packed dirt, some rocks at the top

**HIKING TIME:** 4 hours

**DRIVING DISTANCE:** 70 miles (1 hour 20 minutes) from Pioneer Square

**SEASON:** June–October

**BEST TIME:** June or October

**BACKPACKING OPTIONS:** None

**ACCESS:** No fee

**WHEELCHAIR ACCESS:** None

**MAPS:** USFS Salmon–Huckleberry Wilderness

**FACILITIES:** None at the trailhead

**INFO:** Zigzag Ranger District, (503) 622-3191

---

## *Directions* ⟶

Take **US 26** from **Portland**, driving **36 miles east** of **I-205**. Turn right on **Salmon River Road**, which is 0.1 mile before Lolo Pass Road on the left. Continue 6.5 miles straight down this road; you'll come to a small parking area on the left; the trail enters the trees on the right.

## GPS Trailhead Coordinates

UTM Zone (WGS84) 1oT

Easting 583283

Northing 5o12378

Latitude N 45.25997°

Longitude W 121.93850°

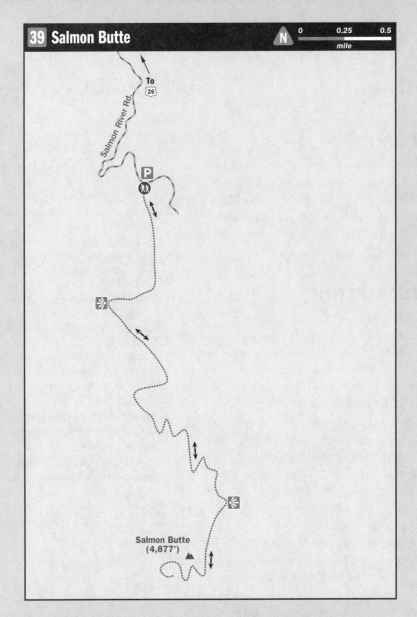

N

0        0.25        0.5
mile

To
26

Salmon River Rd.

P

Salmon Butte
(4,877')

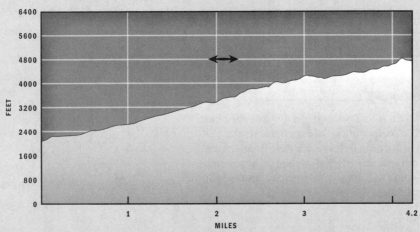

6400
5600
4800
4000
3200
2400
1600
800
0

FEET

1                2                3        4.2
MILES

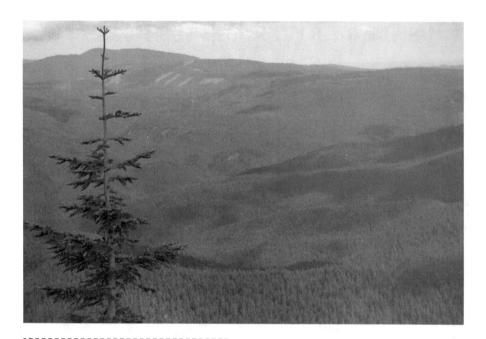

A view of the wilderness from Salmon Butte

opportunity. If you continue on for another mile, you'll gain the ridgeline in an open area loaded with rhododendrons and affording a view to the left of the sweeping Salmon River Valley. You'll now have climbed 2,100 of this hike's 2,800 feet.

Near the top, the trail dead-ends into an old road that once served as a lookout tower; turn right and follow the road to the summit, which is reached by a rocky scramble of about 100 feet. From here you're looking south and east, with Mount Hood 15 miles to your left, Mount Jefferson 35 miles to your right, and Mounts Adams and Rainier off on the horizon. In front of you is the Salmon–Huckleberry Wilderness; what a difference a lack of clearcuts makes, eh? While you're up there, scavenge for old pieces of glass and metal that are part of the burned-down lookout tower. Then cruise back down the same gentle grade you came up.

## NEARBY ACTIVITIES

The Mount Hood Brewing Company in Government Camp (10 miles east on US 26) serves good pizza and generally has about six of the brewery's beers on tap, with cool names like Cloud Cap Amber and Ice Axe IPA.

# 40 SALMON RIVER-DEVILS PEAK

## KEY AT-A-GLANCE INFORMATION

**LENGTH:** Lower section 5.2 miles round-trip, upper section 6.6 miles round-trip

**CONFIGURATION:** Out-and-back

**DIFFICULTY:** Easy all the way to the campsites in the upper section, moderate beyond that

**SCENERY:** Old-growth forest, spawning salmon in the spring and fall, a canyon view at the top

**EXPOSURE:** Shady all the way to the top, exposed rocks at the top

**TRAFFIC:** Heavy all summer long

**TRAIL SURFACE:** Packed dirt, with rocks and roots

**HIKING TIME:** 2 hours for the lower loop, 3.5 hours for the upper

**DRIVING DISTANCE:** 50 miles (1 hour 15 minutes) from Pioneer Square

**SEASON:** Year-round, but might get snow in winter

**BEST TIME:** October, for the colors and salmon

**BACKPACKING OPTIONS:** Nice sites in the upper section

**ACCESS:** Northwest Forest Pass required

**WHEELCHAIR ACCESS:** None

**MAPS:** USFS Salmon–Huckleberry Wilderness

**FACILITIES:** None at trailheads; water and restrooms at Green Canyon campground

**INFO:** Zigzag Ranger District, (503) 622-3191

## IN BRIEF

The Salmon River, which starts on the slopes of Timberline Ski Area, is the only river in the lower 48 states to be classified as a Wild and Scenic River from its headwater to its mouth. (To see its headwater and cross it where you can skip across, do the Barlow Pass trip, hike 30, page 142.) The trail along the Salmon can be thought of as having three sections, two of which are described here. They are extremely easy to get to, and in the fall they host spawning salmon. The uppermost section, accessed by a different road near Trillium Lake, is less interesting than these, tougher to find, and not worth the effort. Its only advantage is that nobody hikes it.

## DESCRIPTION

Start with the lower, easier section, which is Trail 742A, Old Salmon River Trail. From the roadside parking area (the first one you came to while driving in), you'll start out downhill through a beautiful forest of Douglas firs and western red cedars. You'll be close to the river after 0.1 mile and follow it most of the rest of the way. After two little footbridges over side creeks, you'll come to the first of several trails leading down to the river. You will pass two more small bridges, and after

## GPS Trailhead Coordinates

UTM Zone (WGS84) 10T

Easting 582810

Northing 5018016

Latitude N 45.31076°

Longitude W 121.94359°

## *Directions* ⟶

Take US 26 from Portland, driving 36 miles east of I-205. Turn right on Salmon River Road, which is 0.1 mile before Lolo Pass Road, on the left. Continue 2.7 miles straight down this road to reach the lower trailhead (just beyond the Mount Hood National Forest sign), or drive 4.9 miles to the upper trailhead, at a bridge over the river.

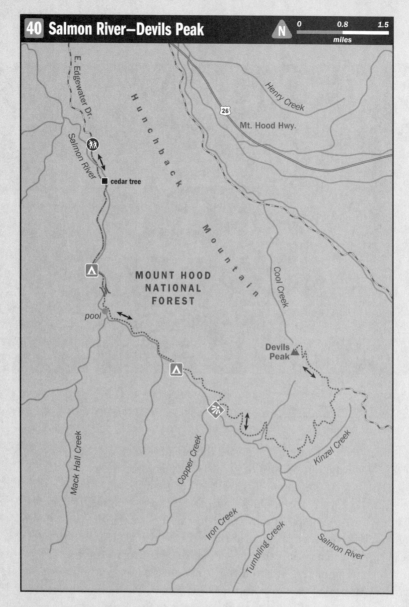

**N**

| 0 | 0.8 | 1.5 |

*miles*

E. Edgewater Dr.

Henry Creek

26

Mt. Hood Hwy.

Salmon River

H u n c h b a c k

■ cedar tree

M o u n t a i n

Cool Creek

**MOUNT HOOD
NATIONAL
FOREST**

*pool*

Devils
Peak

Mack Hall Creek

Copper Creek

Kinzel Creek

Iron Creek

Salmon River

Tumbling Creek

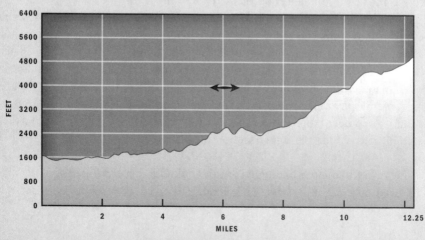

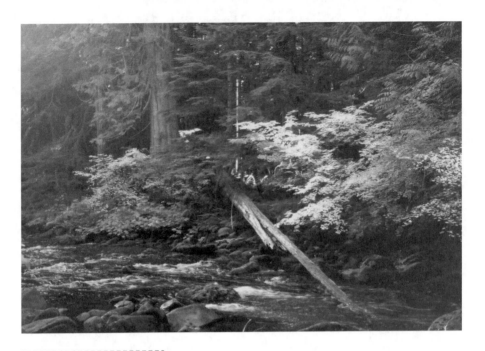

Along the Salmon River in fall

0.4 miles come to a campsite where there's a log sticking out over the river. It's perfectly sturdy, but be sure of your balance before you go out on it.

The best thing about this trail, other than its convenience and the river itself, is the nature of the old-growth forest. Look for "nurse" logs, fallen trees that are now the home of new trees. Just past the campsite with the suspended log, you'll go up a set of steps, at the top of which there's an absolutely massive western red cedar; you can't miss it—it's right next to the trail and about ten feet thick in diameter. At about the 1-mile mark, look for a hollowed-out cedar stump with a new tree growing from it; just past it is the biggest Douglas fir (about eight feet in diameter) on this stretch of the trail.

At about the 1.5-mile mark, you'll come to the first of two sections where the trail briefly joins the road. Take the second trail back into the woods; the first trail is used by anglers and dead-ends at the river. Continue 50 yards back on the trail and look for three large trees—two firs and a cedar—that are almost bonded together. Just past here, where a downed tree lies along the bank, I came across several spawning salmon on a late-September hike. They were in the shallows just a few feet from shore. The fish will actually go several miles farther upstream; if you hike the upper section of this trail in the fall, you'll get more chances to see them.

There are two more highlights to this trail. One is a cedar tree so large that a hollowed-out area in its base is big enough to be called a cave. The other is a

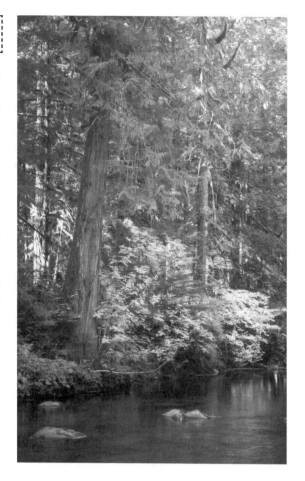

There's plenty of peace along the Salmon River.

"nurse" log, cut into three pieces for trail-construction purposes, which is now host to no fewer than eight saplings.

When you have hiked a little more than 2 miles, you'll come to Green Canyon Campground, which has an outhouse and water. Then, after a second section on the roadside, you'll briefly drop back into the woods before emerging at the upper trailhead, where the road crosses the river.

Now, for the next section up the river, which is the beginning of Trail 742, Salmon River Trail. From the trailhead, walk upstream through a forest of Douglas fir. Just less than a half mile up, you'll pass a deep pool, where anglers often gather. A short distance past this, when you get another view of the river from about 40 feet above it, look (in September and October) for dark shapes swirling about in the pools. Those are salmon; the black-gray ones are chinook, and the less-often-seen gold ones are coho. Consider that they have spent their lives in the ocean and have swum some 75 miles up the Columbia River, about 41 miles up the Sandy, then about 20 miles up the Salmon.

At the 2-mile mark, a series of campsites on the right offers yet more chances to get close to the river and look for fish. Just past a trail that leads right, to a nice little falls and deep pool—both formed by a huge log that fell across the river, you'll embark on just about your only climb of the day, picking up about 600 feet in 1.3 miles as you climb toward an overlook of Salmon River Canyon. After you pop out into the open, make sure you go as far as the rock outcrop for the best view. Just be very careful around here, and don't try any of the trails heading down toward the river. You might descend farther and faster than you ever intended.

That scenic view is your recommended turnaround, as you're now 3.3 miles from the upper trailhead, but the trail actually goes another 10.8 miles upstream to the road near Trillium Lake. If you're feeling truly industrious, or perhaps you camped back along the river and have more time, consider putting in the big climb to the lookout tower at Devils Peak. Just continue 2.3 miles up Salmon River Trail, and turn left to climb Kinzel Lake Trail (665), following it 2.3 miles (and 1,600 feet) up to Hunchback Trail (793), which leads 1.6 miles (and another 700 feet) up to the 5,045-foot lookout. So, if you started at the bridge, you're looking at 9.8 miles *one-way* with a climb of 3,400 feet. Good luck with that. There are other ways to get up there, but this one would be good as part of an overnight trip.

## NEARBY ACTIVITIES

Start your day with breakfast at the Zigzag Inn, 0.1 mile east of Salmon River Road on US 26. They do good things with French toast there.

# TAMANAWAS FALLS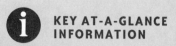

## IN BRIEF

This is a classic falls in a dramatic setting at the end of an easy, beautiful hike. *Tamanawas* (pronounced "ta-MAH-na-was") is a Chinook word for a friendly, guardian spirit, and it's an appropriate name for this nonthreatening, pleasant hike.

## DESCRIPTION

So many people like this trail that even a flood in 2000, which wiped out two trail bridges, didn't keep folks away. Officially, the trail was closed that entire summer, but Oregonians displayed their typical respect for the government by hiking the "closed" trail in such numbers that the Forest Service acquiesced and made the new, hiker-created trail the official one. The Forest Service hasn't rebuilt the bridges, so the trail you hike today is what the locals came up with in 2000.

From the trailhead, walk to your right and cross the East Fork of the Hood River on a one-log bridge with handrails. Note the milky color of this river; that's glacial silt. At the far end of the bridge, join East Fork Trail (650) and follow it downstream, where it bears right to parallel the road for half a mile.

At 0.7 miles, you'll leave East Fork Trail and cross Cold Spring Creek on 650A,

### KEY AT-A-GLANCE INFORMATION

**LENGTH:** 3.4 miles
**CONFIGURATION:** Out-and-back
**DIFFICULTY:** Easy
**SCENERY:** Two mountain streams, one plunging waterfall
**EXPOSURE:** Shady all the way, then open toward the end
**TRAFFIC:** Heavy on summer weekends, moderate otherwise
**TRAIL SURFACE:** Packed dirt and rocks
**HIKING TIME:** 2.5 hours
**DRIVING DISTANCE:** 75 miles (1 hour 40 minutes) from Pioneer Square
**SEASON:** June–November
**BEST TIME:** July–September
**BACKPACKING OPTIONS:** None
**ACCESS:** Northwest Forest Pass required
**WHEELCHAIR ACCESS:** None
**MAPS:** Mount Hood Wilderness; Green Trails #462 (Mount Hood); USGS Dog River
**FACILITIES:** None at trailhead; water and restrooms 0.5 miles south on OR 35, at Sherwood Campground
**INFO:** Hood River Ranger District, (541) 352-6002

## Directions

Take US 26 from Portland, driving 51 miles east of I-205. Turn north on OR 35, following signs for Hood River. Drive 15 miles on OR 35, and 0.2 miles past Sherwood Campground; park at the trailhead, on the left.

## GPS Trailhead Coordinates

UTM Zone (WGS84) 10T
Easting 611811
Northing 5028046
Latitude  N 45.39700°
Longitude W 121.57145°

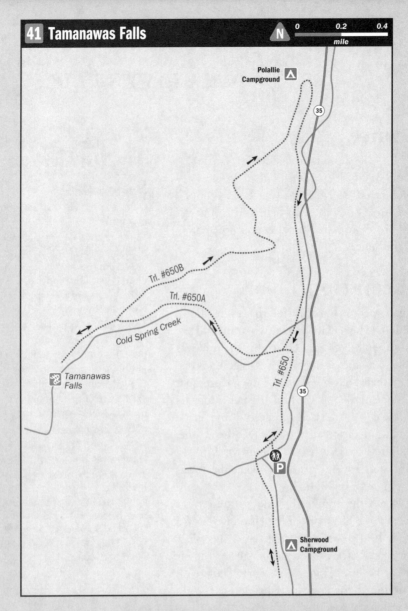

N

0   0.2   0.4
mile

Polallie
Campground

35

Trl. #650B

Trl. #650A

Cold Spring Creek

Tamanawas
Falls

Trl. #650

35

P

Sherwood
Campground

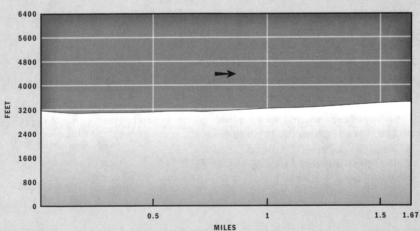

FEET

6400
5600
4800
4000
3200
2400
1600
800
0

0.5   1   1.5   1.67

MILES

The prize at the end of the trail

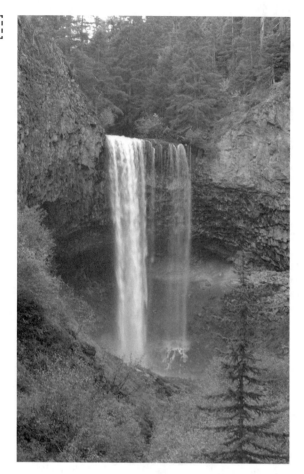

Tamanawas Falls Trail. Now enjoy a lovely stretch right along the creek, passing numerous cascades, creekside picnic areas, and forest features, and in 0.7 miles come to a rockslide area where 650B (also known as Tie Trail) splits off to the right. The original Tamanawas Falls Trail went left here and crossed the creek on a bridge, but that was one of the bridges wiped out in 2000. To follow the new route, walk along 650B for about a minute, until it switches back to the right in the face of a larger, older rockslide. It was here that locals made their new way in 2000.

This larger rockslide has been here for a long time; it is, in fact, the reason the trail crossed the creek in the first place. The path winds through this rockslide; when you get across it, see if you can spot the ruins of the upper bridge down in the creek. From there, it's about 0.2 miles to the falls.

What makes this falls so special is that even in late summer there's plenty of water coming over it, and it's rimmed by basalt walls, much of which are pink because pieces have so recently fallen into the chasm. For this reason, take care if you want to go nearer (or even behind) the falls, as you'll be walking on wet rocks with no official trail and with cliffs above you—cliffs that provide ample evidence that rocks could come crashing down at any time. These are just little reminders from Mother Nature that we are, after all, just visitors in her world.

## NEARBY ACTIVITIES

Drive 7.5 miles north on OR 35, then turn left to visit the Hutson Museum in Parkdale, which features local history, Indian artifacts, and memorabilia of the early settlers.

# 42  TIMBERLINE LODGE

## KEY AT-A-GLANCE INFORMATION

**LENGTH: 13 miles to Paradise Park, 4.8 miles to Zigzag Canyon overlook, 2.2 miles to Silcox Hut, 1 mile to White River Canyon**

**CONFIGURATION: Paradise Park, balloon; Zigzag and White River Canyon, out-and-backs; Silcox Hut, loop**

**DIFFICULTY: Easy–strenuous depending on the length of the hike**

**SCENERY: Flower-filled meadows, deep canyons, overhead glaciers**

**EXPOSURE: Both shady and open**

**TRAFFIC: Heavy all summer long**

**TRAIL SURFACE: Dirt, rock, pavement**

**HIKING TIME: 0.5–5 hours**

**DRIVING DISTANCE: 64 miles (1 hour 30 minutes) from Pioneer Square**

**SEASON: July–October**

**BEST TIME: August**

**BACKPACKING OPTIONS: Good sites in Paradise Park**

**ACCESS: No fees or permits**

**WHEELCHAIR ACCESS: A few patches of road around the lodge**

**MAPS: USFS Mount Hood Wilderness; Green Trails #462 (Mount Hood)**

**FACILITIES: Full services at lodge**

**INFO: Zigzag Ranger District, (503) 622-3191**

**SPECIAL COMMENTS: No matter what the weather looks like, bring warm clothing for this hike.**

## IN BRIEF

If you spend just one day in Oregon, you should spend it at Timberline Lodge. If you go on only one hike, you should go to Paradise Park in August or early September. But, fear not—if you aren't up to a 13-mile loop, options abound at this spectacular mountain palace.

## DESCRIPTION

Timberline Lodge is the greatest man-made thing in Oregon. It was built in 1937 by the Works Progress Administration and dedicated by President Franklin D. Roosevelt the same day that he dedicated Bonneville Dam. But as astounding as the interior is, it's the setting of the place that requires one to spend time there. Only a few peaks in Oregon are above it, and with few trees around, the views are amazing, especially views to the summit of Mount Hood—the highest point in the state—3 miles away, and to Mount Jefferson, 45 miles to the south. In August, wildflowers bloom everywhere.

Let's start with the shortest hike, to the White River Canyon overlook. Follow a sign to the right of the lodge, pointing you to the PCT. You'll walk uphill a couple hundred yards, perhaps wondering why you're suddenly breathing heavily: it's because you

## GPS Trailhead Coordinates

UTM Zone (WGS84) 10T

Easting 601054

Northing 5020504

Latitude  N 45.33076°

Longitude  W 121.71040°

## *Directions*

**Take US 26 from Portland, driving 48 miles east of I-205. Turn left onto the well-marked Timberline Road, 2 miles past Government Camp. Follow Timberline Road 6 winding miles to the parking lot.**

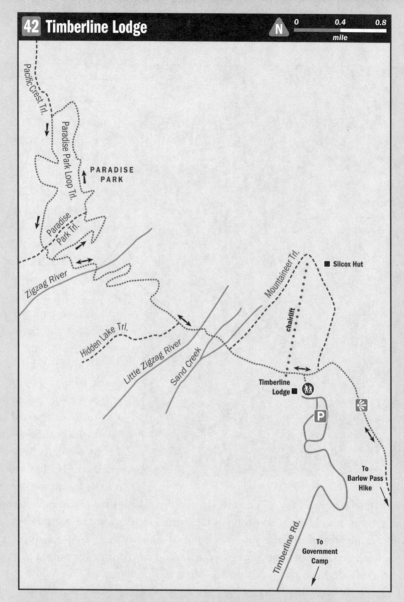

N

0      0.4      0.8

*mile*

Pacific Crest Trl.

Paradise Park Loop Trl.

**PARADISE PARK**

Paradise Park Trl.

Zigzag River

Hidden Lake Trl.

Little Zigzag River

Sand Creek

Mountaineer Trl.

■ **Silcox Hut**

chairlift

**Timberline Lodge** ■

P

To Barlow Pass Hike

Timberline Rd.

To Government Camp

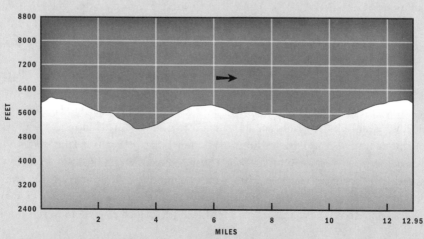

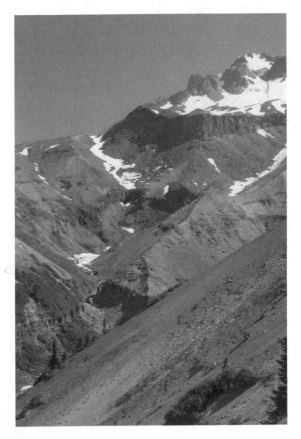

A view of Zigzag Canyon from the PCT

are now at 6,000 feet. At the PCT, turn right (that would be toward Mexico) and walk a half mile to the overlook; note that you'll have to skip over a couple of small creeks along the way.

If you'd like to do a one-way hike with a car shuttle, this trail connects (in another half mile) with the top of the Barlow Pass trip (hike 30, page 142).

For our next-toughest destination, go straight when you get to the PCT and follow the road uphill 1.1 miles to Silcox Hut. There seem to be a lot of small trails, but you can see the hut at the top of the chairlift, so just head for it. The last part of the hike is on a dirt road. Timberline Lodge rents this hut out to groups of 12 or more during the winter. For about $100 per person, they take you to the hut by Snow Cat, cook your dinner, then come back in the morning to cook your breakfast. And in the summer, you can ride the Magic Mile chairlift up here, then walk down.

To loop back to the lodge, go back the way you came or take the service road under the chairlift. For a slightly longer loop, take a trail that goes right (as you look down) from the top of the lift. It drops 1 mile to the PCT west of the lodge, in forest broken up by flowered meadows. Turn left and walk 0.8 miles to the lodge.

But enough with the preliminaries: let's head for Zigzag Canyon and Paradise Park. From the lodge, follow the PCT to your left; it will cross under two chairlifts and start descending slowly as it enters the woods. Hike 0.8 miles, ignoring Mountaineer Trail, which leads up to Silcox Hut. Continue 1.4 miles, ignoring a trail to the left, leading to Hidden Lake (it's a nice lake, but it's 3 miles below you). Just keep on truckin' through meadows and forests, past flowers and little springs. The best of these are around 2 miles out from the trailhead: great vertical bands of grass and color, the farthest one with a cool view of Ski Bowl and Tom, Dick, and Harry Mountain (described elsewhere in this book

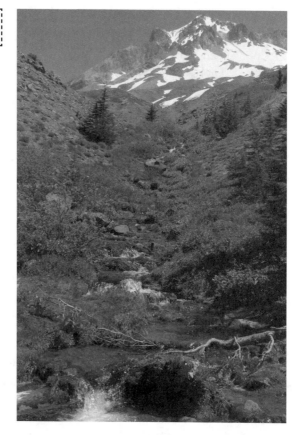

One of several creeks in Paradise Park

as part of the Mirror Lake trip (hike 37, page 172).

At 2.4 miles, you'll find yourself standing agog at the edge of a massive gash in the hillside, with Mount Hood rising to your right. This is Zigzag Canyon. If you've had enough at this point, head back, and you'll have done a 4.8-mile out-and-back trip. But for the real prize of this part of the mountain, keep going.

Now, you may have noticed that Paradise Park is actually below Timberline Lodge, making it sound pretty easy. What you need to know, however, is that in the next 3 miles, while crossing Zigzag Canyon and climbing up to Paradise Park, you will descend 600 feet and then climb 900. Just believe that it's worth it, and press on. You'll have to hop across the Zigzag River (look for the waterfall just upstream) and, 0.7 miles up the other side, take the first right (Paradise Park Loop Trail, 757). Then, yes, keep climbing toward Paradise Park—that's if you want to climb up to the best attractions. You can also stay on the PCT/Timberline Trail 2.1 miles to the lower end of our Paradise Park loop, and you'll save yourself several hundred feet of climbing but still see some great waterfalls.

Heading up Paradise Park Loop (757), things start to get really spectacular. The number and variety of flowers in this area—lupine, daisies, lilies, and those bushy-looking pasque flowers—and, of course, the plump sweetness of huckleberries in late summer make it a prime destination. Hike 1 mile to reach Paradise Park Trail coming in from the left; you can take it 0.6 miles down to the PCT and shorten your walk by 3.8 miles. But those 3.8 miles are fairly flat and very beautiful, so keep going.

Staying on the 757 trail, in a quarter mile you'll cross Lost Creek, spy an amazing campsite on a ledge above it, and 100 yards later come to the site of the old Paradise Park Shelter, one of several built in the 1930s for people hiking Timberline Trail.

The trail makes a right turn just before the shelter foundation and starts a long, wonderful, flat traverse through Paradise Park: heather, flowers, creeks, Mount Rainier, Mount St. Helens, a big cliff above you called Mississippi Head, the Zigzag Glacier above that . . . not bad at all for a flat walk. After 1.2 miles of this, you'll descend into the forest again, where your trail intersects the PCT and Timberline Trail; this area has great views down Sandy River Canyon and across it to Slide Mountain, a literal cross-section of Mount Hood.

Turn left here, and start back toward the lodge. After an easy half mile, you'll come to Rushing Water Creek and its wonderful canyon, where you'll pass just under its waterfall; below you is an amazing slot canyon and a view down into Sandy River Canyon. Hike another half mile, slowly descending now, to return to Lost Creek. Look for a trail that leads uphill just after the crossing; it first passes a little double waterfall, then a magical, hidden cove with yet another waterfall. They're everywhere! It's not hard to find campsites in this area, either.

Another 0.7 miles brings you to the lower end of Paradise Park Trail, where a horse corral will encourage you to keep moving. The descent is steeper now, and in 0.4 miles you'll have returned to the junction where your loop started, Paradise Park Loop Trail (757). Follow the PCT back down into the canyon, and, well, hate to tell you, but from here—with 9.5 miles under your belt—you've 3.5 miles to go, gaining 1,200 feet, and you've seen it all before.

But hey, it was worth it, right? Besides, you've got Timberline Lodge to enjoy now. The hot chocolate and coffee drinks are sublime, the food's not bad (or cheap), there's an interesting film about its construction, and its main lobby is about as nice a place to recover from a hike as you could ask for. And you deserve it.

## NEARBY ACTIVITIES

Though it's crowded, spend some time exploring Timberline Lodge. Watch the film *The Builders of Timberline* to hear the story of how artists and artisans came together during the Depression to create this masterwork. Then learn the details of their accomplishment, especially those of the Head House and its massive central stone tower.

# TRILLIUM LAKE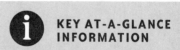

## IN BRIEF

A prime place to take the kids or to stretch your legs after driving up from Portland, Trillium Lake is a tiny body of water with a friendly scene and an impressive and popular view of Mount Hood. In addition to some short, easy hikes, there are opportunities to fish, boat, picnic, or just lie around, catch some rays, and watch the ducks.

## DESCRIPTION

Most outdoorsy Portlanders know Trillium Lake as a cross-country ski area, famed for the terror felt by many beginners on the long hill one drives down from US 26. But in the summer the lake is a beautiful, peaceful place to get a little taste of what the Mount Hood area has to offer. And if you've got kids along, they can swim, fish, and paddle in the lake all day.

To hike around it, start at the day-use area just before the road crosses the dam at the lake's southern end. Stop here and take the picture of Mount Hood that so many other people have taken. In case you're wondering, that square area of snow high up on the mountain is Palmer Glacier, the scene of summer-long skiing and snowboarding at Timberline Ski Area. Walk along the road atop the dam, perhaps ask how the fishing is,

### KEY AT-A-GLANCE INFORMATION

**LENGTH:** 2 miles
**CONFIGURATION:** Loop
**DIFFICULTY:** Easy
**SCENERY:** Marshes, lake, birds, forest
**EXPOSURE:** Shady, except when crossing the dam
**TRAFFIC:** Heavy all summer long, moderate when school is in session
**TRAIL SURFACE:** Packed dirt, boardwalk, pavement
**HIKING TIME:** 1 hour
**DRIVING DISTANCE:** 61 miles (1 hour 20 minutes) from Pioneer Square
**SEASON:** May–November
**BEST TIME:** August–September
**BACKPACKING OPTIONS:** Not great
**ACCESS:** $4 day-use fee per vehicle
**WHEELCHAIR ACCESS:** The area around the campground has several barrier-free trails.
**MAPS:** Mount Hood Wilderness; Green Trails #462 (Mount Hood)
**FACILITIES:** Toilets in day-use area near the dam, water in campground
**INFO:** Zigzag Ranger District, (503) 622-3191

## Directions

Take US 26 from Portland, driving 49 miles east of I-205. Turn right at a sign for Trillium Lake. At the bottom of the hill, proceed straight ahead for the day-use areas. The hiking trail, as described here, starts in the second day-use area you come to.

### GPS Trailhead Coordinates

UTM Zone (WGS84) 10T
Easting 598616
Northing 5013544
Latitude   N 45.26848°
Longitude  W 121.74289°

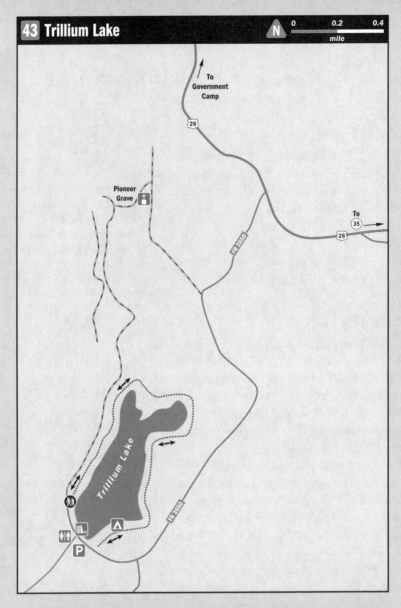

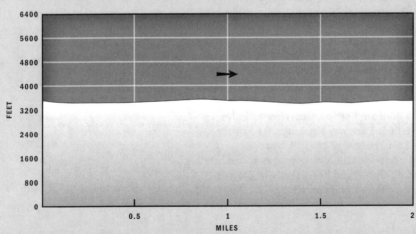

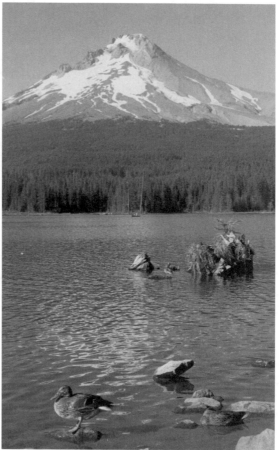

All the locals dig the Mount Hood view

and at the far end of the dam, follow the trail to the right, into the woods.

On the first part of the trail, you won't be right by the lake because the shore on that side is marshy and covered with tall grass. So you'll have to enjoy the forest. At 0.6 miles, a short boardwalk heads right, providing a glimpse of the shoreline. At 0.8 miles, there's a campsite on the right with access to a relatively private lakeshore spot. Beyond this point, the trail becomes a boardwalk that traverses a marshy area thick with vegetation. It will seem like you're swimming through the wildflowers late in the summer.

As you round the northern end of the lake, you'll pass from marsh to meadow, with a view of a corner of the lake that's covered with lily pads. Then, coming back to the more crowded eastern shore, you'll find numerous beaches for the kids to romp on or for you to sun yourself on. At 1.8 miles (just 0.2 miles from where you started, going the other way) there's a boat ramp and another parking lot. Just beyond that is a dock you can walk out onto (it has rails, so you don't have to worry about the kids). I was out there late one summer, with the sun setting and a few pink-hued clouds hanging around Mount Hood across the way, and some grown-ups on the dock were talking about the stock market and housing prices. Some people just don't get it.

When you drive out, drive past the lake for a piece of Oregon history. Head across the dam and go 1 mile on the unpaved road, turn right and go half a mile, and then make another right; park immediately on the right, near a white picket fence. That's a pioneer-era graveyard. Across the road is Summit Prairie, where Barlow Road travelers rested the day before tackling the infamous Laurel Hill.

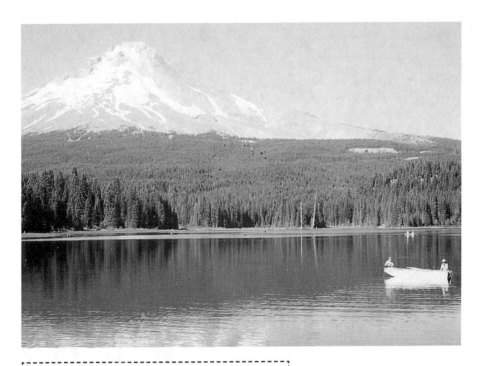

Catching a Hood view, and perhaps dinner, on Trillium Lake

## NEARBY ACTIVITIES

You have to stop at some point at the Huckleberry Inn in Government Camp. They've got huckleberry pies, pancakes, milk shakes, and ice cream, and they serve pretty good cheeseburgers, too. I love that place.

# TWIN LAKES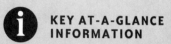

## IN BRIEF

There's not much of a challenge here, either for the day-hiker or for the overnight crowd. The total elevation gain averages less than 200 feet per mile, making this an easy-to-reach, easy-to-do introduction to the PCT and the world of mountain lakes.

## DESCRIPTION

For long-distance hikers on the PCT, the Twin Lakes are a diversion used mainly for water or camping—and, even then, they're often ignored. Long-distance hikers passing through these parts are just a few miles from both a US highway and Timberline Lodge, so there's not much here for them.

In fact, this trail was originally part of Oregon Skyline Trail and, later, the PCT, but the PCT was moved up the hill when the lakes started becoming overused.

What's here now are two lovely lakes and a nice viewpoint, all within easy reach. You can simply hike in to a lakeside campsite with only 4 round-trip miles of hiking and in half a day see all the sights this area has to offer. Another suggestion, before we get started: consider combining this with the hike from Barlow Pass to Timberline Lodge (hike 30, page 142); by adding a car shuttle, you've got a one-way hike of just under 10 miles.

### KEY AT-A-GLANCE INFORMATION

**LENGTH:** 4 miles to Lower Twin Lake, 8.5 miles to both lakes and Palmateer Point

**CONFIGURATION:** Out-and-back, or balloon

**DIFFICULTY:** Moderate

**SCENERY:** Two mountain lakes, old-growth forest, nice view of Mount Hood

**EXPOSURE:** Shady all the way, except at the viewpoint

**TRAFFIC:** Heavy on summer weekends, light otherwise

**TRAIL SURFACE:** Packed dirt, with rocks and roots

**HIKING TIME:** 2 hours to Lower Twin Lake, 5 hours to see it all

**DRIVING DISTANCE:** 58 miles (1 hour and 20 minutes) from Pioneer Square

**SEASON:** June–October

**BEST TIME:** August–September

**BACKPACKING OPTIONS:** Sites at both lakes

**ACCESS:** Northwest Forest Pass required

**WHEELCHAIR ACCESS:** None

**MAPS:** USFS Mount Hood Wilderness; Green Trails #462 (Mount Hood)

**FACILITIES:** Restrooms at the trailhead, water at nearby Frog Lake Campground

**INFO:** Hood River Ranger District, (541) 352-6002

**SPECIAL COMMENTS:** This hike is also a very popular snowshoe and Nordic ski trip.

## Directions

Take US 26 from Portland, driving 55 miles east of I-205 to reach Frog Lake Sno-Park. The trailhead is in the left-hand corner as you enter, and the parking spots left of it will be in the shade all day.

## GPS Trailhead Coordinates

UTM Zone (WGS84) 10T

Easting 602081

Northing 5009151

Latitude N 45.22845°

Longitude W 121.69963°

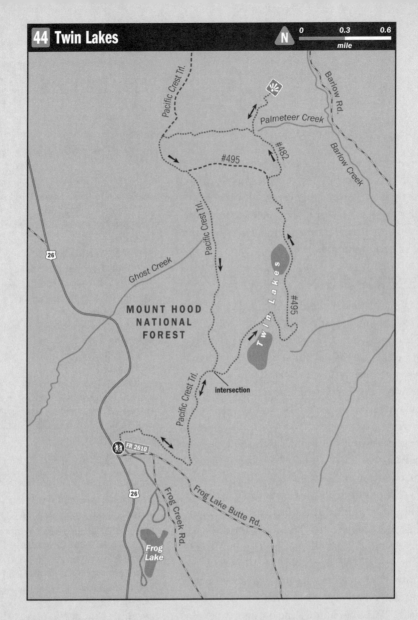

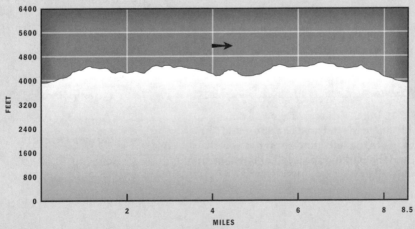

One more thing: I did this hike once in mid-August and was in the middle of a monarch butterfly migration. This is something worth mentioning, because if you find yourself in the middle of this, it's astonishing—hundreds of butterflies fluttering around you, seemingly oblivious to your presence. The migration is fascinating because the butterflies are born in California, fly to Oregon, lay eggs, and die; the ones born in Oregon then fly to Washington, lay eggs, and die; and *those* monarchs fly to Canada, lay eggs, and die. Some of the ones born in Canada then return to California, often flying 100 miles in a day. Unreal.

At the parking lot at Frog Lake Sno-Park, head for the west end of the lot and walk into the woods near a hiker sign. You'll see a picnic table and garbage can here, and two outhouses nearby. Go 100 feet and turn right to take the PCT; you'll notice some evidence of the annual snowfall here, such as the height of the sign on your right, and that of the blue-diamond marker on a nice hemlock on the trail. That's all related to winter sports; this trail is wildly popular with the ski and snowshoe crowds for its easy access and excellent grade.

You'll appreciate that grade as you head uphill on a highway of a trail, wide enough for two people to walk shoulder-to-shoulder, and of such a mellow steepness (gaining 500 feet in 1.5 miles) that you'll hardly notice it—especially if the abundant huckleberries are ripe.

When you reach Trail 495, the beginning of Twin Lakes Trail, turn right on it, and you'll soon descend a hill and spy Lower Twin Lake through the trees on your right. You'll also see a social trail or two plunging down the hillside to the shore, but don't use them; you'll add to erosion, and the main trail goes to the same place. After a total of 2 miles (including a short stretch past the lake, up a drainage), you'll arrive at a junction with Frog Lake Buttes Trail at the northeast shore of the lake. There's camping enough for a village here, and practically nothing alive on the ground, but there's also a trail that goes all the way around the lake, leading to other campsites along the way.

To head for Upper Twin and the rest of the hike, stay on Trail 495. You'll round a bend, climb briefly, and in 0.7 miles come to a rocky area with a view (on the left) looking back down to Lower Twin in its steep-sided, forested bowl. Hike another 0.25 miles to reach Upper Twin Lake and its own round-the-lake trail. Staying on the 495, you'll go along the east side of the lake, passing a big campsite from which a small trail heads into the woods on the right—to a toilet, believe it or not. Not an outhouse, mind you, just a toilet. Bizarre, and quite uncomfortable looking.

Upper Twin, by the way, gets less use, but that might be because it's smaller, much more shallow, and not well suited to swimming.

Half a mile north of "Camp Toilet," you'll come to a trail on the right marked "Palmateer View." Great name, huh? Sounds like a pirate or something, but alas, it's the name of a sheepherder from pioneer days. This trail is a short-cut to Trail 482, which you'll reach in a few minutes; turn left there, and you'll descend to the headwater of Palmateer Creek (probably dry for your visit), then climb briefly to a large meadow called Palmateer Camp. From there, a moderately steep trail on the right leads a third of a mile to the viewpoint.

This view gives you a unique perspective on Mount Hood, from the southeast, and the local stretch of the PCT. Climbing behind the ridge on your left, the PCT drops off its end to Barlow Pass, then climbs to Timberline Lodge, the gray roof of which is visible from your viewpoint.

You're also looking straight across (to the north) at Barlow Butte, which features meadows on the side facing you. The drainage between you and the butte is that of Barlow Creek, traced by the historic Barlow Road, which was an overland portion of the Oregon Trail used by people who didn't want to risk their lives on the Columbia River. You can still drive this road all the way to The Dalles if your car has some clearance; it's accessed just off OR 35, at the trailhead to the Barlow Pass trip (hike 30, page 142).

Descending from the viewpoint, turn right on Trail 482 at Palmateer Camp, and in 0.7 miles you'll be back at the PCT. You're 1.2 miles south of Barlow Pass now, but to return to the car, turn left. You'll pass the upper end of Twin Lakes Trail 495 in 0.3 miles, climb slightly for just less than a mile, then cruise the last 2 miles on the PCT, heading for your car. Pick some more huckleberries, while you're at it.

Nice and easy, huh?

# VISTA RIDGE 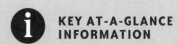 45

## IN BRIEF

A short, easy trail to several flower-filled bowls at the tree line on Mount Hood, this hike is more than worth the tedious drive to the trailhead—especially if you explore a new, volunteer-maintained option. In fact, when people ask me about my favorite hike in the book, I often say, "Vista Ridge in August."

## DESCRIPTION

For years, Vista Ridge Trail was mysteriously underused. It's a long drive, and the last section of the road used to be a hassle, but now that's been smoothed out, and most summer weekends the small trailhead area is jammed with cars. And why wouldn't it be? All you have to do is climb slightly for a couple of miles through quiet woods and you're in wildflower heaven.

The "bad" news is that the beginning and end of this hike can be tedious and buggy; the good news is that when you've gone less

- - - - - - - - - - - - - - - - - - - - - - - - - - - - -

## *Directions*

Take US 26 from Portland, driving 36 miles east of I-205 to Zigzag and turning left on Lolo Pass Road at the Zigzag Store. Drive 10.7 miles and take the second right at Lolo Pass, onto FS 18, which is signed for Lost Lake. After 5.5 miles of gravel you'll be back on pavement, and 5 miles beyond that—having driven a total of 10.5 miles on FS 18—make a hairpin right to take the paved FS 16. (A sign at this intersection points to Vista Ridge Trail 626.) Go 5.4 miles and turn right at a large intersection onto FS 1650, which quickly becomes a good gravel road. The trailhead is 3.6 miles ahead, at the end of the road. Note that twice during this stretch you'll need to stay left and uphill on the bigger of two roads.

### KEY AT-A-GLANCE INFORMATION

**LENGTH:** 6 round-trip miles to Wy'east Basin, 11 miles to see it all
**CONFIGURATION:** Balloon
**DIFFICULTY:** Moderate, with one tricky river crossing
**SCENERY:** Mountain streams, rocks, glaciers, flowers everywhere, and a really big mountain
**EXPOSURE:** Shady for a couple of miles, then in and out of meadows
**TRAFFIC:** Heavy on summer weekends, moderate otherwise
**TRAIL SURFACE:** Packed dirt, roots, rocks
**HIKING TIME:** 3–6 hours
**DRIVING DISTANCE:** 77 miles (2 hours 10 minutes) from Pioneer Square
**SEASON:** July–October
**BEST TIME:** August–September
**BACKPACKING OPTIONS:** Plentiful!
**ACCESS:** Northwest Forest Pass required
**WHEELCHAIR ACCESS:** None
**MAPS:** Mount Hood Wilderness; Green Trails #462 (Mount Hood)
**FACILITIES:** None at trailhead; closest at Zigzag Store
**INFO:** Hood River Ranger District, (541) 352-6002

- - - - - - - - - - - - - - - - - - - - - - - - - - - - -

## GPS Trailhead Coordinates

UTM Zone (WGS84) 10T

Easting 596688

Northing 5031193

Latitude N 45.42757°

Longitude W 121.76401°

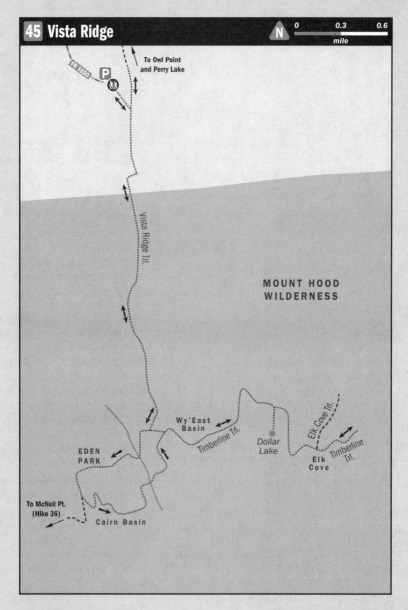

N

0          0.3          0.6
mile

To Owl Point
and Perry Lake

FR 1650

P

Vista Ridge Trl.

MOUNT HOOD
WILDERNESS

Wy'East
Basin

Timberline Trl.

Dollar
Lake

Elk Cove Trl.

Elk
Cove

Timberline
Trl.

EDEN
PARK

To McNeil Pt.
(Hike 36)

Cairn Basin

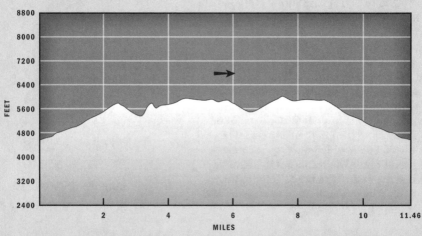

FEET

8800
8000
7200
6400
5600
4800
4000
3200
2400

2          4          6          8          10          11.46
MILES

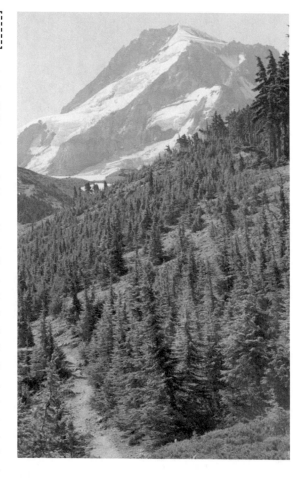

Wy'east Basin at the top of Vista Ridge Trail

than 3 miles, you're basically done climbing for the day and can choose among four spectacular areas of flowers, meadows, creeks, and mountain views.

From the trailhead, go 0.2 miles to a sign at Vista Ridge Trail (626). We'll talk later about what lies to the left. For now, though, turn right. It's not too exciting in here, but when you see Mount Adams through the trees to the left, and the trail gets just a bit steeper, you're almost there. At 2.7 miles from the trailhead, you'll arrive at Timberline Trail (600), in an open area with Mount Hood rising right in front of you. Congratulations: you've now climbed the biggest hill of your day—wasn't much, was it? You can go straight ahead for Wy'east Basin and Elk Cove, turn right for Eden Park and Cairn Basin, or go either way and see them all in a big loop.

But let's turn right on Timberline Trail. You will briefly plunge downhill and then start heading around to the left, crossing babbling brooks and admiring flowers. After 1 mile of this, you'll cross a larger stream, where logs have usually been placed to make a bridge. A quarter of a mile on, you'll be in Eden Park, which might be the loveliest mountain meadow you've seen—so far. To preserve the fragile landscape, stay on the trails.

To continue to Cairn Basin, cross Eden Park and follow the trail through the trees as it turns toward Hood. It will climb a small hill, with a view back down to Eden Park, and then pass through a notch and arrive 0.2 miles ahead at a campsite in Cairn Basin. Here, you can turn right on Timberline Trail to connect with the McNeil Point trip (hike 36, page 168), which is just 0.3 miles and a tricky creek crossing away. Or you can go straight ahead, following a sign for Elk Cove, to complete this loop hike. At the far end of the campsite, you'll wade

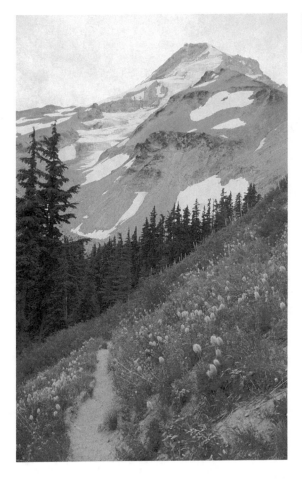

Timberline Trail dropping into Elk Cove

or jump a creek that might be a bit too deep and swift in the early summer, especially; after that, it's basically a flat mile to Wy'east Basin.

Once there, your car is to your left (go 0.3 miles to Vista Ridge Trail and turn right) and Elk Cove is to your right. In just a couple minutes, on the way to Elk Cove, you'll come to a lovely meadow with a creek and views of Mounts St. Helens, Rainier, and Adams. There is a nice campsite up the hill here. Just 1.2 flat miles away, Elk Cove might be the most spectacular of these destinations; it's certainly the largest, and Mount Hood seems to rise out of its far side all at once. Here, you'll find wildflowers throughout August, huckleberries late in the month, and reddish-orange mountain ash in September. I once spoke to a ranger who had seen elk and black bears in Elk Cove. Give them their space, and they won't bother you.

As you head back on Timberline Trail, before you get back to Wy'east Basin, keep an eye out for a side trail leading to Dollar Lake. There's no sign, but it follows a draw uphill in an area of short trees and a tiny stream that's more of a wet spot in the trail. Look for a rocky area uphill of the trail. If you get back as far as Pinnacle Ridge Trail (630), you've missed it by about five minutes. Dollar Lake (so named because it's almost perfectly round, like a silver dollar) probably should be called Half-Dollar Lake; you could wade across it in a minute. You can camp here, or just take a moment to contemplate all the beauty you've seen and say good-bye for now to Mount Hood before heading back to your car.

To do that, just go back down to Timberline Trail, turn left, and stay with it to Vista Ridge Trail; follow that back to the first junction you came to. From there, your car is 0.2 miles to the left. In front of you is a section of trail that for years was not maintained, becoming essentially a "lost" trail.

But in 2007, dedicated volunteers from PortlandHikers.org cleared 178 logs from the trail and restored this 3.2-mile section to tiny Perry Lake. It's now called Old Vista Ridge Trail, 626A, and it offers great views and a rare opportunity for solitude on Mount Hood. Tom Kloster, also known as "Splintercat" on the Web site, deserves credit for much of that work, and this description.

The first 0.8 miles climbs a bit as it traverses the eastern side of Vista Ridge; look in this area for all the sawed-off logs! Look also for remnants of the old phone lines to a fire lookout in the area. There are a couple of viewpoints off to the right. A half mile past this, after you traverse an area of open forest, you'll find huckleberries and beargrass and descend to a small meadow that can be marshy in early summer. The trail crosses the meadow and is marked by flags on both sides.

After a total of 1.8 miles, you'll reach a signed junction with a rustic side path that leads right 0.1 mile to the Rockpile, a Hood viewpoint with quite the reputation for huckleberries. The first 300 feet of this trip is through a heather meadow to a signpost that points right to take you the final 300 feet through beargrass to the Rockpile.

Just 0.1 mile farther, 626A intersects Owl Point Trail, a 0.1-mile spur trail to a viewpoint named for the great horned owls that nest in the area. The path climbs briefly through forest, then emerges to follow the edge of a large talus slope along a 500-foot cairn-marked route. The expansive view here also includes Laurance Lake and the upper Hood River Valley and is probably the best turnaround spot.

Trail 626A continues another 1.2 miles past more viewpoints and on to Perry Lake (more of a pond, really) and the foundation of an old guard station and lookout tower. But since this involves another 500 feet of elevation gain getting back, and since Owl Point is the local highlight, this section could probably be skipped, unless you are looking for a longer hike.

# 46  WILDWOOD RECREATION AREA

## KEY AT-A-GLANCE INFORMATION

**LENGTH:** Two loops totaling 1.75 miles, 10.6 miles to Huckleberry Mountain

**CONFIGURATION:** Loops, out-and-back

**DIFFICULTY:** Easy for loops, strenuous to Huckleberry Mountain

**SCENERY:** Wetlands, meadows, streams, a big-time summit viewpoint

**EXPOSURE:** Alternately shady and open on loops, sunny on mountain hike

**TRAFFIC:** Moderate–heavy on summer weekends, light otherwise

**TRAIL SURFACE:** Gravel, pavement, boardwalk (loops); packed dirt (hike to mountain)

**HIKING TIME:** 2 hours to do both loops, 5 hours for Huckleberry Mountain

**DRIVING DISTANCE:** 43 miles (1 hour) from Pioneer Square

**SEASON:** Year-round; see note in directions about parking. The trail up the mountain is generally snow-free June–October.

**BEST TIME:** Late summer–fall, for the salmon runs

**BACKPACKING OPTIONS:** None in the park; if you're going up into the wilderness, tell park staff which car is yours

**ACCESS:** $5 parking fee per vehicle

**WHEELCHAIR ACCESS:** Both lower loops

**MAPS:** Free maps in parking-area kiosk

**FACILITIES:** At parking area

**INFO:** BLM Salem District, (503) 622-3696

## GPS Trailhead Coordinates

UTM Zone (WGS84) 10T

Easting 578689

Northing 5022447

Latitude  N 45.35112°

Longitude  W 121.99545°

## IN BRIEF

As much an educational experience as a hiking one, this hike offers a glimpse into the Pacific Northwest world of birds, fish, plants, and water. The crown jewel of Wildwood is its underwater-viewing structure, especially when various species of salmon and trout are returning to the area to spawn.

## DESCRIPTION

The 33-mile-long Salmon River is the only river in the lower 48 states that is designated as a National Wild and Scenic River from its headwater to its mouth, in this case, from Mount Hood to the Sandy River, 3 miles below Wildwood. As far from the sea as it is, it still gets several runs each year of anadromous fish—fish that are born in freshwater, go to the ocean, and return to the freshwater of their birth to spawn and die. Although salmon are the most famous of these—and this bend of the Salmon River does get runs of salmon—steelhead do the same thing. Moreover, there are native trout in this stretch of the river.

To sample this natural wonderland, hike two loop trails, the 1-mile Wetland Trail and the 0.75-mile Cascade Streamwatch Trail. To

## *Directions* ———————————→

**Take US 26 from Portland, driving 33 miles east of I-205; turn right at a large sign reading "Cascade Streamwatch." It's half a mile past the Mount Hood RV Village. Drive a mile past the trailhead sign to the parking area for both trails. The road is gated from the weekend after Thanksgiving until the third Monday in March. During that time, you'll have to park at the gate (free) and walk in; restrooms in the park are left open.**

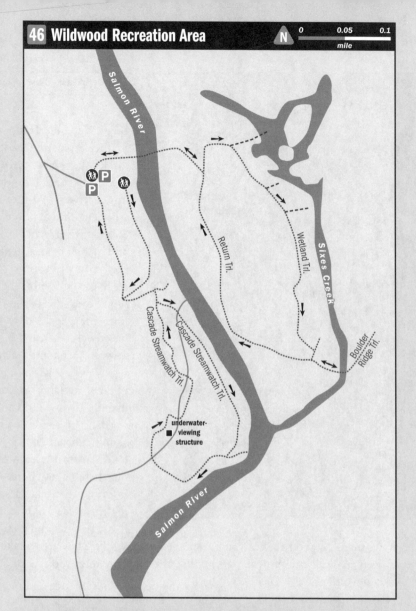

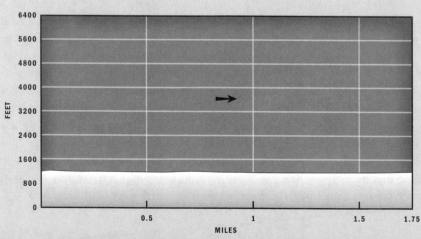

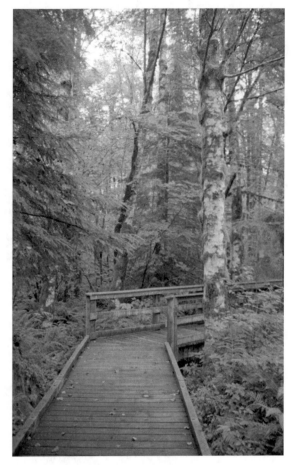

take Wetland Trail, start to the left of the parking-lot kiosk, where there are restrooms and free maps. You'll cross a 190-foot-long wooden bridge over the Salmon River, where in fall and winter you just might see chinook salmon and steelhead spawning below. Once over the bridge, follow the signs onto the boardwalk. You'll visit several lookouts affording views of various parts of the wetland: a cattail marsh, an overgrown beaver dam, an area filled with skunk cabbage, and a wetland stream. At each lookout there's a notebook-style informative display describing the area's wildlife. And if you're quiet and go in the morning, there's a good chance you'll even see some wildlife. Be sure to take the gravel Return Trail back to the parking lot, if only to admire the size of some 80-year-old stumps.

Cascade Streamwatch Trail starts at the same kiosk and takes you on a tour of the world of an anadromous fish. In fact, to navigate the trail you just follow the metal fish in the pavement. Along this trail, you'll visit an overlook of the river, a three-dimensional model of the Mount Hood area, several great picnic areas with grills, and then the fantastic underwater-viewing structure. Here, you can see tiny fish most times of the year and try to identify them using the chart on the wall. From late October to mid-December you might even catch a glimpse of an adult Chinook salmon. You have a better chance of seeing bigger spawning fish a little later on the trail, when it drops to the riverside. Look for winter steelhead in January, spring chinook salmon in March and April, summer steelhead in May, and coho and fall chinook from late September to mid-November. In case you're wondering, the Salmon River is closed to salmon fishing; you can fish for native trout at limited times, but it's all catch-and-release, with artificial lures only.

Now, if it's exercise and a view you're after, take Boulder Ridge Trail up to Huckleberry Mountain—and I do mean up: it climbs 4,100 feet in 5.3 miles to a tremendous viewpoint. Starting at the far end of Wetland Trail, you'll climb a series of switchbacks for just less than 2 miles to reach a spot with a nice view of Mount Hood. From here, it's a slightly less severe grade. Another half mile of climbing puts you at another view from a saddle; from there you'll put in 2 more miles to another saddle, then make a right onto Plaza Trail, heading 1 mile to the summit.

## NEARBY ACTIVITIES

Wildwood is actually a full-service 600-acre recreation area, with picnic areas for rent (some can be reserved), in addition to ball fields, basketball courts, horseshoe pits, and a play area. For rental information, call the Bureau of Land Management reservation line at (877) 444-6777.

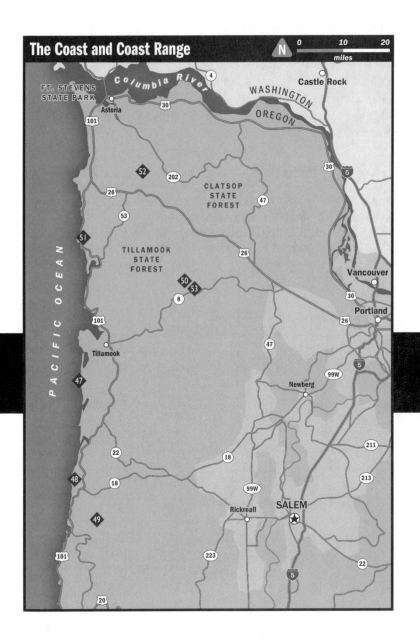

# The Coast and Coast Range

N

0　　　10　　　20
miles

FT. STEVENS STATE PARK

Columbia River

Castle Rock

WASHINGTON

OREGON

Astoria

4

30

101

52

202

CLATSOP STATE FOREST

47

26

53

51

TILLAMOOK STATE FOREST

26

50

53

8

Vancouver

101

30

Portland

Tillamook

47

26

47

99W

Newberg

5

PACIFIC OCEAN

22

18

211

48

18

99W

213

49

Rickreall

SALEM

22

101

223

5

20

30

5

# THE COAST AND COAST RANGE

# 47  CAPE LOOKOUT STATE PARK

## KEY AT-A-GLANCE INFORMATION

**LENGTH:** 4.8 miles round-trip to end of cape, 3.6 miles round-trip to South Beach, 4.6 miles round-trip to picnic area
**CONFIGURATION:** 3 out-and-backs
**DIFFICULTY:** Moderate
**SCENERY:** Old-growth forest, high cliffs, whales in winter and spring
**EXPOSURE:** Shady, open at end, cliff-top walking
**TRAFFIC:** Heavy on summer weekends, moderate otherwise
**TRAIL SURFACE:** Gravel, dirt, mud
**HIKING TIME:** 2 hours to end of cape, 2 hours to South Beach, 2 hours to picnic area
**DRIVING DISTANCE:** 85 miles (1 hour 40 minutes) from Pioneer Square
**SEASON:** Year-round, with mud and storms in winter and spring
**BEST TIME:** July–September for the weather, March–April for the whales
**ACCESS:** No fees or permits needed, but parking in day-use area is $3 per day
**WHEELCHAIR ACCESS:** No trails
**MAPS:** USGS Sand Lake
**FACILITIES:** Portable restroom at trailhead May–September; restrooms, showers, and water at campground
**INFO:** (503) 842-3182
**SPECIAL COMMENTS:** This park gets an average of 90 inches of rain annually—compared with Portland's 37.5 inches. You've been warned.

## GPS Trailhead Coordinates

UTM Zone (WGS84) 10T
Easting 423656
Northing 5021330
Latitude  N 45.34132°
Longitude  W 123.97445°

## IN BRIEF

This park offers everything you'd want from the Oregon coast: old-growth forest, secluded beaches, cliff-top views, and wildlife on land, wing, and water. You've got three options from the trailhead, and with a little energy you could do them all.

## DESCRIPTION

When you park at this trailhead, you will have three options to choose from, and it's all downhill from here. Of course, you'll have to come back uphill to get to the car, but even the 800-foot climb from the beach is so well graded you'll hardly be winded when it's done. On our elevation profile for this hike, I've included both the beach route and the cape route.

Start with the best of the trails, the one that goes out to the cape. Taking the trail behind the sign at the far end of the lot, continue straight when you get to a junction 100 yards ahead. You'll be hiking through that rarest of treats: a coastal old-growth forest.

## *Directions*

Take US 26 from Portland, driving 20 miles west of I-405, then bear west on OR 6, following a sign for Tillamook. Drive 51 miles to Tillamook, and continue straight through the intersection with US 101. From there on, you will be following signs for Cape Lookout State Park and the 3 Capes Scenic Route. After crossing US 101, go two blocks and turn left on Stillwell Street. Drive two more blocks and turn right on 3rd Street. Travel 4.9 miles and turn left. After 5.3 miles you'll pass the state-park campground and day-use area; this is where you can stash a second car to do the shuttle. The free trailhead is 2.7 miles past the campground, on the right.

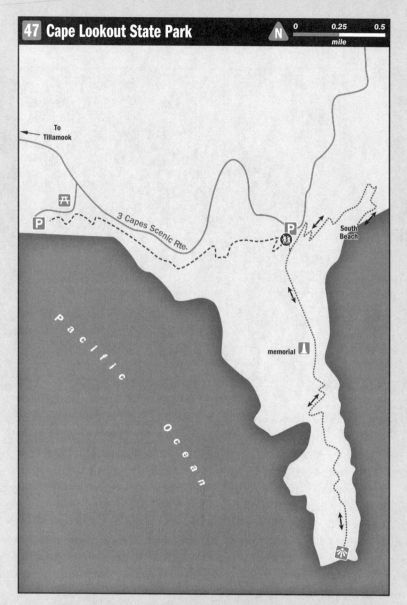

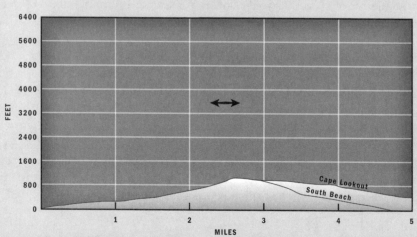

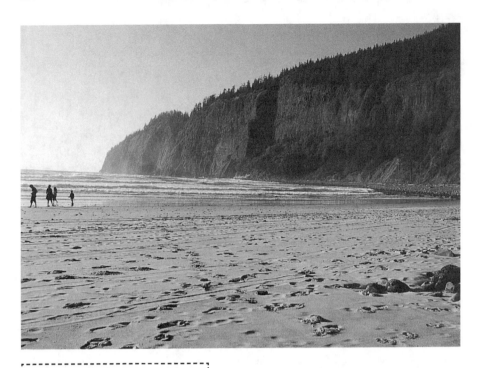

South Beach with Cape Lookout beyond

There are some nice Sitka spruces and hemlocks in here, and the whole thing is as peaceful as can be.

Just past half a mile out, you'll come to a plaque honoring the flight crew of a B-17 bomber that crashed into the cape just to the west in 1943. After another half mile you'll get a view north; look for the three rocks just off Cape Meares and the town of Oceanside. You can make out an arch in the middle rock; in fact, all three have such arches, and they're called Three Arch Rocks. When you get to some moderately nerve-racking dropoffs on the left, along with inspiring views south, you're almost done.

At the tip of the cape, you're looking 270 degrees around and 400 feet straight down at the crashing sea. There is a protective cable at the end of the cape, but in other places you'll be right at the top of a cliff. On a calm day—which is rare in a place that gets around 90 inches of rain per year—it's not uncommon to see seals or sea lions down there. But the main attraction is the gray whales. Thousands of them make the trip each year from the Bering Sea in Alaska to Baja, California, a swim of some 6,000 miles. In late December and early January, when they go south, they tend to be farther out. But in March and April, they're on their way back north with newborn calves, so they go slower and stay closer to shore. At these times of year, bring binoculars (and a raincoat), and you might see dozens of whales in a day. For the best viewing, go early in the day, when the sun will be behind you as you look out.

On your way back to the trailhead, when you reach the junction, turn right (downhill) and follow this trail to South Beach. Avoid the temptation to take all the various cutoff trails, as they add to erosion. If the 1.5-mile, 800-foot descent seems a little tedious (like when the beach looks as though it's just right there below you but you're walking more sideways than down), just believe that you'll be thankful for this easier grade on your way back up.

You can also hike down the beach, which extends 4 miles south to Sand Lake, but eventually you'll get into an area where cars are allowed, which sort of detracts from the wilderness feeling.

The last option from the trailhead is across the lot, going north on the Oregon Coast Trail. It's 2.3 miles, all downhill, to the picnic area and the nature trail, which is by the campground. You'll pass a couple of viewpoints on the way and probably have the trail largely to yourself.

If you have two cars, put one down at the campground–picnic area. You'll have to pay a $3 day-use fee there, but at the end of the day you can walk downhill just 2.3 miles from the trailhead back to your second car (a total of 11.3 manageable miles for the day). There's also a short nature trail there. If you have only one car, you'll have to come back up to the car at the end of the day, stretching it to almost 13 miles, so it might not be worth it.

## NEARBY ACTIVITIES

As long as you're in Tillamook, take advantage of its tourist stops, most notably the collection of World War II airplanes at the Air Museum south of town and the two cheese factories to the north. The Tillamook Cheese Factory is the best known, but there are slightly more exotic choices at the Blue Heron Cheese Factory.

# 48  CASCADE HEAD

### KEY AT-A-GLANCE INFORMATION

**LENGTH: 5.4 miles round-trip to Harts Cove, 2.5–4.5 miles round-trip to Nature Preserve**

**CONFIGURATION: Out-and-back**

**DIFFICULTY: Moderate, with an easy option**

**SCENERY: Old-growth forest, waterfalls, sea cliffs, wildflowers, wildlife**

**EXPOSURE: In forest at first, then open**

**TRAFFIC: Heavy on summer weekends, moderate otherwise**

**TRAIL SURFACE: Packed dirt, some roots**

**HIKING TIME: 3 hours to Harts Cove, 1–2.5 hours for Nature Preserve**

**DRIVING DISTANCE: 79 miles (1 hour 45 minutes) from Pioneer Square**

**SEASON: The road to the upper trailheads is open July 16–December 31. The lower trailhead is open year-round.**

**BEST TIME: July–September**

**BACKPACKING OPTIONS: None**

**ACCESS: No fees or permits**

**WHEELCHAIR ACCESS: None**

**MAPS: USGS Neskowin**

**FACILITIES: Outhouse at Knight Park but no facilities at upper trailheads, no drinkable water on the trail**

**INFO: The Nature Conservancy, (503) 802-8100, or the Hebo Ranger District, (503) 392-3161**

**SPECIAL COMMENTS: Dogs are not allowed on either trail at Cascade Head.**

## GPS Trailhead Coordinates

UTM Zone (WGS84) 10T

Easting 421883

Northing 4988122

Latitude N 45.04225°

Longitude W 123.99187°

## IN BRIEF

Imagine standing high atop a windswept, flower-covered meadow, with the sea and the coast spread out below you and not a tree to block the view. Or imagine peeking into a hidden cove where sea lions bark, a waterfall plunges, and waves crash. Well, you don't have to imagine either scene: you can go to Cascade Head.

## DESCRIPTION

First, Harts Cove Trail. At the start, you might think you've got it made, because it's all downhill and steep—it loses about 500 feet in the first half mile. Too bad you have to walk back up that at the end of the hike. The forest here is a young one of mostly Sitka spruce; notice that only the tops of the trees are green—that's because these lower portions don't get

## *Directions*

Take I-5 from downtown Portland, driving 6 miles south to Exit 294/Tigard/Newberg. Bear right on OR 99 West and follow it 22 miles. Just before the town of McMinnville, turn left on OR 18 (following signs for the coast) and follow it 53 miles to its intersection with US 101. Turn right (north) on US 101. For the lower, year-round trailhead to the Nature Preserve, go 1 mile north and turn left on Three Rocks Road. Follow this 2 miles, turn left, and park at Knight Park. To reach the trailhead, follow a trail along the road.

For the two upper trailheads, go 3.8 miles north of OR 18 on US 101 and turn left onto the unsigned FS 1861, just before the top of a hill on US 101. Stay left at 2.4 miles, still on FS 1861. The upper Nature Preserve trailhead is 0.8 miles past this turn, on the left. The Harts Cove trailhead is at the end of the road, 1 mile on.

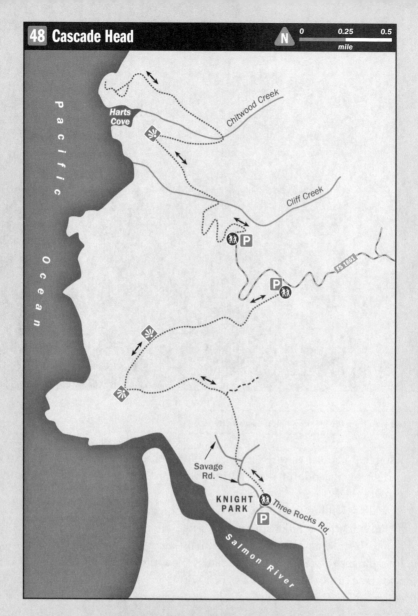

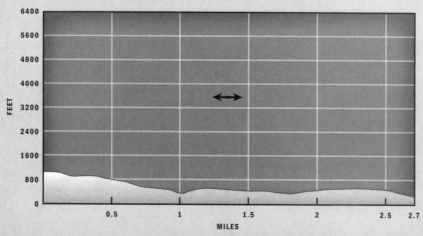

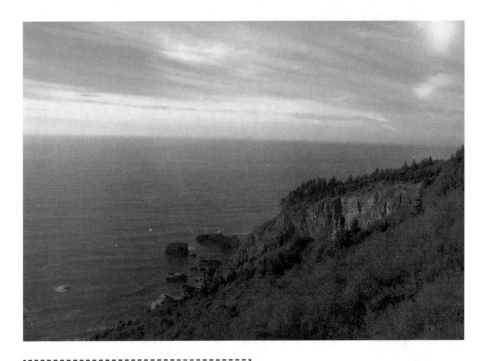

The view from the Meadows atop Cascade Head

any sun, not because they're unhealthy. Notice also the very large stumps; there's one right on the side of the trail that you can get on top of and measure for yourself.

Walk 0.7 miles to cross Cliff Creek and enter a different world. Here you can find out what a Sitka spruce looks like after about 300 years. You'll probably also hear what hundreds of sea lions sound like—they're to the left, and you might get to see some of them later. Now the hiking gets flatter, as you go out to the end of the ridge to a bench with a view of Harts Cove ahead. Wrap back around to the right, through the drainage of Chitwood Creek. Half a mile past the bench, walk under a massive blown-down spruce and then out into the meadows atop the bluff—yet another world.

It's important to stay on the trails here; this area is fragile. If you come in July or August, you'll be part of a landscape that looks like it was lifted from the upper reaches of Mount Hood, with goldenrod, lupine, Indian paintbrush, and violets in abundance. Follow the trail that heads for the trees on the left; there's a wonderful spot to sit there, and it has a front-row view into Harts Cove. The waterfall you see is on Chitwood Creek, which you just crossed. As for the louder-than-ever sea lions, they are mostly around the point to the south, but if you have binoculars you might be able to see some of them lounging on rocks or the far beach.

There's no real beach to access here, but you can get close to the water. From the trees, walk west and keep left. There's a steep trail there, almost a slide in spots, that you can descend to the rocky shore. This rock, and all of Cascade Head, in fact, is lava that flowed up through the water. If you make your way to the right 100 yards or so on the rock, you'll have a fabulous view of the headland, Cape Kiwanda to the north, and, farther off, Cape Lookout.

Now, for the Cascade Head Nature Preserve. If the upper road is open and you want an easy, flat, 2.5-mile round-trip hike, start up there. The trail, actually an old roadbed, traverses a young and unexciting forest to the main-attraction meadow.

My advice is to start down below; it's a better, more scenic walk, and effort always makes one more appreciative. From the parking lot at Knight Park, start near the interpretive sign; you'll spot the trailhead directly across Three Rocks Road. The first 0.4-mile stretch crosses private property, switching from board-walks to trail and occasionally crossing a road, so make sure you stay on the path and don't disturb the landowners or get run over.

Finally heading into the woods, the trail briefly steepens, over steps and roots, then mellows after 0.1 mile, where a massive spruce guards the path. Enjoy typical coastal scenery—spruces and ferns, skunk cabbage and devil's club, and a small meadow filled with foxglove—as you cross several small streams on boardwalks and continue climbing, now on a more moderate grade. When you reach a trail junction just less than a mile out, keep left, and in a few moments you'll reach a sign telling you you're entering National Forest property. At 1.2 miles you'll come to a registration station and donation box.

At this point, you'll probably have been hearing the ocean for a while, and at 1.3 miles you'll finally emerge from the tunnel of vegetation to see the Pacific and the mouth of the Salmon River, some 600 feet below you. The trail is flat and wonderful for 0.25 miles—look for elk on the bluffs and bald eagles in the sky. At a switchback to the right, the path starts to climb more steeply.

In summer, you'll climb through waist-high flowers, with birds chirping, swallows swooping, and butterflies and bumblebees buzzing. From any of the switchbacks, wander out, carefully, toward the cliff edge to peer north; you might spot sea lions below. When you see a sign reading, "Danger: Hazardous Cliffs," you've gone 2 miles and gained 1,000 feet. Only 0.25 miles and a couple hundred feet to the top! The spot where the upper trail emerges from the woods is 0.3 miles past the summit.

As you take it all in from the top of the hill, consider this: more than 30 years ago, this meadow was slated to become a housing development, but conservation-minded folks banded together, bought it, and donated it to The Nature Conservancy. Now also designated as a United Nations Biosphere Reserve, it's protected as the home of the Oregon silverspot butterfly, whose caterpillar will eat only a rare violet that lives in these meadows. That's why FS 1861 and the upper part of the trail is closed from January 1 through July 15. The silverspots emerge in late August and flutter here for about a month.

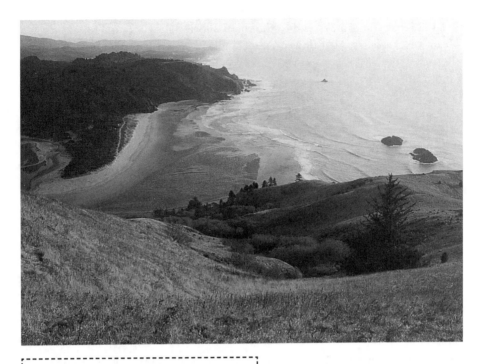

The mouth of the Salmon River, from Cascade Head

## NEARBY ACTIVITIES

Back on OR 18, a mile before you reached US 101, you went through the town of Otis. You might not have noticed it (it has only about a dozen buildings), but it's the home of an Oregon coast tradition, the Otis Café, where you'll find 28 seats, a line outside, and the biggest portions this side of a logging camp. Famous for sourdough pancakes, German potatoes, and whole-wheat molasses toast, the café also makes wonderful pies.

# DRIFT CREEK FALLS 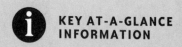 49

## IN BRIEF

This is a long drive, best done as part of a day at the coast, and there is just about nothing to this hike. If it weren't for the suspension bridge it crosses, nobody would ever hike it. But what a bridge! There are a couple of places to hang out by the stream, and a nice waterfall . . . but what a bridge!

## DESCRIPTION

It's a long drive to this trail, so do it on a day when you're headed to the coast anyway—especially in spring, early summer, or late fall, when there will be plenty of water in the creek. It's all about the bridge.

From the trailhead, you descend and, a little more than 200 yards ahead come to . . . a trash can! It (and the sign and restroom at the trailhead) owe their existence to the fact that you need a pass to park at this trailhead, and new regulations require such amenities where a pass is required. The reason it's this far down the trail is to keep folks driving by from filling it with their garbage.

You'll see a bench at 0.4 miles as you wind down through a young forest that may remind you of Forest Park in Portland. At half

### KEY AT-A-GLANCE INFORMATION

**LENGTH: 3.5 miles**
**CONFIGURATION: Out-and-back**
**DIFFICULTY: Easy**
**SCENERY: Forest, creek, waterfall, one amazing bridge**
**EXPOSURE: All in the woods**
**TRAFFIC: Light**
**TRAIL SURFACE: Packed dirt, muddy in winter and spring**
**HIKING TIME: 2 hours**
**DRIVING DISTANCE: 91 miles (2 hours) from Pioneer Square**
**SEASON: Year-round, but there could be snow in winter**
**BEST TIME: Spring or early summer**
**BACKPACKING OPTIONS: None**
**ACCESS: Northwest Forest Pass required**
**WHEELCHAIR ACCESS: None**
**MAPS: Siuslaw National Forest**
**FACILITIES: Toilets at trailhead**
**INFO: Hebo Ranger District, (503) 392-5100**
**SPECIAL COMMENTS: In late 2009 the Forest Service was working on a printable interpretive guide to this trail, which they intended to post on their Web site; check www.fs.fed.us/r6/siuslaw.**

## Directions

Take I-5 from Portland, driving 6 miles south to Exit 294/Tigard/Newberg. Bear right on OR 99W and drive 23 miles. Just before McMinnville, turn left on OR 18 to follow an Oregon Coast sign. Travel 49 miles and turn left on Bear Creek County Road (following a sign for Drift Creek Falls Trail). Two miles ahead, the pavement ends. At 3.3 miles, continue straight, again following a sign for the trail; you're now on FS 17. The trailhead is 10 miles ahead, on the left.

## GPS Trailhead Coordinates

UTM Zone (WGS84) 10T
Easting 429525
Northing 4974174
Latitude N 44.91750°
Longitude W 123.89290°

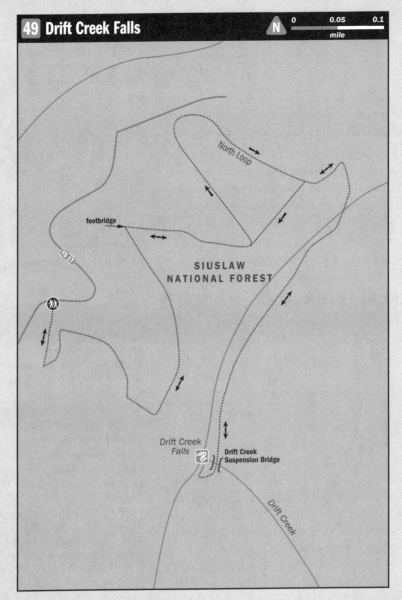

# 49 Drift Creek Falls

N

0    0.05    0.1

*mile*

North Loop

footbridge

FS 17

S I U S L A W
N A T I O N A L   F O R E S T

Drift Creek
Falls

Drift Creek
Suspension Bridge

Drift Creek

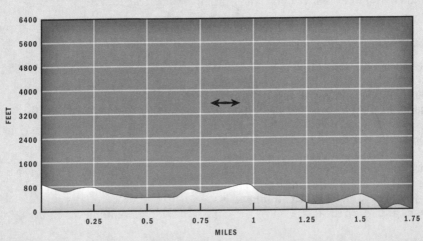

6400
5600
4800
4000
3200
2400
1600
800
0

FEET

0.25    0.5    0.75    1    1.25    1.5    1.75

MILES

The Drift Creek Falls Suspension Bridge

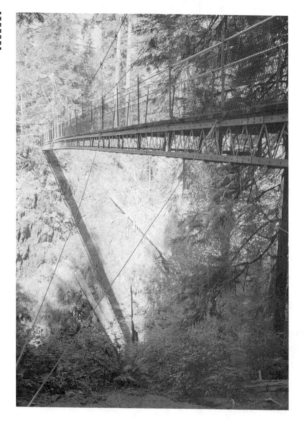

a mile, you'll cross a small footbridge that was built in 2003, replacing one that was wiped out in the floods of February 1996. That was when, in a four-day period, 30 inches of warm rain fell on top of two feet of snow in the coastal mountains; when it all came down, all hell broke loose. Tillamook County alone suffered more than $50 million in damage.

Just past this bridge, you'll reach a new "North Loop," the sign for which does not really indicate where it goes. What the trail does is loop out to the north, then back to this trail, adding about 0.5 miles to the trip. But it's easy, and it visits the only (tiny) patch of old forest around, so I recommend it.

At the far end of North Loop, a total of 1.4 miles into your hike, return to the original trail on the shores of the north fork of Drift Creek, in a mossy, fern-filled bottomland. Cross this creek 0.1 mile down, then, 0.25 miles farther on, you'll come to the real bridge.

Built between 1993 and 1997, the Drift Creek Falls Suspension Bridge is 240 feet long, 3 feet wide, and 100 feet above the canyon floor. It cost $170,000 to build, and came in 0.2 inches short. The falls to your right are 75 feet high—and you're above them! A few more technical details: the towers are 29 feet tall and made of Douglas fir beams that are 12-by-18-inches thick. The anchors include 28 cubic yards of concrete and 10-foot rock bolts. The mainlines are 1.25-inch galvanized wire rope. Also of note is that the same company that built this bridge built the one over Lava Canyon, another hike in this book (hike 17, page 80).

And how do they build such a thing? You might wonder. (I did.) They flew in materials with a helicopter and built the main span from a "skyline" more than 100 feet off the ground—not a business for anyone afraid of heights.

Enough with the technical talk. It's a wonderful bridge, spanning the canyon and at the same time visiting the tree canopy. And, if you're into such things,

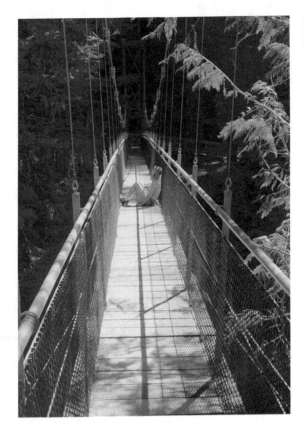

A peaceful moment high above Drift Creek

you can get it rocking back and forth. Just put a foot on each side and have at it. Some of your friends might not appreciate it, though.

The bridge is dedicated to the late Scott Paul, a Forest Service trail builder who was the foreman of this job and died in an accident during the bridge's construction. As to why it was built, I haven't been able to figure it out. The trail and bridge were built at roughly the same time (the trail was finished in 1994), and the total cost was $225,000. So I guess the trail was built to show off the bridge, which was built to get the trail across the creek. I think they just built it because it was a darn cool thing to do.

If you continue 0.25 miles past the bridge, you can get down to the creek and look up at both the falls and the bridge. There's a nice little pool where I saw some tiny trout swimming around, and somebody carved a picnic table out of a log down there.

## NEARBY ACTIVITIES

Perhaps you noticed another bridge on the way down Bear Creek Road. The Drift Creek Covered Bridge is one of only four in Lincoln County, and it has an interesting history; for starters, it was built in 2001, and it's not over Drift Creek. There was a Drift Creek Covered Bridge (over Drift Creek) built in 1914 (hence the date on the sign), but it turns out the one still in existence in 1997 was built in 1933, after the original two got washed out. The county voted to tear it down, because it was beyond repair, but a Mr. and Mrs. Sweitz offered to haul away the pieces and rebuild it here, over Bear Creek. The rest is a truly amazing story, related in a flyer on the bridge, complete with miracles and a near-divorce and more miracles. Seriously—you should read it. The bridge reopened on July 14, 2001, and is open to the public, though not to cars. The place across the way is the Sweitz home.

# KINGS MOUNTAIN-ELK MOUNTAIN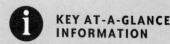

## IN BRIEF

There are four options here: a steep hike up Kings Mountain, a *really* steep scramble up Elk Mountain, a killer loop that includes both, and a casual (though long) stroll up Elk Creek. With a campground at one trailhead, why not spend the night and do a couple of hikes?

## DESCRIPTION

All these hikes are in the Tillamook State Forest; this might not sound impressive compared with a national park or wilderness area, but there is a fascinating story behind this forest.

On a hot August day in 1933, a fire started at a logging operation in Gales Creek Canyon. The temperatures had been in the 90s for weeks, and humidity was at an all-time low. The forest, therefore, was a bomb waiting to go off. The Gales Creek fire started as a fairly standard fire, but then a hot, dry wind came in from the east, and the 40,000-acre fire turned, in less than 24 hours, into a 240,000-acre fire. This "explosion" threw up a mushroom cloud 40 miles wide that rained two feet of debris on a 30-mile stretch of the Oregon coast. There was a major fire every six years until 1951, by which time 355,000 acres and 13 billion board

### KEY AT-A-GLANCE INFORMATION

**LENGTH:** Options from 5–13 miles
**CONFIGURATION:** Loop, or out-and-back
**DIFFICULTY:** Difficult
**SCENERY:** Second-growth forest, regrowth after fires, wildflower meadows, a couple of panoramas on top
**EXPOSURE:** Shady on the way up, open on top; some dangerous sections up above, especially if it's wet
**TRAFFIC:** Moderate on summer weekends, light otherwise
**TRAIL SURFACE:** Packed dirt, with some rock; sheer rock and steep scrambles on Elk Mountain
**HIKING TIME:** 3.5 hours to Kings Mountain, 8 hours for longer loop
**DRIVING DISTANCE:** 47 miles (55 minutes) from Pioneer Square
**SEASON:** Year-round, but there will often be snow on top in winter; recent rains make some slopes very slippery
**BEST TIME:** May–June, for wildflowers
**ACCESS:** No fee
**WHEELCHAIR ACCESS:** None
**MAPS:** USGS Jordan Creek
**FACILITIES:** Toilets and water in campground at Elk Creek, vault toilet at Kings Mountain trailhead
**INFO:** Tillamook State Forest, (503) 357-2191
**SPECIAL COMMENTS:** If it's raining, or there's snow on the ground, avoid the mountain hikes described here.

## Directions

Take US 26 from Portland, driving 20 miles west of I-405; then bear west on OR 6, following a sign for Tillamook. To start at Elk Mountain, go 23 miles to Elk Creek Campground, on the right just past milepost 28. The road will be gated in winter, but it's only 0.25 miles to the trailhead, which is on the right just beyond the campground. For Kings Mountain, continue 3 more miles to the trailhead, on the right just before milepost 25.

### GPS Trailhead Coordinates

UTM Zone (WGS84) 10T
Easting 460826
Northing 5052627
Latitude  N 45.62608°
Longitude  W 123.50254°

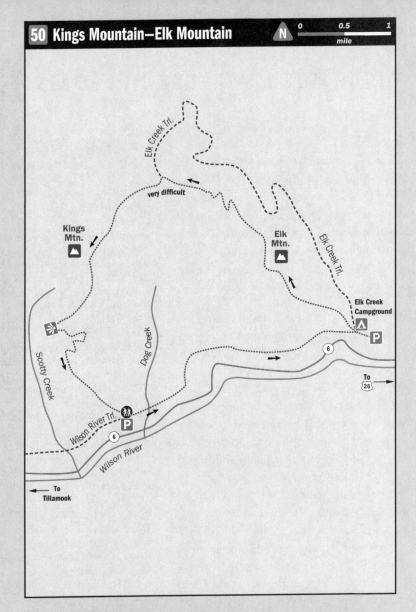

N

0        0.5        1
*mile*

Elk Creek Trl.

very difficult

Kings
Mtn.

Elk
Mtn.

Elk Creek Trl.

Elk Creek
Campground

P

6

To
26

Dog Creek

Scotty Creek

Wilson River Trl.

P

6

Wilson River

To
Tillamook

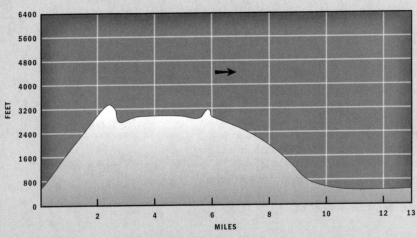

feet of timber (enough for more than 1 million large homes) had been completely destroyed. Logging came to a halt, wildlife was decimated, rivers were choked with sediment and debris, and, most importantly for the forest, seed cones were annihilated, meaning that the forest wouldn't grow back on its own.

But a recovery effort was launched with a bond measure in 1949. Eventually, more than 72 million seedlings were hand-planted, and in 1973 what had been known as the Tillamook Burn was renamed Tillamook State Forest. Now the question facing the state is whether or not to start logging it again. These hikes offer you a chance to explore one or two of the highest points in the forest and have a look at how the place has recovered. Keep an eye out for charred logs, for example, and remember that 50 years ago most of this area was bare.

I'm laying out four options for you here, so I'll give mileages and difficulty for each one.

**KINGS MOUNTAIN TRAIL (5.2 MILES ROUND-TRIP; DIFFICULT):** This hike gives you the most reward for your effort. It's 5 miles up and down, and it's tough, but compared to Elk Mountain it does have the advantage of taking you along a legitimate trail the whole time.

From the Kings Mountain trailhead on OR 6, you set out through a forest of alder and fern—replanted after the big burns—with a small, unnamed creek off to your right. At 0.1 mile, you'll see (but not take) Wilson River Trail on your right; if you're interested in that one, its entire 21-mile length is described in this book starting on page 238.

Around 1 mile, things get nasty steep; the next mile gains about 1,300 feet, as opposed to the 800 feet you've gained in the first mile. When your trail makes a sharp turn to the right, look for a small trail to the left leading to a peak called "Kings Jr." Go a few feet out there for your first real view to the north. Lester Creek, below you, flows into the Wilson River to your left; Kings Mountain is directly behind you, higher than the rocky peak you can see from here. There are also some large, charred stumps on this ridge. The live trees were all planted after the big fires, and some of the seeds up here were dispersed by helicopter.

The last 0.6 miles of this hike gain about 900 feet, so just take your time and believe it's worth the effort. If you're here in May or June, you'll have no doubt about that when you walk past a picnic table (many thanks to Troop 299 from Tigard!) and out into the meadows, which in early summer are filled with beargrass, lupine, Indian paintbrush, and seemingly a billion other tiny flowers. The summit is now just 0.3 miles straight ahead, marked by a sign. The view stretches from the ocean to the Cascades; be sure to sign the register, one of the few in Oregon.

If you want to do both peaks, I strongly suggest starting with Elk Mountain and coming back this way.

**ELK MOUNTAIN TRAIL (3 MILES ONE-WAY; DIFFICULT):** This is the steepest, roughest trail in this book in one stretch. It climbs 1,900 feet in 1.5 miles, making it considerably steeper than Dog Mountain, for example. If you ascend this trail, don't come back down it. To make a loop that includes Kings Mountain or Elk Creek, see below.

From the trailhead at Elk Creek, head up Wilson River Trail 0.2 miles, then take off up Elk Mountain Trail. I don't know what to tell you about the next mile and a half, except that the view is worth it. You'll pass a false summit on the way; the real one has a register and, in early summer, plenty of beargrass and paintbrush. If you face the river on the summit, Kings Mountain is the peak off to your right.

If you really want to descend down that way, have at it. My advice is to continue on the trail, which dives off the summit and becomes a little rocky and steep in places—as a State Forest brochure puts it, "the next mile is loose scree that often requires using your hands to guide you along the craggy ridge route." After that, the trail follows an old road for another mile to a junction with Kings Mountain Trail.

If you're headed down the easy way, turn right here and follow the path 0.7 miles to Elk Creek Trail. Turn right again, and after 4 less-than-exciting (but easy) miles, you'll be back at the car, having made an 8.4-mile loop.

The **ELK–KINGS LOOP** is some pretty serious business. If you have a second car at the Kings Mountain trailhead, the loop is only 7.5 miles. Without that shuttle, you'll have to hike 3.7 more miles to return on Wilson River Trail. Either way, it's a challenge.

As if going up Elk Mountain and then scrambling over to Kings Mountain Trail wasn't enough work, you're now faced with a 1.3-mile ridgetop traverse that even in dry weather could stir up a fear of heights. The spookiest section is along the top of cliffs on the north side of the ridge, where snow will linger later than in other places.

The good news is, there's only one trail and it sticks to the ridge, so you won't get lost. When you get to Kings Mountain, enjoy that view, then head down the steep trail described above. If you have a car at that trailhead, good for you; if not, turn left on Wilson River Trail to follow it 3.7 miles back to the starting point.

**ELK CREEK TRAIL (4 MILES ONE-WAY; MODERATE):** This is the least challenging one around, of interest mostly as a safer, saner return trip from Elk Mountain. If you want to ascend it, follow the road from the trailhead up past the gate. You'll walk along the main creek— it has a steelhead run, and river otters have reportedly been sighted here.

At 0.5 miles, you'll come to the confluence of the main creek and its West Fork; head up the West Fork a mile before starting your climb out of the canyon. After 2.5 miles of gradual uphill walking, you'll arrive at the junction with Elk Mountain Trail. To visit that summit, hike 0.7 miles left, then make another left and continue 2 miles to the summit.

Doing the summit loop up and down this way is 13.4 tedious miles, so go ahead and tackle the steep part going up.

Whichever hike you choose, I say you deserve the next day or two off!

# OSWALD WEST STATE PARK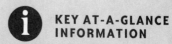

## IN BRIEF

This ultra-popular state park includes two of the best hikes on the northern Oregon coast: a flat stroll through old-growth forest to a cliff-top ocean view, and a vigorous hike to a peak with a grand panorama.

## DESCRIPTION

**CAPE FALCON:** About five steps from the parking lot, you'll find yourself in a rare old-growth coastal forest, walking a wide, mostly flat path to a wonderful destination. You'll cruise 0.4 miles to a junction, where Short Sand Beach will be to your left and downhill about 0.3 miles; Cape Falcon will be to the right. Straight ahead is a nice view of Smugglers Cove.

Turn right, cross a small creek, and start winding along the contours of the land. Around 1.3 miles, where the trail makes a sharp left turn, a downed tree on the right has left a large, disfigured stump. Some more-imaginative hiking friends of mine dubbed this stump the Throne of the Forest King. Assume the throne to survey your kingdom, which includes a nice little grove of Sitka spruce and hemlock.

### KEY AT-A-GLANCE INFORMATION

**LENGTH:** 5 miles to Cape Falcon, 2.5 or 9 miles to Neahkahnie Mountain

**CONFIGURATION:** Out-and-back

**DIFFICULTY:** Easy to Cape Falcon, strenuous to Neahkahnie Mountain

**SCENERY:** Old-growth forest, waterfalls, several cliff-top vistas of the sea

**EXPOSURE:** Shady, except for cliff tops at the cape and a rocky scramble at the mountain

**TRAFFIC:** Heavy all summer, especially weekends; moderate otherwise

**TRAIL SURFACE:** Packed dirt, with some gravel; brief rock scrambling on Neahkahnie

**HIKING TIME:** 2.5 hours to Cape Falcon, up to 4 for the mountain

**DRIVING DISTANCE:** 89 miles (1 hour 40 minutes) from Pioneer Square

**SEASON:** Year-round, but wet in winter

**BEST TIME:** Whenever it's not raining

**BACKPACKING OPTIONS:** None

**ACCESS:** No fees or permits

**WHEELCHAIR ACCESS:** None

**MAPS:** USGS Arch Cape

**FACILITIES:** Toilets and drinking water near trailhead

**INFO:** Managed by Nehalem Bay State Park, (503) 368-5943

### Directions

Take US 26 from Portland, traveling 74 miles west of I-405; turn south on US 101. The trailhead is 14 miles ahead on the right. There are actually four parking areas in succession here. The first (unmarked) one on the right is for Cape Falcon, distinguished by a small median strip along the highway. The second one, 0.1 mile ahead on the left, is where the restroom is. For the shortest trip to Neahkahnie Mountain, drive 2 miles past the restroom and turn left onto a gravel road by a brown hiker sign. The trailhead is 0.4 miles up on the left.

### GPS Trailhead Coordinates

UTM Zone (WGS84) 10T

Easting 425767

Northing 5068218

Latitude N 45.76353°

Longitude W 123.95462°

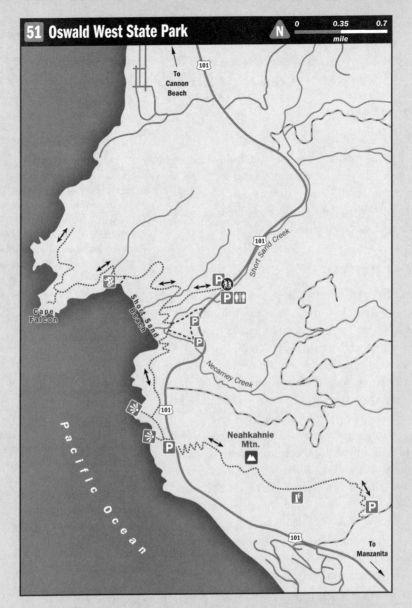

N

0          0.35          0.7

mile

To
Cannon
Beach

101

Short Sand Creek

101

Cape
Falcon

Short Sand
Beach

P

P

P

P

Necarney Creek

101

Neahkahnie
Mtn.

P

P

Pacific Ocean

101

To
Manzanita

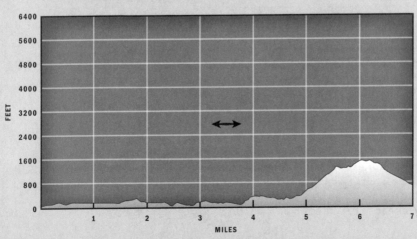

6400

5600

4800

4000

3200

2400

1600

800

0

FEET

1          2          3          4          5          6          7

MILES

Half a mile past that goofiness, ignore a series of trails that plunge down to the left. They access the beach, but they're too steep to fool with—especially at the end. On the main trail, just before a footbridge over a creek, a brushy path to the left leads 100 feet to a tiny, hidden waterfall. If you take it another 100 yards or so, often having to nearly crawl through the brush, you'll find yourself at the top of an even larger falls that goes right down to the ocean. Just be careful of your footing, or you'll wind up in a heap on the rocks some 50 feet below.

A short distance later, back on the main trail, you'll start out toward the end of Cape Falcon itself. You'll get nice views back into Smugglers Cove and up to Neahkahnie Mountain, then you'll descend through the trees once more to a junction at the edge of a brushy, largely treeless area. For the end of the cape, turn left, and walk about 0.2 miles through the gauntlet of brush. Out at the end, you'll be 200 feet above the sea, with Falcon Rock out in front of you; you'll also be at the top of an unrailed 200-foot cliff. There are some good picnicking spots under the trees. In late May and early June, the grassy bluffs here are awash in Indian paintbrush and irises. Look for seals and sea lions below.

When you head back to the main trail, walk left for a bit to add more scenery to your day. This is the Oregon Coast Trail, which stretches (in one form or another) from California to the Columbia River. In this next mile or so, you'll get three more views of the sea. When the trail starts climbing inland, you might as well turn back, unless the old-growth magic has you in its grip. There are no more ocean views for a while, but there are plenty of big trees and not many people.

**NEAHKAHNIE MOUNTAIN:** Perhaps all these trailheads have you confused. Well, don't be. It's really very simple. Neahkahnie Mountain has a killer view from 1,600 feet above the ocean, and you have two good options for getting there: the simplest is a 2.5-mile round-trip from the southernmost trailhead, gaining 850 feet; the longer option starts at the beach and offers more to see as it gains 1,600 feet in 3.3 miles. With two cars, you could do both and put in only 4.5 miles.

First, the shortest option, starting at the southernmost trailhead. Switchback up through open areas filled with tasty red thimbleberries in late summer, and, after 0.7 miles, you'll reach a junction with a road that leads left to some radio towers. Cross the road and follow the trail. You'll climb gradually another 0.3 miles, pass to the north of (and below) the radio towers, and then, in 0.2 miles, come to the summit trail. Right where you pop out into the open, after you cross to the west side of the ridgeline, you'll see a little trail heading up and to your right: that's it. It's a little rocky scramble, nothing intense.

For the beach option, which is the best and most scenic route, start at the parking lot for Oswald West State Park Campground. Walk 0.1 mile down the trail, among some awesome Sitka spruces, toward Short Sand Beach to reach a junction offering a choice between beach and campground; choose beach. Walk 0.1 mile, turn left at another junction, and this time cross a wonderfully bouncy suspension bridge over Necarney Creek. Take a few minutes to explore the lovely beach, which has some pretty decent tidepools around to the left.

Now, back on the trail to Neahkahnie Mountain, you'll climb up a ridge covered with fantastic trees. About 0.2 miles up the trail, you'll actually go *through* a Sitka spruce. When that tree is 0.3 miles behind you, look for a large western red cedar just by the trail on the left; just beyond that are two ridiculously large Sitka spruces, with foot-thick branches that have turned upward to become trees in their own right. If you think they can't get any bigger, just wait: the largest spruce of the hike, which has several trunks, is 0.2 miles ahead.

When you pop out into the open, in a meadow more than 200 feet above the sea, you'll have come 1.3 miles since leaving your car. Just ahead you'll see two trails splitting off to the right. Ignore the first one you come to; the second one leads to a cliff-top viewpoint among the trees, looking down at Devils Cauldron. And don't wander around in these meadows. I know a guy who fell into a 15-foot hole here and had to be pulled out with a rope.

When you reach US 101, cross it carefully, and start into the woods at a trail sign. Climb 0.6 miles in the open before reentering the trees. At this point, you're about 1,000 feet above sea level. You'll climb gradually after this; if the trail then seems to dip, don't worry—you're just walking around to the far side of the mountain, where the view is. When you reach a junction where two large trees fell, stay right. Eventually, you'll be back in the open and see a small trail heading up to the left; that's the summit.

From the top of Neahkahnie, you can see all the way south to Cape Meares; look for Three Arch Rocks offshore there. If it's a really clear day, you might make out Cape Lookout, south of Cape Meares. The beach town seemingly at your feet is Manzanita, and the body of water beyond it is Nehalem Bay. During the invasion-scare days of World War II, the Coast Guard had a lookout up here, while soldiers patrolled the beaches on horseback, and blimps from Tillamook cruised offshore.

If you have a car at the southern trailhead, time your arrival on the summit for just before sundown. It's quite a show from up there, and even at dusk it's no problem getting back to your car, especially if you came the short way.

## NEARBY ACTIVITIES

I have a soft spot for the family-operated Ecola Seafood Market in Cannon Beach, 11 miles north of the trailhead on US 101. The name, by the way, is the native word for "whale." I feel quite strongly that they serve the best clam chowder around, and they always have lots of fresh seafood. It's at the corner of Second and Spruce, right across from the visitor center.

# SADDLE MOUNTAIN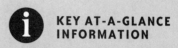

## IN BRIEF

The highest point in northwest Oregon, Saddle Mountain is also one of the most popular hiking trails in the state. Traversing flower-filled meadows unparalleled in this part of the state, it affords a view from the top that stretches from the ocean to the mouth of the Columbia River to the Cascades.

## DESCRIPTION

Saddle Mountain just doesn't seem to belong in its surroundings. It's the highest point in this part of the state; the hills around it aren't even close. It doesn't even resemble them, with its two-headed, rocky summit of "pillow lava," which looks like that because it erupted under water, millions of years ago when this area was the sea floor. When you get on top of Saddle Mountain, you might think you're on Mount Hood, with the faraway views and abundant wildflowers. Of course, as crowded as it gets on summer weekends, you might think you're in a city park right after quitting time on a weekday. Whatever—it's a great hike, so start early in the morning and get there before everybody else.

When you get out of your car, you might be a little intimidated as you look up at the mountain. You might even see some speck-

### KEY AT-A-GLANCE INFORMATION

**LENGTH: 5.2 miles**

**CONFIGURATION: Out-and-back**

**DIFFICULTY: Strenuous**

**SCENERY: Deep forest, wildflowers, panoramic view**

**EXPOSURE: In the forest, then out in the open on top; occasionally steep on some loose rocks and metal fencing—slippery if there's been rain or snow**

**TRAFFIC: Very heavy on summer weekends, heavy on other summer days, moderate otherwise**

**TRAIL SURFACE: Packed dirt with rocks, then just rocks**

**HIKING TIME: 3.5 hours**

**DRIVING DISTANCE: 74 miles (1 hour 30 minutes) from Pioneer Square**

**SEASON: Year-round, but it does get snow in the winter**

**BEST TIME: June–July, for the flowers**

**BACKPACKING OPTIONS: None; campground at trailhead is open March–October**

**ACCESS: No fees or permits**

**WHEELCHAIR ACCESS: None**

**MAPS: USGS Saddle Mountain**

**FACILITIES: Restroom at trailhead (closed November–February)**

**INFO: Managed by Nehalem Bay State Park, (503) 368-5943**

---

## Directions

**Take US 26 from Portland, traveling 66 miles west of I-405, and turn right at a sign for Saddle Mountain State Park. The trailhead is 7 miles ahead, at the end of the road.**

### GPS Trailhead Coordinates

UTM Zone (WGS84) 10T

Easting 446552

Northing 5090147

Latitude  N 45.96281°

Longitude W 123.68979°

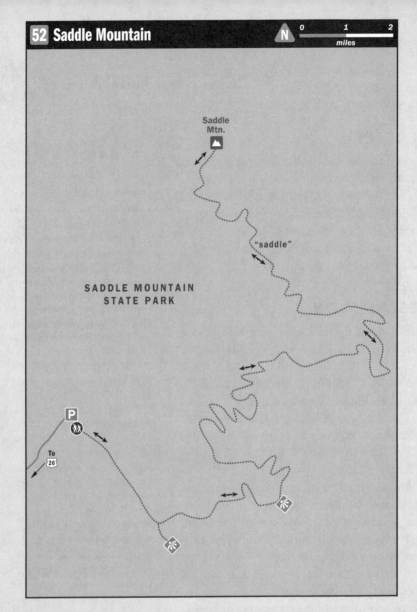

Saddle
Mtn.

"saddle"

SADDLE MOUNTAIN
STATE PARK

P

To
26

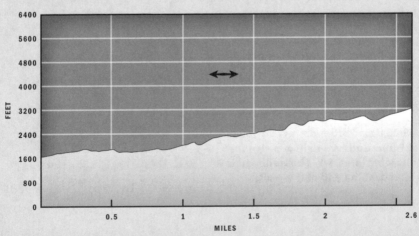

FEET

6400
5600
4800
4000
3200
2400
1600
800
0

0.5     1     1.5     2     2.6

MILES

sized people up there. The good news is, you'll be up there soon enough; the bad news is, that's not the summit.

Things start out mellow, in a young forest filled with big, old stumps—relics of logging in the 1920s and fires in the 1930s. After you've hiked 0.2 miles, you'll see a side trail to the right, which leads 0.1 mile to a great view of all of Saddle Mountain—the only one in the park, oddly enough. Then you'll start climbing, gaining about 1,100 feet in the next 1.4 miles, and occasionally walking on a combination of rocks and metal grating put in for traction. When the trail turns back to the left and flattens, you'll be at 2,900 feet, just 300 feet below the summit.

Now you're out in the flower meadows. There are several rare species here, such as the Saddle Mountain saxifrage and Saddle Mountain bittercress—species that survived the last Ice Age. Stay on the trail and on the footbridges, and remember it's illegal to pick the flowers. You'll descend briefly and cross the saddle—this is the point you can see from the car, which is now visible, if very small, on your left—and then climb the last, steep scramble to the summit, in places with handrails to hold onto.

On a clear day, you can see from the volcanoes of the Cascades to the Pacific, and to the mouth of the Columbia just beyond Astoria to the north. On a really clear day, you can make out the mountains of the Olympic Peninsula beyond that. I also once, on a *really* clear day, spotted Saddle Mountain from Chinidere Mountain in the Columbia River Gorge (hike 4, page 25); needless to say, I've never seen Chinidere from Saddle Mountain.

## NEARBY ACTIVITIES

You no doubt noticed Camp 18 a few miles before the turnoff from US 26. How could you not? It might look like a logging museum, and it is, but it's also a restaurant with a famously filling Sunday buffet served from 10 a.m. to 2 p.m., and it includes prime rib! As one newspaper story put it, "you can throw on one serious feedbag." It's not a bad way to prepare for (or recover from) an assault on Saddle Mountain.

# 53  WILSON RIVER

## KEY AT-A-GLANCE INFORMATION

**LENGTH: 20.6 miles, with sections 3.5–7.4 miles in length**

**CONFIGURATION: Out-and-back, with shuttles available**

**DIFFICULTY: Easy–difficult, it's up to you**

**SCENERY: Second-growth forest, a river, occasional views from up high**

**EXPOSURE: In the forest the whole way**

**TRAFFIC: Moderate on summer weekends, light otherwise**

**TRAIL SURFACE: Packed dirt, some rocks**

**HIKING TIME: 12 hours for the whole thing**

**DRIVING DISTANCE: About 50 miles (1 hour) from Pioneer Square, depending on which trailhead you choose**

**SEASON: Year-round, but might get snow in winter, especially the Kings–Jones section**

**BEST TIME: March–April for flowers, or October for fall colors**

**BACKPACKING OPTIONS: None**

**ACCESS: No fee**

**WHEELCHAIR ACCESS: None**

**MAPS: Brochures available from Tillamook State Forest**

**FACILITIES: In the campgrounds at Elk Creek and Jones Creek, both closed in winter**

**INFO: Tillamook State Forest, (503) 357-2191**

### GPS Trailhead Coordinates

UTM Zone (WGS84) 10T

Easting 463617

Northing 5050856

Latitude N 45.61030°

Longitude W 123.46660°

## IN BRIEF

This relatively new trail explores the canyon of the Wilson River, where salmon and steelhead come to spawn. For many years, it was known to those who don't fish as "that river along Highway 6 on your way to Tillamook," but with a trail and a forest center now in place, the Wilson is a destination all its own.

## DESCRIPTION

This is a great, year-round hike that's close to Portland and offers something for everybody: steep hills, flat sections, solitude, picnic areas, forests, views, you name it. There's a pretty good chance that the Kings–Jones or Footbridge–Keenig sections will have snow in winter, but otherwise it should be open. Come in spring for flowers and maximum water flow, or in October for amazing fall colors.

If you want to do this whole 21-mile thing at once, stash a car at Keenig Creek, start your hike at Elk Creek, and know that

---

## Directions

Take US 26 from Portland, driving 20 miles west of I-405, then bear west on OR 6, following a sign for Tillamook. The trailheads are all along the right side of the highway. For Elk Mountain, go 23 miles to Elk Creek Campground, just past milepost 28. Kings Mountain is 3 miles farther along, just before milepost 25. Jones Creek is in a day-use area between mileposts 22 and 23; head for the campground, then turn left just after a bridge. Footbridge is a parking area on the right at milepost 20. For Keenig Creek, go 2 miles past Footbridge, turn right on Cedar Butte Road, cross the bridge, and go left onto Muesial Creek Road. The trailhead is 0.2 miles ahead, on the right.

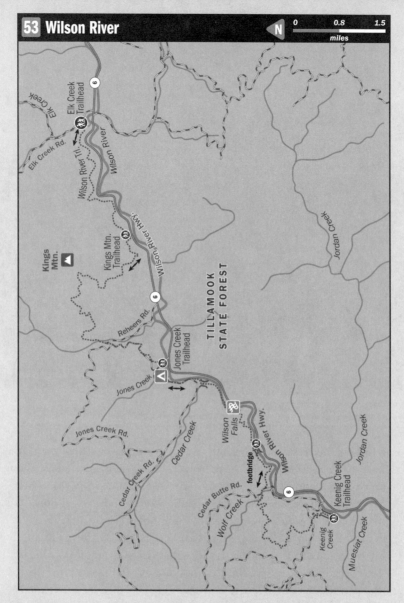

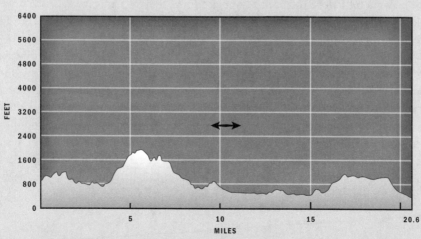

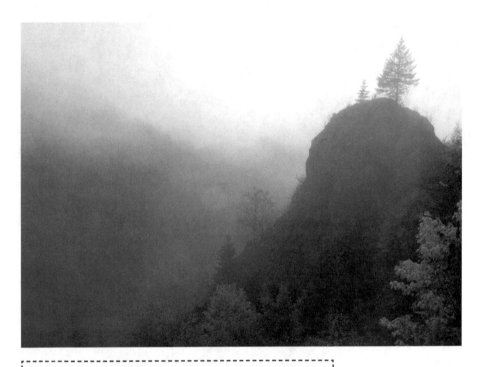

Rock formation between Kings Mountain and Jones Creek trailheads

you will have my respect and admiration, for whatever it's worth. Otherwise, pick one of these sections and have at it. I do advise a car shuttle, though; it's easy to work out and means you don't have to backtrack.

**Elk Creek to Kings Mountain** is a 3.7-mile stretch most often done as part of the dreaded Elk Mountain–Kings Mountain loop, described in this book starting on page 227. But it's a nice forest stroll on its own, with the highlight being a series of meadows just a half mile from the Kings Mountain trailhead.

From the Elk Creek trailhead, you'll ascend 0.2 steep miles to reach the even steeper Elk Mountain Trail. Continue on Wilson River Trail, and the grade will let up a bit before the path becomes a long, mostly flat traverse. At 2 miles, just after a switchback that seems like a dramatic change, descend to a bridge over Dog Creek.

The next mile is more of the same, until you descend to the meadows at 3.2 miles. Try to get here in the morning or late afternoon, and if you're quiet you might see some elk. Another half mile brings you to Kings Mountain Trail, where you can turn left and descend 0.1 mile to that trailhead. Or keep going.

**Kings Mountain to Jones Creek,** at 7.4 miles, is the toughest, highest, and most scenic section of Wilson River Trail. It also, somewhat ironically, never visits the Wilson River. The reason is that a bloc of private land along the river necessitates a big climb up the slopes of Kings Mountain, but you get some nice views from up there.

Bridge over North Fork Wilson River

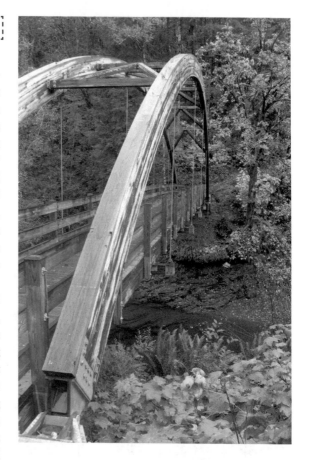

Leaving Kings Mountain Trail, which is 0.1 mile up from Kings Mountain trailhead, you'll first cross a jeep track with a sign reading "Kings Mt. Jr." then start to climb. You'll put in 1,200 feet in 1.5 miles on a steady grade. Just before the hilltop is a nice lunch spot, a trailside log where some old roadbeds intersect.

Past there, you'll start generally downhill, making lots of tiny creek crossings. You're going around a side canyon, that of Lester Creek. Around 3 miles, you'll come to a big rock formation with a tree growing atop it. My friends and I joked that, despite all the forest scenery so far, this was The Only Interesting Thing On The Hike. (But that's true only if you're doing this in the rain and didn't expect that 1,200-foot climb!) There are two good viewpoints here, and a chance to head out (carefully) to the rock itself.

Half a mile later, hike down steeply, and at 4 miles total, traverse a tiny meadow where several more old roads intersect. Those roads are *steep*, aren't they? Imagine driving a truck loaded with logs down one of those things.

Keep moseying along, drop through a particularly lush area with a sea of sword ferns, and at 5.5 miles cross the North Fork of the Wilson River on a large, scenic bridge. At the far end, there's a picnic table and a side trail leading down to the river. You'll see a sign here for Tillamook County Water Trail. This is a combined effort of local citizens with the Tillamook Estuaries Partnership to develop maps and guides for the whopping 1,800 miles of navigable water in the county. Check out **www.tbnep.org** to see how they're doing.

You may also, in this area, hear offroad vehicles. Fear not: they can't come on your trail. Follow the path downstream, and after 100 yards pass Lester Creek Falls across the Wilson, finely adorned with a bright-orange No Trespassing sign.

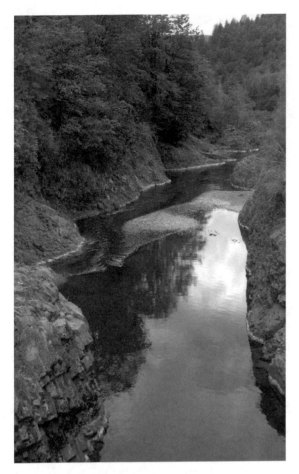

Over the next 1.9 miles, you'll cross two roads and a small ridge, then pop out at Jones Creek Trailhead. Keep an eye out in this section for some amazing anthills and "legacy" trees that survived the forest fires last century.

**Jones Creek to Footbridge,** at 3.5 miles, is the most popular section, owing to its ease of access, lack of big hills, and proximity to the river. The Jones Creek area has a campground nearby and a series of picnic sites along the first stretch of the trail.

After a third of a mile—some of which will certainly go into the river one day—you'll reach a big bridge leading over to Tillamook Forest Center, which has exhibits about the forest and its history. The trail stays on the north side of the river, occasionally on roads, and after a mile swings away from the river a bit to cross Cedar Creek on a one-log bridge over a deep pool that looks like a good place for a dip.

Just past the bridge, keep left to avoid power lines, and at 1.3 miles look for a social trail leading down to a rocky area along the river. A quarter mile ahead is a better trail to a sandier beach. Soon after, there's a bit of a hill to get up. You'll climb for about 1 mile to pass the 100-foot Wilson Falls, which may seem overrated if it hasn't rained lately.

The last 1.5 miles of this section traces a fern-filled bowl, then makes a long, gradual descent to the trail over to Footbridge. Even if you intend to keep going, it's worth a trip down to the river here. There's a huge logjam there—and a nice swimming hole, with a rock outcropping and a swing rigged from a log—and the footbridge itself, which crosses the Wilson at a deep, placid pool in a small gorge.

To get to the trailhead from there, turn left at the far end of the bridge and walk 100 (protected) yards along the shoulder of the highway.

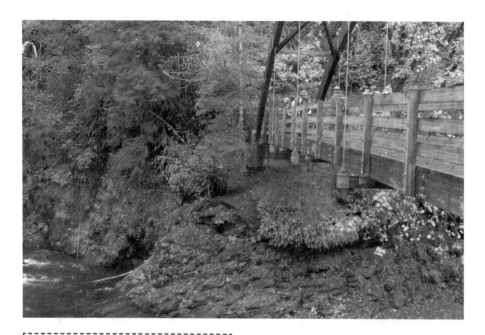

A viewpoint of North Fork Wilson River

**Footbridge to Keenig Creek** is a 6.1-mile, lonesome stretch with another big hill but lots of cool scenery. If you're starting at Footbridge, walk up the road from the parking lot, cross the bridge, and follow the trail across the creek bed and into the woods. Turn left on Wilson River Trail, and you're on your way.

In the first mile, you'll cross a log bridge and then head up to a rock bluff with views of the Wilson. At 1 mile, you join Wolf Creek Road for about 500 feet; head to the right, up the road to the north, to find the trail. At the creek just below, there's a nice log bench for a break—which you'll need.

After Wolf Creek, things get steep for a mile, then the grade relents a bit. You'll have some waterfalls and creeks to break up the monotony before you cross over a ridge at 2 miles to start a 3-mile traverse in and out of side canyons.

When you hit Cedar Butte Road, you have only 1.5 downhill miles through switchbacks and a recent clearcut. Nothing much to see, in other words, but by this time you're probably just ready to be done—especially if you're one of those 21-miles-in-one-day folks!

## NEARBY ACTIVITIES

Tillamook Forest Center is open March through November, Wednesday to Sunday, from 10 a.m. to 4 p.m. Admission and programs are free. One thing to remember, though: if you park here and go hiking, your car will be stuck if you don't return before they lock the gates at closing time. See **www.tillamookforest center.org** for more info.

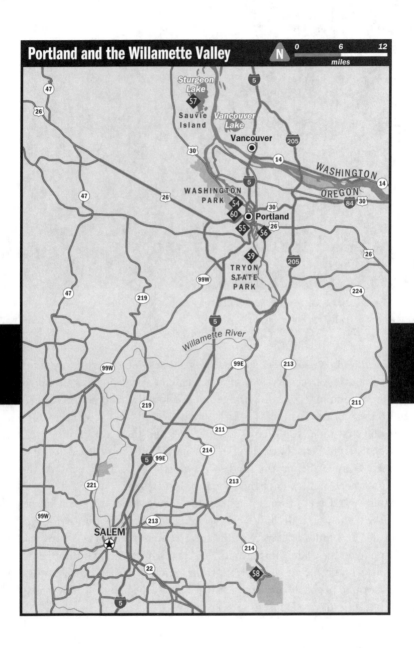

Portland and the Willamette Valley

# IN PORTLAND AND
# THE WILLAMETTE VALLEY

# 54 MACLEAY TRAIL

## KEY AT-A-GLANCE INFORMATION

**LENGTH:** 2.2 miles to Upper Macleay Park and Audubon Society, 4.5 miles to Pittock Mansion

**CONFIGURATION:** Out-and-back

**DIFFICULTY:** Easy to Upper Macleay Park and Audubon Society, moderate to Pittock Mansion

**SCENERY:** Quiet woods, predatory birds (in cages), three must-see trees

**EXPOSURE:** Shady all the way, one road crossing

**TRAFFIC:** Light on the trail weekdays, moderate on weekends; heavy at mansion

**TRAIL SURFACE:** Packed dirt, with some gravel

**HIKING TIME:** 1 hour to Audubon Society, 2.5 hours for the whole thing

**DRIVING DISTANCE:** 3 miles (10 minutes) from Pioneer Square

**SEASON:** Year-round

**BEST TIME:** Any clear day, for the view

**BACKPACKING OPTIONS:** None

**ACCESS:** No fees or permits

**WHEELCHAIR ACCESS:** Paved lower 0.25 miles, mansion area entirely accessible

**MAPS:** Forest Park maps at Audubon Society

**FACILITIES:** Water and toilets at trailhead, Audubon Society, and mansion

**INFO:** Portland Parks and Recreation, (503) 823-7529

## GPS Trailhead Coordinates

UTM Zone (WGS84) 1oT

Easting 522366

Northing 5042286

Latitude N 45.53375°

Longitude W 122.71355°

## IN BRIEF

If you just take the easier trip to the Audubon Society, you'll get some quiet time in the woods, where you'll see two monumental trees, and enjoy close-up views of (caged) wildlife. If you put in a little more effort, you'll get that and some history with a great view—and another monumental tree. And it's all right in the middle of town!

## DESCRIPTION

First, if the headquarters of the Forest Park Ivy Removal Project (at the trailhead) is open, it's worth a look inside. The project has cleared hundreds of acres and saved thousands of trees in Forest Park from invasive English ivy, which creates "ivy deserts," where no native plants can survive. In this building the crews house some of their "trophies," ivy roots bigger than you can imagine such things being. Gawk, get some water, and head up the trail.

What you're walking up here is Balch Creek, named for the man who once owned this land—also the first man in Portland to be tried and hanged for murder. Small as it

## Directions

From downtown Portland, drive 1 mile west on Burnside Street and turn right on NW 23rd Avenue. Proceed 0.8 miles and turn left on Thurman Street. Go six blocks to NW 28th Avenue and turn right. Go one block, turn left on NW Upshur, and follow it three blocks to the trailhead, at the end of the road. This trailhead can also be reached via Tri-Met. From downtown, take the #15 bus (NW 23rd Avenue), but make sure it's headed for Thurman Street and not Montgomery Park. Get off at Thurman and 28th, walk one more block, and descend a flight of steps beside the bridge.

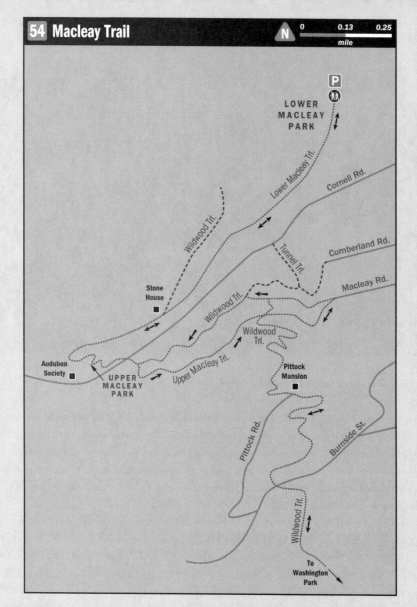

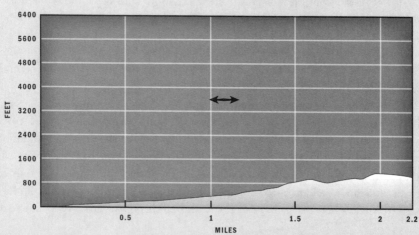

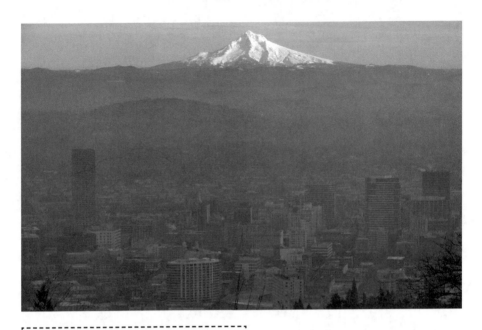

Mount Hood and Portland from Pittock Mansion

is, the creek was the original water supply for the city of Portland. And if that doesn't amaze you, consider that in 1987 the Oregon Department of Fish and Game discovered a native population of cutthroat trout living in this tiny stream. It is one of only two year-round streams in all of Forest Park. Check some of the deeper pools, and you just may see some of the fish. Please keep your dog on a leash and out of the water.

At 0.4 miles, look for a Douglas fir on your left that is marked with a plaque identifying it as a Portland Heritage Tree, one of some 300 such trees around town to be forever protected from the saw. This one happens to be the tallest tree in the city of Portland, at 241 feet, and is thought to be the tallest in any major U.S. city.

At 0.9 miles, you'll join the 30-mile Wildwood Trail at an old stone building that was a restroom until the early 1960s, when a storm destroyed its pipes by uprooting numerous trees. In fact, legend has it that this house is also the scene of nocturnal battles between the ghosts of Danford Balch and his victim, Mortimer Stump. And if there's a better Old Portland name than Mortimer Stump, I want to know what it is.

Stay straight (upstream), now joining Wildwood Trail, and over the next half mile you'll climb to Upper Macleay Park. Whether you're headed for Pittock Mansion or not, make a right here and walk 100 yards to the Portland Audubon Society. They rehabilitate injured owls and hawks here, and you can view the caged birds for no charge; they also have an extensive collection of mounted animals and an excellent gift shop plus bookstore. Three loop trails explore sanctuaries from here; free maps of those and all of Forest Park are available at

Falls on Balch Creek

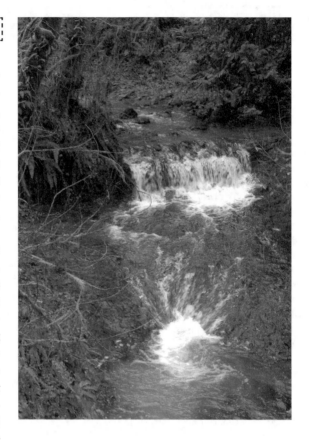

the gift shop. Particularly worth visiting is a shelter overlooking a pond, just below the headquarters. You can impress your friends by telling them that the massive sequoia beside the parking lot is actually less than 100 years old. They grow quickly at first.

To do just a 2.2-mile hike, head back to the car. To add another 2.7 miles (and just over 400 feet in elevation), stay on Wildwood Trail by walking along Macleay Park's parking lot, crossing the sometimes-busy Cornell Road at a crosswalk, and reentering the forest. After 100 yards, turn right on Upper Macleay Trail. This trail climbs about 0.2 miles, then flattens out. At 0.5 miles, you'll find a wooden bench with a cool pattern on it. Just past that, rejoin Wildwood Trail, turning right and uphill for the final 0.6 miles to the Pittock Mansion parking lot.

The home (see Nearby Activities, below) is to your left. Wander out to the front yard to enjoy the roses and a view of city and mountains, and admire yet another spectacular tree: a European white birch that offers enough shade for a small town.

If you took the bus, you don't have to walk back down the trail. You can, instead, walk down the road from the mansion to Burnside Street, about 0.3 miles away, cross it (carefully!), and take the #20 (Burnside) bus downtown. You can also continue 1 mile on Wildwood Trail (descending 300 feet) to connect with the Washington Park–Hoyt Arboretum hike (hike 60, page 268).

## NEARBY ACTIVITIES

Pittock Mansion, built in 1914 by the owner–publisher of the *Oregonian* and founder of the Portland Rose Festival, is open for tours daily. For more information, call (503) 823-3623.

# 55 MARQUAM TRAIL TO COUNCIL CREST

## KEY AT-A-GLANCE INFORMATION

**LENGTH: 3.7 miles**

**CONFIGURATION: Out-and-back, with a side loop**

**DIFFICULTY: Easy on Nature Loop Trail, moderate to Council Crest**

**SCENERY: Woods, impressive homes, and a sweeping vista on top**

**EXPOSURE: Shady all the way up, open on top, a couple of street crossings**

**TRAFFIC: Heavy on weekends and workday evenings, moderate otherwise**

**TRAIL SURFACE: Packed dirt, gravel**

**HIKING TIME: 2 hours**

**DRIVING DISTANCE: 1 mile (5 minutes) from Pioneer Square**

**SEASON: Year-round**

**BEST TIME: Any clear day**

**BACKPACKING OPTIONS: None**

**ACCESS: No fees or permits**

**WHEELCHAIR ACCESS: None**

**MAPS: Available at trailhead**

**FACILITIES: Water at trailhead and at Council Crest**

**INFO: Portland Parks and Recreation, (503) 823-7529**

GPS Trailhead
Coordinates

UTM Zone (WGS84) 10T

Easting 524271

Northing 5038778

Latitude  N 45.50211°

Longitude W 122.68933°

## IN BRIEF

This pleasant trail through a wooded canyon just minutes from downtown leads to the highest point in Portland, where you can take in a view of four volcanoes. What a city we live in!

## DESCRIPTION

Council Crest got its name in 1898 when a group of visiting ministers met there after a two-hour wagon drive. They assumed the Native Americans must have held many a council there. It turns out they probably didn't, but the name stuck. In the early and mid-20th century you could ride a trolley to the top and visit an amusement park. Today you can get there by car or bus, but the best way is to walk up Marquam Trail through a wooded ravine.

At the trailhead shelter, two signs lead you to Marquam Trail, a 7-mile stretch of the 40 Mile Loop that passes through Marquam Nature Park, running from Willamette Park to Washington Park. The Nature Trail is a 1.2-mile interpretive loop trail that meets Marquam Trail and returns to the shelter. If

### *Directions*

From downtown Portland, drive south on Broadway Avenue. After it crosses I-405, take the second right onto SW 6th Avenue, following the blue H signs leading to the hospital. (Don't take the right signed "Council Crest.") Continue straight through three lights in the next half mile, passing two large concrete water towers on your right. When the road cuts back to the left, turn right on SW Marquam Street to enter a parking lot. You can also take Tri-Met bus #8 to the third light, Sam Jackson and Terwilliger, and walk 200 yards to the trailhead.

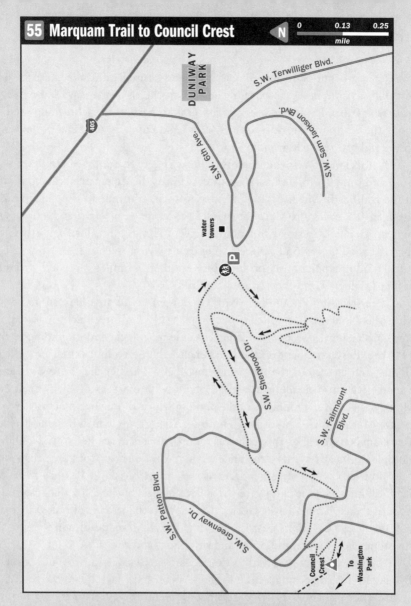

DUNIWAY PARK

S.W. Terwilliger Blvd.

S.W. Sam Jackson Blvd.

405

S.W. 6th Ave.

water towers

P

S.W. Sherwood Dr.

S.W. Fairmount Blvd.

S.W. Patton Blvd.

S.W. Greenway Dr.

Council Crest

To Washington Park

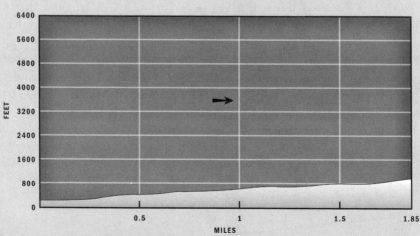

6400
5600
4800
4000
3200
2400
1600
800
0

FEET

0.5        1        1.5        1.85

MILES

you got a brochure and feel like adding the Nature Trail, take the path on the left that says 0.7 miles, instead of the one on the right that says 0.4 miles. This leads you 0.3 miles up the creek to a junction; here, turn right; numbered signs along the way point out various local flora and fauna as you head 0.4 miles back to the right to reach Marquam Trail.

At this junction, if you don't feel like going up the hill, bear right on Shelter Trail and walk 0.4 miles back to your car (this is the right-hand trail you skipped at the trailhead). But for the best view in town, continue to the left and follow the trail 0.5 miles up Marquam Gulch, then make a left turn, following the signs to Council Crest. At this point the trail climbs a bit. Just before you cross the next road (Sherwood), there's an extremely cool treehouse on your left. Oh, to be a kid in a neighborhood like this! Another 0.4 miles on, you'll cross Fairmount Boulevard and then continue uphill.

After crossing yet another road (Greenway), in an area planted decades ago with May-blooming rhododendrons, you'll walk uphill to reach the wide, open area atop Council Crest, where couples come to snuggle and kids come to throw a Frisbee. Rest a moment on the two benches there to admire the view of Mount Hood—and check out the dates inscribed here. The benches were dedicated to a couple who both made it to age 98, dying within a year of each other. Nadia Munk was one of the founders of the park, in whose dining room plans were made to save Marquam Gulch 40-plus years ago. That group, which became Friends of Marquam Nature Park, stopped plans for apartments in the ravine and lobbied for multiple trailheads to make the area accessible as a retreat from the urban world.

Now, climb to the stone circle at the top of the park. Plaques there point out the four volcanoes and give the native name for each. To the east you can see into the Columbia River Gorge. The view to the west goes out to Beaverton and, on a clear day, the Coast Range. Find the small metal disc in the middle of this stone enclosure, stand on it, and say, "Portland rocks."

You can connect this trail to the Washington Park trip (hike 60, page 268), if you're up for something a little longer. As you start back down the trail, take a left just after you enter the trees, turning to the northwest. This trail will traverse the hill briefly before descending to the right, eventually reaching the intersection of SW Talbot and SW Fairmount. Walk down Talbot about 0.3 miles to the intersection with SW Patton. Cross Patton, then turn right, onto the sidewalk; 200 feet ahead you'll see a trail descending to the left. Follow it 1 mile through the forest until you reach an access road along US 26. Walk left 50 yards, cross the bridge over the expressway, then look on the left for a trail going up the hill, into the trees again. This will lead you through a meadow, behind the World Forestry Center, and eventually (in 0.2 miles or so) to an intersection with Wildwood Trail. (This is also the end of Marquam Trail.) Turn right on Wildwood Trail, and in 0.1 mile you'll be at the parking lot; across that is the MAX station, where you can catch a train back to town if you don't want to keep hiking.

To return from Council Crest, head 1.3 miles back down the trail, following signs for Marquam Shelter, and when you get to a junction pointing left 0.4 miles to Marquam Park, take it. That's the shorter route back to the car that you skipped earlier in favor of Nature Loop Trail.

## NEARBY ACTIVITIES

If it's a Saturday between late March and early December, don't miss the Portland Farmer's Market at Portland State, just a few blocks north. It runs from 9 a.m. to 2 p.m. on Saturdays. From April to October it's open from 10 a.m. to 2 p.m. on Wednesdays, a bit to the north in the Park Blocks.

# 56 OAKS BOTTOM WILDLIFE REFUGE/ WILLAMETTE RIVER

**KEY AT-A-GLANCE INFORMATION**

**LENGTH:** 3 miles for Oaks Bottom; 11 more miles for the Willamette Greenway Trail

**CONFIGURATION:** Balloon

**DIFFICULTY:** Easy

**SCENERY:** Wildlife, woods, wetlands, water, and even an amusement park

**EXPOSURE:** Shady, occasionally open

**TRAFFIC:** Heavy on weekends, moderate otherwise

**TRAIL SURFACE:** Packed dirt, and gravel

**HIKING TIME:** 2 hours, but only because you'll want to bird-watch

**DRIVING DISTANCE:** 4 miles (10 minutes) from Pioneer Square

**SEASON:** Year-round, but muddy in winter and spring

**BEST TIME:** Winter for waterfowl on the pond; spring–summer for migratory songbirds

**BACKPACKING OPTIONS:** No camping or fires permitted

**ACCESS:** No fees or permits

**WHEELCHAIR ACCESS:** Some of Oaks Bottom, and all of Springwater on Willamette Trail, is paved and accessible.

**MAPS:** USGS Lake Oswego; there's also a map on a sign at the trailhead

**FACILITIES:** Water at trailhead, closest restroom at Sellwood Riverfront Park

**INFO:** Portland Parks and Recreation, (503) 823-7529

## IN BRIEF

This trail goes through the heart of a refuge built around a wetland and pond. The bike–hike path essentially forms a viewing platform through this watery wildlife preserve, which is home to dozens of bird species, especially in spring and fall, and it couldn't be more conveniently located.

## DESCRIPTION

It is so easy, when living in a city, to think that we are "here" and nature is out "there" somewhere, in the hills or on the coast. Occasionally you'll be walking down the street and see some Canada geese fly overhead, and you'll remember that nature is actually all around us. Whenever you need a reminder of this, just go down to Oaks Bottom.

Oaks Bottom is approximately 170 acres of wildlife habitat just a few miles from downtown. It supports some 140 species of birds at various times of the year, especially in the spring and fall migration seasons. At any time of year, you can expect to see herons and ducks, and if you're lucky, you might catch a glimpse of beavers, deer, cormorants, woodpeckers, ospreys, kingfishers, or bald eagles.

From the trailhead off of SE Milwaukie Avenue, walk downhill on the moderate-

GPS Trailhead
Coordinates

UTM Zone (WGS84) 10T

Easting 527341

Northing 5036982

Latitude N 45.48583°

Longitude W 122.65013°

*Directions* ⎯⎯⎯⎯⎯⎯⎯⎯➤

From downtown Portland, go south on Broadway Avenue and follow the signs for Ross Island Bridge (US 26 East). After crossing the bridge, turn right at the first light (Milwaukie Avenue). Go south 1.1 mile on Milwaukie and park at the signed trailhead on the right, just past Mitchell Street. You can also take Tri-Met's #19 Woodstock bus from downtown to the trailhead.

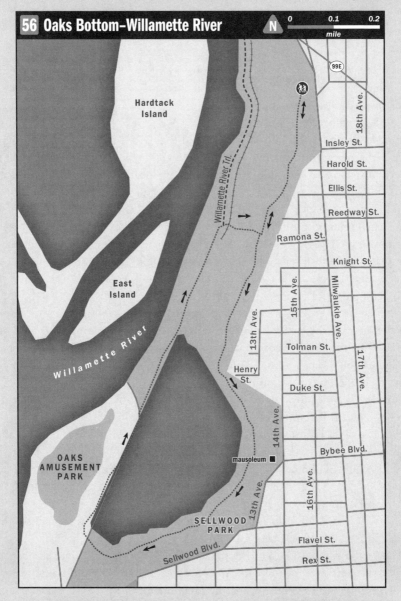

Hardtack
Island

99E

18th Ave.

Insley St.

Harold St.

Ellis St.

Reedway St.

Ramona St.

Willamette River Trl.

Knight St.

East
Island

15th Ave.

Milwaukie Ave.

13th Ave.

Tolman St.

17th Ave.

Willamette River

Henry
St.

Duke St.

14th Ave.

mausoleum

Bybee Blvd.

OAKS
AMUSEMENT
PARK

16th Ave.

13th Ave.

SELLWOOD
PARK

Flavel St.

Sellwood Blvd.

Rex St.

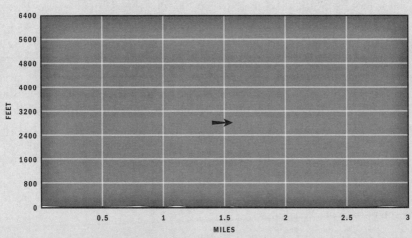

6400

5600

4800

4000

3200

FEET

2400

1600

800

0

0.5          1          1.5          2          2.5          3

MILES

grade Oaks Bottom Access trail. Within the first 0.25 miles, you'll see a trail leading right and into the meadows; ignore it. This area is closed to the public for research and restoration.

Staying on the main trail, you'll reach a fork at 0.3 miles. The trail to the right leads under the railroad tracks and to a paved section of the Springwater on Willamette Trail (see more details below). Staying left at the fork, you'll traverse an active stewardship area managed by local schoolkids. The work began in 2000 with an ivy-removal project; English ivy, not native to the Pacific Northwest, has taken over many of Portland's parks, creating "ivy deserts," where no native plants can grow. So the students, with the help of the city, went in, removed ivy from this section, and planted native conifers and deciduous trees (especially western red cedar and maple) and many native shrubs such as snowberry, elderberry, and hawthorne, in an attempt to reestablish the native plants. You can judge for yourself how it worked.

The trail crosses a bridge and begins to skirt a marsh area (or meadow, depending on the time of year) of willow, red twig dogwood, and reed canary grass. On the slopes above, city crews are restoring oak habitats. After a few minutes you'll reach a large pond that was part of the Willamette River before the construction of the railroad cut it off from the main river in the late 19th century. The meadow at the south end of the pond was used as a construction-debris landfill before becoming the wildlife refuge in 1988.

The pond is best viewed in spring and late fall, when the maximum amount of water is present—both in the pond and on the trail, by the way. Wear sturdy boots and bring binoculars. At all times of the year, look for great blue herons standing still in the water, awaiting a meal; in the summer, Canada geese swoop in for a landing on their way north or south.

When the trail reaches the south end of the pond, one branch cuts right and heads for Oaks Amusement Park. Another continues straight ahead to a trailhead at the southern end of the park. A third, the smallest one, climbs a small hill to the left to Sellwood Park, where there are water fountains and restrooms. Turn right here to head toward the amusement park, then consider making a loop of it by turning right on the paved trail along the railroad tracks. This is the Springwater on Willamette Trail, and in just less than a mile, you'll see the underpass leading to the right and back toward your trailhead. There's also, on the river side of the underpass, an interesting area of artwork in the woods, and a Willamette River overlook.

If you're looking for a much longer walk, the 11-mile Willamette Greenway Trail makes a loop around downtown Portland. From the lower end of this hike, take Spokane, Sixth, and Tacoma streets up onto Sellwood Bridge, and at the west end of that, turn right to follow Willamette Greenway. That will take you north past condos and office buildings, a butterfly park, and Willamette Park, then into downtown and to Tom McCall Waterfront Park. Continue to Steel Bridge, cross that, head south on East Bank Esplanade, and just keep on truckin' until you're back at Oaks Bottom.

*AWFUL*

# SAUVIE ISLAND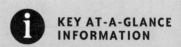

## IN BRIEF

Two casual strolls on the edge of the city offer a glimpse into the local world of wildlife—and back into the past. Both of them are easy to reach and easy to do, and there's plenty of other stuff to do on the island while you're out there.

## DESCRIPTION

First, let's go to Oak Island, which is actually a peninsula in a lake on an island in a river.

Some hikes are in the wilderness, some are walks through history, some are educational, some offer a distant view. This one is out in the country, or so it feels. You'll even pass crops! The whole scene might remind

--------------------------------------

### *Directions* ⟶

Take US 30 from Portland, driving 10 miles west of I-405. Turn right to cross Sauvie Island Bridge. Sauvie Island Market (where you buy your parking pass) is on the left, 0.1 mile beyond the far end of the bridge. Go 2 more miles and turn right on Reeder Road.

For Oak Island: Drive 1.3 miles on Reeder Road, then turn left on Oak Island Road—although, since Reeder heads right here, it's more like continuing straight. After 1.9 miles you'll leave the pavement, and 0.8 miles farther you'll cross a dike. At the bottom of the dike, go left; the trailhead is 0.4 miles ahead at the end of the road.

For Warrior Rock: After 10 miles on Reeder Road, you'll leave the pavement and reach a series of parking areas for Welton Beach, just over the dike to your right. Past that is parking for Collins Beach, which happens to be clothing-optional but is blocked from the road by forest. At 2.3 miles after you leave the pavement, the road ends at the parking area for Warrior Rock.

### ⓘ KEY AT-A-GLANCE INFORMATION

**LENGTH:** 3 miles for Oak Island, 7 miles for Warrior Rock
**CONFIGURATION:** Oak Island is a loop, Warrior Rock an out-and-back.
**DIFFICULTY:** Easy
**SCENERY:** Lakeshore, woods, meadows, beaches, and birds
**EXPOSURE:** Oak Island is mostly open, Warrior Rock mostly wooded.
**TRAFFIC:** Moderate on summer weekends, light otherwise
**TRAIL SURFACE:** Packed dirt, grass, and some beach
**HIKING TIME:** 1 hour for Oak Island, 3 hours for Warrior Rock
**DRIVING DISTANCE:** Oak Island is 19 miles (30 minutes) from Pioneer Square, Warrior Rock 22 miles (45 minutes).
**SEASON:** Oak Island open April 16–September 30, Warrior Rock year-round
**BEST TIME:** Mid-April–May for Oak Island, fall for Warrior Rock
**ACCESS:** $3.50 daily or $11 annual parking pass required; for sale at Sauvie Island Market
**WHEELCHAIR ACCESS:** None
**MAPS:** USGS St. Helens; free map on site
**FACILITIES:** Outhouse at each trailhead, nearest water at Sauvie Island Market
**INFO:** Sauvie Island Wildlife Area Headquarters, (503) 621-3488

--------------------------------------

GPS Trailhead
Coordinates
UTM Zone (WGS84) 10T
Easting 513951
Northing 5062107
Latitude  N 45.71238°
Longitude W 122.82076°

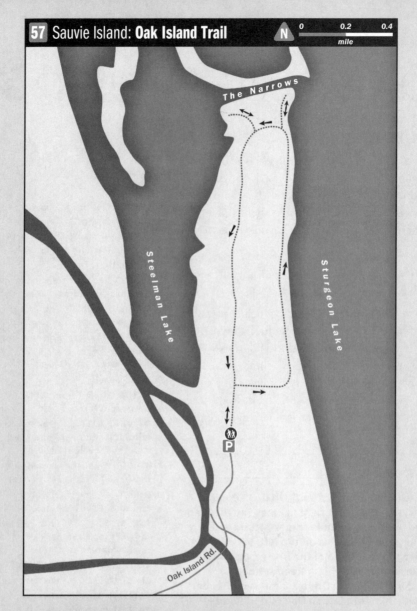

The Narrows

Steelman Lake

Sturgeon Lake

Oak Island Rd.

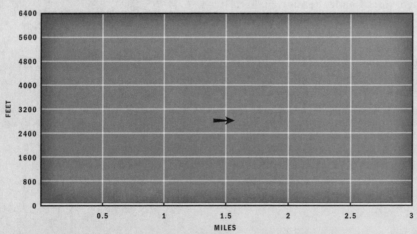

you of visiting your grandparents in the country. But even the crops are part of a plan by the Oregon Department of Fish and Wildlife to manage waterfowl in this area—and waterfowl are what Oak Island is all about.

Sauvie Island (named for a French-Canadian employee of the Hudson's Bay Company) has, for thousands of years, been a rest stop for migratory birds. At the peak of the fall migration, some 150,000 ducks and geese alight here. Several thousand sandhill cranes come, as well. In all, about 250 species of birds spend time on the island each year, including bald eagles by the score in the winter. So if you were to go to Oak Island in the middle of a summer day, you might wonder what the big deal is. But if you come in the spring or fall, or early on a summer day when the animals haven't hidden from the heat yet, you just might see a whole different world. And, in fact, even though the bulk of the migratory birds are gone when the trail is open, there are numerous songbirds here, in addition to ducks, geese, and even bald eagles that spend the whole summer.

From the trailhead, walk a few minutes on the mowed roadway–trail to a junction. Be sure to grab a guide from the box; it explains several signs around the trail. Head in either direction, or strike off into the grassy meadows or woods. If you stay on the trail, going right will take you to a view of Sturgeon Lake, which at some times of the year might be a long way off because it's so shallow. Turn left here, hike 0.9 miles and, when the signed trail turns left, follow another trail to the right, continuing 200 yards to the Narrows, a—you guessed it—narrow body of water that connects Sturgeon Lake to the east with Steelman Lake to the west.

Continuing on the loop trail, you'll head back to the left and walk along a plowed area; Fish and Wildlife actually farms some 1,000 acres of its land on Sauvie Island as part of a cycle that brings alfalfa, corn, millet, and other foods to migratory birds in the winter and cattle in the summer.

And now for the other stroll—Warrior Rock.

In the fall of 1805 Lewis and Clark's Corps of Discovery floated down the Columbia River and managed to miss the Willamette River entirely. It wasn't that they were fools; it's just that the Willamette's entry was blocked from view by the forested wetland now called Sauvie Island. While much of it has long since been diked, and some is now farmed, about half of it is managed by the Oregon Department of Fish and Wildlife.

Lewis and Clark, while exploring the island that was the summer and fall home of the Multnomah Indians, camped on the beach that is just beyond the parking area. If for some reason you would like to skip the beach entirely, walk over a low point in the fence at the southern end of the parking lot, then walk through the pasture, parallel to the river, to the trees. You'll find the road there.

To start on the beach, follow the trail out onto it and stroll along, considering what it must have looked like in 1805, but also how quiet it is today. Look also for animal tracks leading from the woods to the water; raccoons and deer are all common here. But those critters move around mostly at night, and if the hunters and fishermen aren't out, you may have the place to yourself.

If it's late summer or early fall when the river is low, you can make it almost the whole 3 miles to the lighthouse on Warrior Rock by walking the beach. Otherwise, go as far as you can, or wish to, and then look for a place to head up into the woods. Up on the bluff, you'll encounter a trail that once served as a service road to the lighthouse. Follow it through a world of blackberry, oak, alder, and maple. After about 2.5 miles, at a point where the trail is right at the top of the bluff, look to the right for an old shipwreck on the beach. Just a few minutes later, you'll come to a large meadow; keep right 0.2 miles to the lighthouse.

Warrior Rock got its name when members of a 1792 English expedition up the Columbia (the party that named the river for their ship, and Mount Hood for the head of the English navy) found themselves surrounded on this rock by dozens of native warriors. They cleverly made peace and lived to tell the tale. The lighthouse is maintained by the U.S. Coast Guard. And speaking of ships, there's a decent chance you'll see an oceangoing vessel making its way roughly 70 river miles from Portland to the Pacific Ocean at Astoria.

A hundred yards up the sandy beach to the left, somebody cut a perfect little bench into a large piece of driftwood; with any luck, the river will not have reclaimed it before you get there. A few minutes beyond that, at the northwestern tip of Sauvie Island, you'll come to old pilings that no one seems able to explain. Leading theories are that it was a fish-processing plant, a boat works, or a loading dock for shipping milk from island dairies. Whatever it was, it offers a viewpoint of the town of St. Helens, Oregon, which was founded in 1845—and in case you're wondering why the town and the nearby mountain are called St. Helens, well, the same English sailors who named Hood and the Columbia named Mount St. Helens for the English ambassador to Spain at the time, a certain Baron St. Helens. His real name was Fitzherbert; thank goodness they chose his official name.

Nothing like some useless trivia to contemplate while you're walking back to the car. Speaking of which, if you stay on the trail the whole way, you'll come to the cow pasture above the beach where you started. Just walk across it—careful where you step—to the fenced parking area and step over the low portion of the fence to your right, next to the hunters' check-in stand.

And, for the record, Lewis and Clark saw the Willamette on the way home, in the spring of 1806. Clark stood on a bluff where the University of Portland is today; from there, he saw and named Mount Jefferson.

## NEARBY ACTIVITIES

Many of the farms on Sauvie Island are "you pick 'em" operations, with treats like berries, flowers, pumpkins, and corn. One of them, on Reeder Road, has a corn maze (or a maize maze). You can't miss it. Stop and get a little something for dinner on your way home, if you don't get lost.

# SILVER FALLS STATE PARK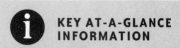

*\* wonderful hike \* !*

## IN BRIEF

If it's waterfalls you're after—especially the chance to get behind them—this is the hike of your dreams. It's an easy loop that's known as Trail of Ten Falls. There are also shorter loops available, all of which take in views of one or more waterfalls.

## DESCRIPTION

This is the crown jewel of the Oregon State Parks system; it's also one of the most visited parks in the state. Unless it's a rainy weekday in the winter, you probably won't be close to alone here, but it hardly matters. It's one of the finest walks around, especially if you're into waterfalls. By the way, Silver Creek was named not for its color but for a pioneer who settled here in the 1840s. He was known as "Silver" Smith because it was said he brought a bushel of silver dollars with him from back East.

Be sure to visit South Falls Lodge, 0.1 mile from the parking lot. It was built of native stone and wood by the Civilian Conservation Corps (CCC) in 1941. Warm yourself by two massive fireplaces, enjoy photos of the park and some of the tools used by the CCC, and take advantage of that most modern of conveniences: a

### KEY AT-A-GLANCE INFORMATION

**LENGTH:** Up to 7 miles
**CONFIGURATION:** Loop
**DIFFICULTY:** Easy–moderate
**SCENERY:** Every type of waterfall, in a forested canyon
**EXPOSURE:** Shady all the way
**TRAFFIC:** Heavy spring, summer, and fall; light–moderate otherwise
**TRAIL SURFACE:** Pavement, gravel, dirt
**HIKING TIME:** Up to 4 hours
**DRIVING DISTANCE:** 61 miles (1 hour 30 minutes) from Pioneer Square
**SEASON:** Year-round, but wet in winter and spring with occasional snow or ice
**BEST TIME:** March–April for big water, September–October for fall colors
**BACKPACKING OPTIONS:** Not allowed
**ACCESS:** $3 day-use fee per vehicle
**WHEELCHAIR ACCESS:** Much of the recommended loop is not accessible, but some falls are, as are many other trails.
**MAPS:** USGS Drake Crossing; free maps in South Falls Lodge and at trailheads
**FACILITIES:** Water, restrooms, snack bar, and gift shop at South Falls trailhead
**INFO:** Silver Falls State Park, (503) 873-8681
**SPECIAL COMMENTS:** Dogs, even on a leash, are not allowed on Canyon Trail, which is the one described here. They are welcome (if leashed) on other trails in the park.

### Directions

Take I-5 from Portland, driving 17 miles south of I-205 to Exit 271/Woodburn. Turn left and drive 14 miles on OR 214 to Silverton. Note that you'll be turning right at 2.7 miles, then left at 3.9 miles. Both intersections have signs; watch for them. In Silverton, follow signs for Silver Falls State Park, continuing 15 miles on OR 214. After entering the park, drive 2.3 miles on OR 214 and park on the right, at the South Falls parking area.

### GPS Trailhead Coordinates

UTM Zone (WGS84) 10T
Easting 526954
Northing 4969993
Latitude N 44.88285°
Longitude W 122.65871°

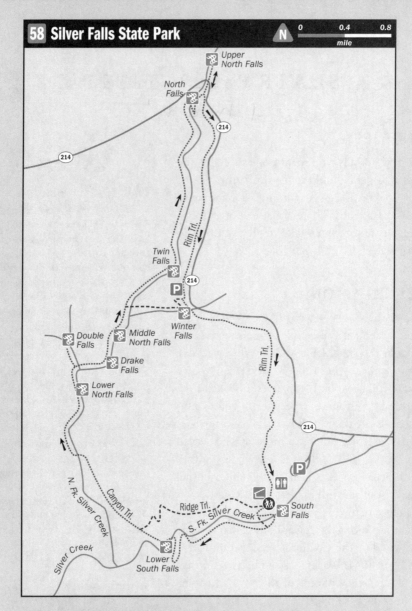

N

0    0.4    0.8
mile

Upper
North Falls

North
Falls

214

Rim Trl.

Twin
Falls

214

P

Double
Falls

Middle
North Falls

Winter
Falls

Drake
Falls

Rim Trl.

Lower
North Falls

214

P

Canyon Trl.

N. Fk. Silver Creek

Ridge Trl.

S. Fk. Silver Creek

South
Falls

Silver Creek

Lower
South Falls

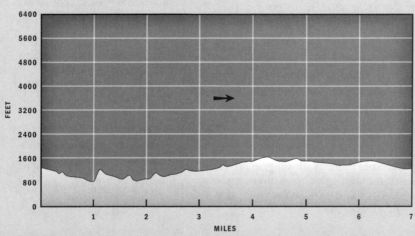

FEET

6400
5600
4800
4000
3200
2400
1600
800
0

1    2    3    4    5    6    7

MILES

South Falls

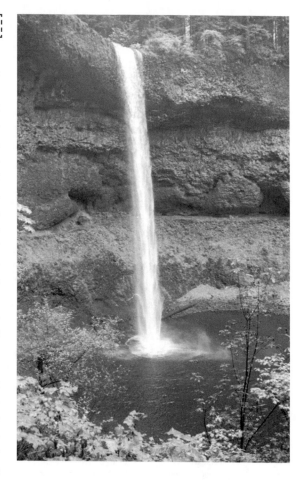

snack bar with an espresso stand.

With your hot drink in hand, walk toward 177-foot South Falls, take in the view from the top, and contemplate the fact that in the 1920s a man named D. E. Geiser used to send old automobiles over the falls as a Fourth of July stunt. It's said that fishermen were pulling car parts out of the pool for decades. Now, take the trail behind the sign. (*Note:* This is as far as your dogs can go, even if they're on a leash.) The trail will switchback down 0.2 miles, then go behind South Falls. The cavelike setting was created over the millennia by water seeping through the rocks above, freezing and expanding, and then cracking away the rocks that now lie at your feet.

When the trail comes to a bridge 100 yards ahead, you can cross it to finish a 0.6-mile loop—the first of several opportunities to cut the loop short. But continue 0.7 miles to see the 93-foot Lower South Falls. The trail descends a number of steps, often wet even in summer, and passes behind this falls, which is a combination of curtain and cascade falls.

After another 0.2 miles, you'll come to your second chance to cut the loop short. Turn right, and it's 1 mile along Ridge Trail back to the lodge; continue straight, and it's 0.7 miles to the 30-foot Lower North Falls. At this point you've left the South Fork of Silver Creek for the North Fork; the two combine downstream from here to form Silver Creek—this is why you're suddenly walking upstream rather than down. (I like to pose this "mystery" to fellow hikers, to see who's paying attention.) Keep an eye out for deer and beaver, both of which live in the park. Human tree-cutters left their mark, too; on some of the big cedar stumps, you can still make out springboard slots, where loggers stood to cut the trees by hand.

Just past Lower North Falls, make sure to go left for a 0.1-mile side trip to see Double Falls, at 178 feet. Its shallow splash pool, which you can get in, if you'd like, almost always hosts a rainbow when the sun is out. Back on the main trail, you'll pass the 27-foot Drake Falls (named for a photographer whose images were instrumental to the creation of the park), and 103-foot Middle North Falls (which you can go behind to visit a small cave) in the next 0.4 miles. When you get to a bridge (the halfway point for the full loop), you can turn right for one last chance to cut the loop short. Take this trail 0.3 miles to Winter Falls, and then continue past it; turn right on Rim Trail and walk 1.2 miles back to the lodge to end your day at 4.2 miles.

If you ignore the bridge and continue straight, you'll walk 0.3 miles to reach the 31-foot Twin Falls, which at low-water times of the year is just one falls, but which does have the hike's best picnic spot, right at the creek's edge. Another 0.9 miles along (look for the rocks in the creek with ferns growing on top), you'll reach North Falls, which you'll see before you get there and which is probably the most spectacular falls in the park. Once again, the trail takes you behind the falls. Back there, look for the columns in the rock overhead, left when lava cooled around trees and then the trees rotted—15 million years ago!

After examining that, climb some steps, then head up along a railing with another view back down to North Falls. When you get to Rim Trail, on the right, go ahead and put in the 0.4-mile loop to Upper North Falls, a seldom-visited 65-foot drop in an area with ample opportunity to rock-hop and explore.

On Rim Trail's 2.3-mile trip back to the lodge, you'll pass by the top of Winter Falls (more of a damp spot in the late summer and fall, but worth descending to) and through some pleasant forest, where I have encountered deer on three occasions. When you get to the picnic area, continue straight on a nice new trail, and you'll be back at the lodge in no time. I recommend another coffee drink.

## NEARBY ACTIVITIES

Just upstream from the South Falls parking area, there's an official swimming area in Silver Creek. The kids will love it, and if it's a hot day, grown-ups might like to take a dip in the creek as well. The park also has campsites and cabins you can rent for the night; horses can be rented between May and September.

# TRYON CREEK STATE PARK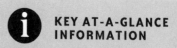

## IN BRIEF

Tryon Creek—Oregon's only state park in a major city—is the kind of place you want to visit over and over, just to see what's going on. Are the steelhead in? Are the trees wearing their fall colors yet? Are the trilliums in bloom? Any beavers around?

## DESCRIPTION

An iron company logged this whole area in the 1880s to provide fuel for their smelter, so what you see today is what's known as second-growth forest. But it's certainly not a second-*class* forest; if nothing else, some of those old tree trunks are amazing! This 670-acre park, in a ravine between Portland and Lake Oswego, hosts 50 species of birds, plus deer, beaver, fox, coyote, barred owl, and a winter steelhead trout run, in addition to resident steelhead and cutthroat trout.

Numerous hiking options start at the Nature Center, so pick up a free map and make your own way, or call the park for a schedule of ranger-led activities. For our suggested loop, when you come out of the Nature Center, turn left, walk past Jackson Shelter, and start on Maple Ridge Trail. As the name implies, this area is home to many

### KEY AT-A-GLANCE INFORMATION

**LENGTH:** 3 miles, total 8 miles of hiking trails in park

**CONFIGURATION:** Loop

**DIFFICULTY:** Easy

**SCENERY:** A woodsy ravine with a creek, lots of springtime wildflowers

**EXPOSURE:** Shady

**TRAFFIC:** Heavy on weekends, moderate otherwise

**TRAIL SURFACE:** Packed dirt, gravel

**HIKING TIME:** 1 hour for this loop

**DRIVING DISTANCE:** 6 miles (15 minutes) from Pioneer Square

**SEASON:** Year-round

**BEST TIME:** April, for the trillium bloom

**BACKPACKING OPTIONS:** None

**ACCESS:** No fees or permits

**WHEELCHAIR ACCESS:** The 0.4-mile Trillium Trail offers two barrier-free loops.

**MAPS:** Free maps at Nature Center

**FACILITIES:** Water and toilets at Nature Center

**INFO:** Tryon Creek State Park, (503) 636-9886

**SPECIAL COMMENTS:** The nonprofit Friends of Tryon Creek puts on numerous events in the park, from day camps to nighttime hikes to classes and lectures. To find out what's going on, call (503) 636-4398, or visit tryonfriends. org.

---

## *Directions*

Take I-5 south from Portland, driving 3 miles to Exit 297/Terwilliger. Turn right at the end of the ramp, then take the first right on Terwilliger Boulevard. Stay on Terwilliger 2.5 miles; the main entrance to the park is on the right.

## GPS Trailhead Coordinates

UTM Zone (WGS84) 10T

Easting 525433

Northing 5031994

Latitude N 45.44101°

Longitude W 122.67480°

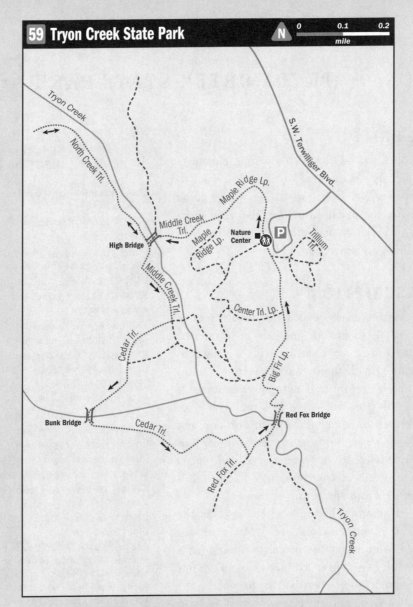

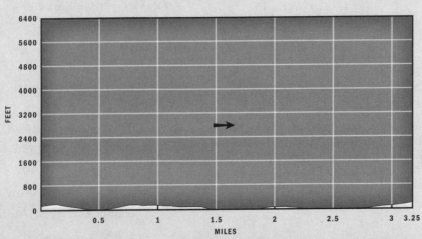

vine maples, which put on quite a red-and-orange show in late October and early November.

Hike 0.2 miles, then take a right on Middle Creek Trail. Descend 0.2 miles to cross Tryon Creek at High Bridge. It's worth it to turn right here and explore up the 0.4-mile North Creek Trail, if only to see the astonishing fields of impatiens (also known as jewelweed) and a few places to access the creek, one of them a deep pool at a bend. Return to Middle Creek Trail and follow it 0.2 miles to an intersection with Cedar Trail. Follow this trail to the right as it crosses a horse trail (careful where you step!) and then climbs a short ways into a more open forest. Keep an eye out for a downed cedar trunk on the right that has obviously been explored by many an adventuresome child.

Cedar Trail crosses Bunk Bridge, then continues 0.8 miles to a junction with Red Fox Trail. Turn left here and cross Red Fox Bridge; if it's winter, keep an eye out for spawning steelhead. Climb briefly to Old Main Trail, and then turn right and follow it back to the Nature Center.

## NEARBY ACTIVITIES

The Original Pancake House, founded in 1953, is not far away at 8601 SW 24th Avenue. A third-generation family business that has spawned more than 80 franchises in 22 states, this one won the 1999 James Beard America's Regional Classics Award. Go there, get an apple pancake or a Dutch baby, and discover the joy of breakfast. It's cash only, though.

# 60 WASHINGTON PARK– HOYT ARBORETUM

## KEY AT-A-GLANCE INFORMATION

**LENGTH:** 4 miles

**CONFIGURATION:** Loop

**DIFFICULTY:** Easy

**SCENERY:** 950 species and varieties of plants, more than 5,000 labeled trees and shrubs

**EXPOSURE:** Shady, with the occasional open spot for city views

**TRAFFIC:** Heavy on weekends, moderate during the workday or bad weather

**TRAIL SURFACE:** Pavement, packed dirt, gravel

**HIKING TIME:** 2 hours for the recommended loop

**DRIVING DISTANCE:** 2 miles (5 minutes) from Pioneer Square

**SEASON:** Year-round

**BEST TIME:** Spring, for the blooms

**BACKPACKING OPTIONS:** None

**ACCESS:** No fees or permits

**WHEELCHAIR ACCESS:** There are several barrier-free trails in the area; ask at the visitor center.

**MAPS:** Trail guide at Hoyt Arboretum Visitor Center

**FACILITIES:** Water and restrooms throughout park

**INFO:** Portland Parks and Recreation, (503) 823-7529

## GPS Trailhead Coordinates

UTM Zone (WGS84) 10T

Easting 522065

Northing 5039824

Latitude   N 45.51160°

Longitude  W 122.71752°

## IN BRIEF

A family could spend a weekend in Washington Park and never run out of things to do. The park has a zoo, a children's museum, the World Forestry Center, the Oregon Vietnam Veterans Memorial, a world-class Japanese garden, the Hoyt Arboretum, and miles of hiking trails. TriMet runs a shuttle bus that connects it all. The loop described here is only a suggestion.

## DESCRIPTION

This loop hike can be your base for exploring and an introduction to all that Washington Park has to offer. From a hiker's perspective, the heart of the park is Hoyt Arboretum (literally meaning "tree museum"), founded in 1928 on land that was completely clearcut in the early 20th century. Be sure to stop in the visitor center (which is on this loop) for a helpful map.

Beginning your walk at the Oregon Vietnam Veterans Memorial, follow the trail under and then across the bridge and through a circular series of memorials describing events at

## Directions

The best way to get to this trailhead is to take the MAX Light Rail. It takes you to the deepest transit station in North America (at 260 feet, the second-deepest in the world), which features artwork and displays on the geological history of the region. An elevator puts you right next to the World Forestry Center; turn right from there for the trailhead. To drive here from downtown Portland, head west on US 26 and take Exit 72/Zoo after 1.3 miles. At the end of the ramp, turn right on SW Canyon Road. Then stay to the left, circling the parking lot, and turn left at the MAX station. The trailhead is at the Vietnam Veterans Memorial on your left 0.1 mile ahead.

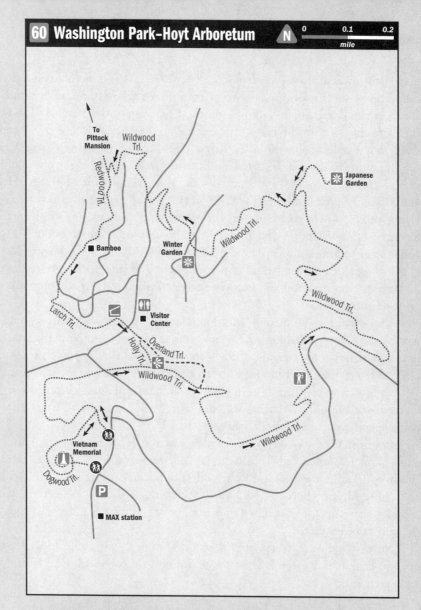

**To Pittock Mansion**

Wildwood Trl.

Redwood Trl.

Japanese Garden

Bamboo

Winter Garden

Wildwood Trl.

Larch Trl.

Wildwood Trl.

Visitor Center

Overland Trl.

Holly Trl.

Wildwood Trl.

Wildwood Trl.

Vietnam Memorial

Wildwood Trl.

Dogwood Trl.

P

MAX station

0    0.1    0.2

mile

N

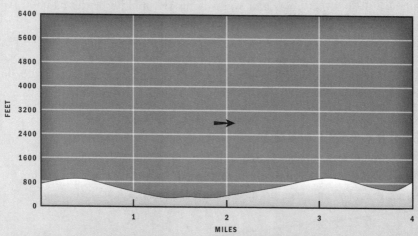

FEET

6400
5600
4800
4000
3200
2400
1600
800
0

1          2          3          4

MILES

home and in Southeast Asia from 1959 to 1972. At this point, you're in the arboretum—specifically, on Dogwood Trail. (Each arboretum trail is named for the trees that dominate it.) Follow Dogwood Trail out of the memorial, and then turn left onto Wildwood Trail. (To your right is the beginning of this "wonder trail" that wanders some 30 miles through Washington Park and Forest Park.

Stay on Wildwood Trail 0.4 miles as it circles to the right and climbs a small hill to a viewpoint between two water towers. Look for Mount St. Helens and Mount Rainier, and then turn left on Holly Trail and walk 100 yards to the visitor center, where there's water, restrooms, and a mountain of information. Return to the viewpoint and turn left on Wildwood Trail. In about 200 feet you'll come to Magnolia Trail on the left; take it 0.3 miles to the Winter Garden if you'd like to cut about 1.6 miles off your hike and stay in the arboretum. For a pleasant, woodsy stroll and access to other Washington Park attractions, stay on Wildwood Trail.

The wide, flat Wildwood Trail loops out 1.5 miles, with access along the way to the Cherry, Walnut, and Maple trails. At the 1.2-mile mark, you will have a view down to the right of the waterfall area of the Japanese garden; just after that, a trail on the right leads to the garden, the largest in the world outside Japan and a must-see. Just down a hill beyond that is the International Rose Test Garden, with 8,000 rosebushes in more than 550 varieties. Did I mention you could spend quite a while in Washington Park?

Back on Wildwood Trail, 0.3 miles past the Japanese Garden Trail, you enter Winter Garden, where Magnolia Trail reenters. Just 0.6 miles later on Wildwood Trail, take a left on Redwood Trail for an exploration of the sequoia collection. Shortly beyond that, you'll enter the redwood collection, which includes a specimen of the dawn redwood, which, until a few decades ago, was thought to be extinct.

*Note:* If you were to stay on Wildwood Trail here, you could add a 2.4-mile out-and-back trip to Pittock Mansion, which is at the top of Macleay Trail (hike 54, page 246).

Back on Redwood Trail, when you come to a trail on the right marked "To Creek Trail," take that, and you'll be in the middle of the bamboo collection. From redwoods to bamboo—culture shock is now a possibility. Creek Trail dead-ends at a road; pick up Redwood Trail at the far side and you'll pass through the larch collection on your way to the picnic shelter. Cross the road, and you're back at the visitor center. Turn right, take Holly Trail back to Wildwood Trail, turn right on it, and follow it a half mile back to your car.

## NEARBY ACTIVITIES

The Children's Museum features hands-on exhibits in a "center for creativity, designed for kids age 6 months through 12 years old." Kids can climb, swim, toss balls, act in a play, and even produce a movie there.

# APPENDIXES
# AND INDEX

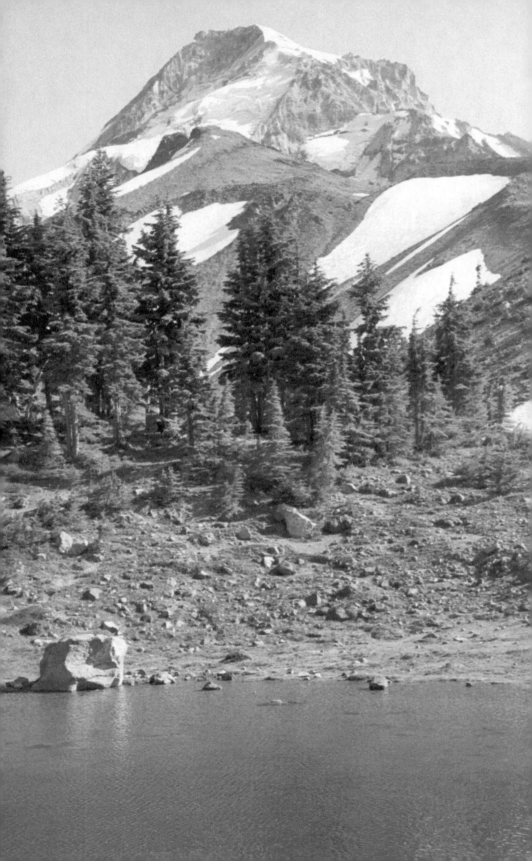

# APPENDIX A:
## HIKING STORES

**Columbia Sportswear**
911 SW Broadway
(503) 226-6800, **columbia.com**

**Next Adventure** (*includes used items*)
426 SE Grand Avenue
(503) 233-0706, **nextadventure.net**

**Oregon Mountain Community**
2975 NE Sandy Boulevard
(503) 227-1038, **e-omc.com**

**Patagonia**
907 NW Irving Street
(503) 525-2552, **patagonia.com**

**REI (rei.com)**
Clackamas
12160 SE 82nd Avenue
(503) 659-1156

Portland
1405 NW Johnson Street
(503) 221-1938

Tigard
7410 SW Bridgeport Road
(503) 624-8600

**The Mountain Shop**
628 NE Broadway
(503) 288-6768, **mountainshp.net**

# APPENDIX B:
## PLACES TO BUY MAPS

**Oregon Mountain Community**
2975 NE Sandy Boulevard
(503) 227-1038, **e-omc.com**

**REI (rei.com)**
Clackamas
12160 SE 82nd Avenue
(503) 659-1156

Portland
1405 NW Johnson Street
(503) 221-1938

Tigard
7410 SW Bridgeport Road
(503) 624-8600

> **Dollar Lake at Mount Hood,**
> **on the Vista Ridge hike**

# APPENDIX C:
## WHERE TO GET THE NORTHWEST FOREST PASS

Many of the trailheads in this book require a Northwest Forest Pass. All of the outdoor shops listed in Appendixes A and B sell the pass, which is $5 for one day and $30 for a year. They are also available online at **discovernw.org**.

There are other passes available, such as an Interagency Senior Pass and various national passes, so make sure to get the one that best meets your needs. Visit the Forest Service passes and permits Web site at **www.fs.fed.us/passespermits** for more information.

# APPENDIX D:
## HIKING CLUBS

**Bergfreunde Ski Club**
503-245-8543
**www.bergfreunde.org**

**Columbia River Volkssport Club**
**www.crvcwalking.org**

**Forest Park Conservancy**
1505 NW 23rd Avenue
503-223-5449
**www.forestparkconservancy.org**

**Friends of the Columbia Gorge**
522 SW Fifth Avenue, Suite 720
503-241-3762
**www.gorgefriends.org**

**Mazamas**
527 SE 43rd Avenue
503-227-2345
**www.mazamas.org**

**Oregon Chapter Sierra Club**
1821 SE Ankeny Street
503-238-0442
**oregon.sierraclub.org**

**Portland Parks and Recreation**
503-823-7529
**www.portlandonline.com/parks**

**Trails Club of Oregon**
503-233-2740
**www.trailsclub.org**

# APPENDIX E:
## ONLINE RESOURCES

**PortlandHikers.org** is an invaluable resource of up-to-date conditions, trail descriptions, and people to go hiking with in the Portland area. (Say hello to OneSpeed on there; he wrote this book.)

**NWHiker.com** is an online guide to area hikes, with photos.

**wta.org** is the online home of Washington Trails Association, which promotes hiking, leads trips, and coordinates trail maintenance.

**trailkeepersoforegon.org** is the home of Trailkeepers of Oregon, a new nonprofit dedicated to protecting and enhancing the Oregon hiking experience through advocacy, stewardship, outreach, and education. If you ever wanted to do some work on an Oregon trail to keep it in shape—and that would be a fine thing to do—these are the folks to get in touch with.

**nwhikers.net** is a discussion board with thousands of members posting trip reports and trail conditions from all over the Pacific Northwest.

**summitpost.org** is a massive board discussing mountain ranges all over the world, from the Absarokas in Wyoming to the Zlatibor Massif in Serbia. Seriously.

**www.fs.fed.us/gpnf-** is the Web site for Gifford Pinchot National Forest in southwest Washington.

**www.fs.fed.us/r6/mthood** is the online home of Mount Hood National Forest.

**www.fs.fed.us/r6/willamette** is the Web site for Willamette National Forest.

**hikeyeah.com** is the home page for an online radio show about hiking in the Portland area. It's broadcast by PDX.FM once a week.

# INDEX

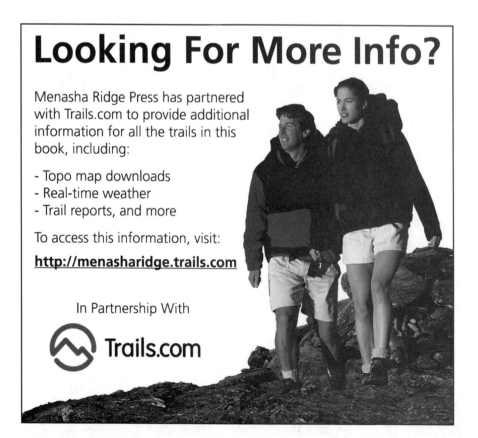

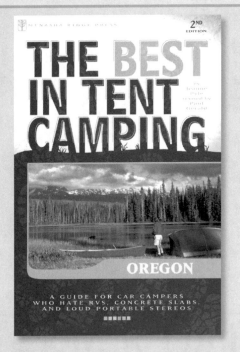
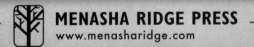

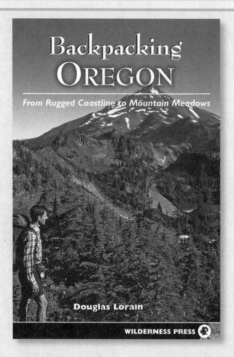
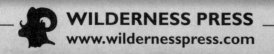

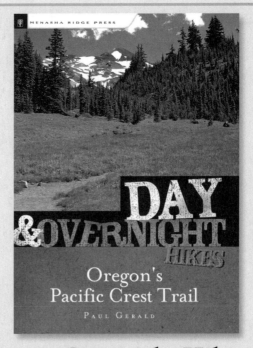

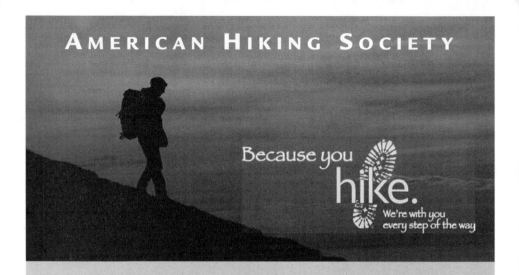
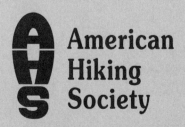

**DEAR CUSTOMERS AND FRIENDS,**

**SUPPORTING YOUR INTEREST IN OUTDOOR ADVENTURE**, travel, and an active lifestyle is central to our operations, from the authors we choose to the locations we detail to the way we design our books. Menasha Ridge Press was incorporated in 1982 by a group of veteran outdoorsmen and professional outfitters. For many years now, we've specialized in creating books that benefit the outdoors enthusiast.

Almost immediately, Menasha Ridge Press earned a reputation for revolutionizing outdoors- and travel-guidebook publishing. For such activities as canoeing, kayaking, hiking, backpacking, and mountain biking, we established new standards of quality that transformed the whole genre, resulting in outdoor-recreation guides of great sophistication and solid content. Menasha Ridge continues to be outdoor publishing's greatest innovator.

The folks at Menasha Ridge Press are as at home on a white-water river or mountain trail as they are editing a manuscript. The books we build for you are the best they can be, because we're responding to your needs. Plus, we use and depend on them ourselves.

We look forward to seeing you on the river or the trail. If you'd like to contact us directly, join in at www.trekalong.com or visit us at www.menasharidge.com. We thank you for your interest in our books and the natural world around us all.

**SAFE TRAVELS,**

*Bob Sehlinger*

**BOB SEHLINGER**
**PUBLISHER**